Advances in Preventing and Treating Violence and Aggression

Series Editor

Peter Sturmey
City University of New York
Queens College City University of New York
Flushing, NY, USA

The series publishes books focused and developed across three domains. The first is understanding and explaining violence and aggression. Books in this domain address such subject matter as genetics, physiology, neurobiology, cultural evolution, biobehavioral, learning, cognitive, psychoanalytic, sociological and other explanations of violence. The second domain focuses on prevention and treatment for individuals and couples. Examples of books in this domain include cognitive behavioral, behavioral, counseling, psychopharmacological, psychosocial, couples, and family therapy approaches. They also explore extant treatment packages for individually focused treatments (e.g., mindfulness, cognitive analytic therapies). Within this domain, books focus on meeting the information needs of clinicians and professionals who work in youth facilities, emergency rooms, special education, criminal justice, and therapy settings. Finally, books in the third domain address prevention and treatment for groups and society, including topical focus on early intervention programs, school violence prevention programs, policing strategies, juvenile facility reform as well as socio-legal and ethical issues. Books in this series serve as must-have resources for researchers, academics, and upper-level undergraduate and graduate students in clinical child and school psychology, public health, criminology/criminal justice, developmental psychology, psychotherapy/counseling, psychiatry, social work, educational policy and politics, health psychology, nursing, and behavioral therapy/rehabilitation.

More information about this series at http://www.springer.com/series/15332

Ruud H. J. Hornsveld
Floris W. Kraaimaat
Luk A. C. L. Gijs
Emma J. Palmer
Editors

Assessment and Obligatory Treatment of Violent and Sexually Violent Offenders

Integrating Research and Practice

Springer

Editors
Ruud H. J. Hornsveld
Erasmus University Medical Center
Rotterdam, The Netherlands

Floris W. Kraaimaat
Radboud University Nijmegen
Nijmegen, The Netherlands

Luk A. C. L. Gijs
KU Leuven
Leuven, Belgium

Emma J. Palmer
University of Leicester
Leicester, UK

Advances in Preventing and Treating Violence and Aggression
ISBN 978-3-030-27839-7 ISBN 978-3-030-27840-3 (eBook)
https://doi.org/10.1007/978-3-030-27840-3

This Springer imprint is published by the registered company Springer Nature Switzerland AG
The registered company address is: Gewerbestrasse 11, 6330 Cham, Switzerland

To the late Arnold P. Goldstein who paved the way for the development of treatment programs for adult violent and sexually violent offenders with a high recidivism risk.

Preface

This book presents an innovative group treatment approach that targets changeable (i.e., dynamic) risk factors of violent and sexually violent offenders. The clinically evaluated treatment programs comprise modules which can be combined by any clinician according to the needs of the offenders. For each module, a session plan is provided including material for conducting various interventions.

The described modules are primarily intended for violent and sexually violent offenders as well as violent and sexually violent forensic psychiatric patients with a cluster B personality disorder or a conduct disorder as their primary diagnosis. In a preliminary comparative study, we found that the differences between both populations in dynamic criminogenic needs were marginal. Because most of the research into assessment and treatment was performed at offenders, we refer to them in this book as offenders, unless in a study it concerns forensic psychiatric patients specifically. Some studies have been carried out on chronic psychotic patients who have been treated for their psychotic symptoms so that their cluster B personality disorder has become prominent.

The book comprises a theoretical part (Chaps. 1–5), a practical part (Chaps. 6–9), and a manual part (Chaps. 10 and 11). All three parts are formulated from a cognitive behavioral therapeutic frame of reference. It is our opinion that this frame of reference provides the best ground for the assessment and treatment of violent and sexually violent offenders. The book is primarily intended for clinicians who want to develop a new program for violent offenders or sexually violent offenders or to adapt their current program. That is why every theoretical chapter ends with conclusions and recommendations for clinicians.

Chapter 1 starts with information on the prevalence and costs of violence, followed by definitions of the aggression-related concepts that are frequently used in this book. Then, theories are described on aggression in general, on sexual aggression particularly, and the relation between personality domains and psychopathy on the one hand and aggressive behavior on the other. Definitions of forensic psychiatric patients are provided as they are used in several Western countries. Chapter 2 offers a model for aggressive behavior and two models for sexually aggressive behavior, which are based on our research and the literature on the dynamic criminogenic needs of violent offenders and sexually violent offenders. In Chap. 3, an overview is provided of the "internal" and "external" factors that affect the responding to self-report questionnaires in populations of offenders and forensic psychiatric patients. For clinicians and researchers, conclusions and recommendations are presented for the use of self-report questionnaires in these populations. Chapter 4 addresses the assessment of violent offenders and sexually violent offenders by presenting in our view the current best applicable risk assessment instruments, neuropsychological tests, observation scales, and self-report questionnaires. Next, it offers practical guidelines on the formulation of functional analyses for individual treatment plans. In Chap. 5, recent literature on treatment programs for violent offenders and sexually violent offenders is described and evaluated. Based on the literature and our own clinical experience, requirements are formulated that have to be met in order for treatment programs to be effective.

The practical part of the book starts with Chap. 6, which describes a program for violent offenders and a program for sexually violent offenders as these have been tested in Dutch forensic psychiatric hospitals and forensic psychiatric outpatient clinics. For each module, aim and method are provided in great detail. Two flowcharts are presented which make it possible for clinicians to compose their treatment programs. In Chap. 7, a module that facilitates the generalization and maintenance of treatment results is described. Both are particularly important for offenders who have followed a treatment program in a closed setting (prison or forensic psychiatric hospital) and who are going on leave or are referred to an ambulant facility for further treatment. The educational level and practical experience that effective trainers need to have at their disposal and the way treatment programs should be implemented in prisons, forensic psychiatric hospitals, probation agencies, and forensic psychiatric outpatient clinics are described in Chap. 8. In Chap. 9, we reflect on what has been described in Chaps. 1–8, and we outline various possibilities for new developments in the assessment and treatment of violent offenders and sexually violent offenders. Then, we present suggestions for further research into the determinants of violent and sexually violent behavior and the design of further research into the effect of new and current treatments.

In Chap. 10, we offer clinicians modules and additional tools for the composition of treatment programs for violent offenders, including session plans, information brochures, various to be practiced interpersonal problem situations, and aims and criteria of prosocial skills. Chapter 11 provides clinicians with modules and additional tools for the composition of treatment programs for sexually violent offenders, including session plans, information on sexuality, problem situations on distorted cognitions, various to be practiced interpersonal problem situations, and aims and criteria of prosocial skills. The book ends with a Glossary in which definitions are given of the terms and concepts, which are most frequently used.

In this book, both the term therapists and trainers are used. By therapists, we mean professionals with academic education and further education as a psychotherapist or clinical psychologist. Trainers are seen as professionals with a higher professional education who are supervised by an experienced therapist in the performance of their duties. Both groups of professionals can be expected to have experience in group treatments for poorly motivated clients or patients. The topics in this book are primarily related to heterosexual, male offenders. However, many interventions can easily be adapted by experienced professionals for offenders of different gender and different sexual orientation. Where "he" is used, this means that the subject can also relate to female professionals or female offenders.

Through this book, we intend to give insight in the way how to formulate cognitive-behavioral models by thorough assessment and how to compose treatment programs with modules that target dynamic criminogenic needs. We hope that it will inspire and help clinicians who want to treat difficult populations as violent and sexually violent offenders. We owe many debts of gratitude to the offenders and staff of the penitentiary and forensic psychiatric institutions who have provided us with valuable comments.

Although this book is primarily intended for clinicians involved in the assessment and treatment of offenders, it also provides useful information for other mental health professionals and, for instance, criminologists. Also, the book can be informative for students who are in training within the aforementioned fields.

Rotterdam, The Netherlands — Ruud H. J. Hornsveld
Nijmegen, The Netherlands — Floris W. Kraaimaat
Leuven, Belgium — Luk A. C. L. Gijs
Leicester, UK — Emma J. Palmer

The original version of this book was revised. The correction is available at https://doi.org/10.1007/978-3-030-27840-3_12

Contents

About the Editors and Authors

Luk A. C. L. Gijs, Ph.D., is an Associate Professor affiliated with the Interfaculty Institute for Family and Sexuality Studies, Department of Neurosciences, KU Leuven, Belgium. He is a healthcare psychologist, sexologist, and supporter of the scientist-practitioner ideal. His main interests are risk assessment of sex offenders, treatment programs for sex offenders, and paraphilia.

Ruud H. J. Hornsveld, Ph.D., is a registered clinical psychologist and supervisor of the Dutch Association for Behavioral and Cognitive Therapy (VGCt). From 1997 to 2013, he was associated as a clinical psychologist and researcher with Forensic Psychiatric Center de Kijvelanden at Poortugaal, Netherlands. During this period, he assessed and treated violent and sexually violent forensic psychiatric in- and outpatients. Also, he developed and evaluated treatment programs for these populations. At the moment, he is affiliated with the Department of Psychiatry of Erasmus MC, University Medical Center Rotterdam, Netherlands. He regularly publishes on his work in national and international journals. E: ruud.hornsveld@ziggo.nl

Floris W. Kraaimaat, Ph.D., is emeritus professor of medical psychology at Radboud University Nijmegen, Netherlands. He has published widely on clinical psychology, behavior therapy, and behavioral assessment. His current research includes topics such as the development of cognitive-behavioral interventions for patients with chronic disorders. Areas of special interest are emotion regulation and aggression.

Henk L. I. Nijman, Ph.D., is Professor of Forensic Psychology at the Behavioural Science Institute, Radboud University, Nijmegen, Netherlands, and senior researcher at forensic psychiatric institute Fivoor, Den Dolder, Netherlands. He is a mental health scientist, and his main area of research is the causes and prevention of aggression of psychiatric patients.

Kevin L. Nunes, Ph.D., is Associate Professor and Director of the Aggressive Cognitions and Behaviour Research Laboratory, Department of Psychology,

Carleton University, Ottawa, Canada. The main focus of his research is on the conceptualization and measurement of cognitions (attitudes, beliefs, expectancies, etc.) thought to be relevant to sexual and nonsexual violent behavior and the role these cognitions may play in violent behavior.

Emma J. Palmer, Ph.D., is Reader in Forensic Psychology, Department of Neuroscience, Psychology, and Behavior, University of Leicester, UK. Her research focuses on offending behavior with specific interests such as the development of offending behavior (particularly social cognition and family/parenting), risk and needs assessment of offenders, and the design and evaluation of interventions with offenders.

Sabine J. Roza, M.D., Ph.D., is Associate Professor of Forensic Psychiatry at the Department of Psychiatry, Erasmus University Medical Center, Rotterdam, Netherlands. She is a psychiatrist and serves as expert witness for courts in youth and adult criminal law. Her scientific interest involves the biopsychosocial development of psychiatric disorders across a lifetime in persons with violent and aggressive behavior.

Part I
Theory

Chapter 1
Prevalence, Risks, Costs, Theories, and Legal Aspects

Ruud H. J. Hornsveld, Floris W. Kraaimaat, Luk A. C. L. Gijs, Kevin L. Nunes, and Emma J. Palmer

1.1 Introduction

In 1996, the World Health Assembly declared violence a major public health issue. To follow-up on this resolution, the WHO released in 2002 the first World Report on Violence and Health. The report analyzed different types of violence such as child abuse and neglect, youth violence, intimate partner violence, and sexual violence. For all these types of violence, the report explored the magnitude of the health and social effects, the risk and protective factors, and the types of prevention efforts that have been initiated (Krug, Mercy, Dahlberg, Mercy, & Zwi, 2002). In the report, it was estimated that 1.6 million people died from violence in 2000, which corresponds to 28.8 per 100,000 population. Almost half of these deaths were suicides, nearly a third were homicides, and a fifth was war-related. Rates appeared to vary considerably between and within countries. Although global estimates for the

The original version of this chapter was revised. The correction to this chapter is available at https://doi.org/10.1007/978-3-030-27840-3_12

R. H. J. Hornsveld (✉)
Erasmus University Medical Center, Rotterdam, The Netherlands
e-mail: ruud.hornsveld@ziggo.nl

F. W. Kraaimaat
Radboud University Nijmegen, Nijmegen, The Netherlands

L. A. C. L. Gijs
KU Leuven, Leuven, Belgium

K. L. Nunes
Carleton University, Ottawa, Canada

E. J. Palmer
University of Leicester, Leicester, UK

R. H. J. Hornsveld et al. (eds.), *Assessment and Obligatory Treatment of Violent and Sexually Violent Offenders*, Advances in Preventing and Treating Violence and Aggression, https://doi.org/10.1007/978-3-030-27840-3_1

different types of violence were difficult to make, it was clear that violence is a worldwide problem. More specifically, in 48 population-based studies from around the world, between 10% and 69% of women reported having been physically assaulted by an intimate partner during their lifetime and about 20% of women reported having been sexually abused as children.

1.1.1 Legal Aspects of Sexual Offending

Sexual offending is generally defined as performing sexual activities with an individual who does not give consent or is deemed incapable of giving consent (Abel, Becker, & Cunningham-Rathner, 1984). There are several circumstances in which an individual can be considered as incapable of consenting to sexual contact, of which being under the "age of majority" is most common. The age of majority is the legally defined minimum age at which an individual is considered to have the full competency to make decisions, such as voluntarily agree to engage in sexual behavior or to get married without parental consent. The age of majority is set in the range of 14–16 years for most countries in Europe, while the North American jurisdictions have set limits between 16 and 18 years.

Sexual assault is sexual behavior without consent and can be divided into hands-on (contact) and hands-off (noncontact) offenses. Hands-on offenses include rape, attempted rape, harmful genital practices, forced oral-genital contact, prostitution of a victim, sadistic sexual activity, or intrusive sexualized kissing. Hands-off offenses include exhibitionism, unrecognized sexual jokes and comments, the unintended showing of pornography to a victim, and voyeuristic activities (Ramsey-Klawsnik, 2003).

In this book, we are mainly concerned with medium- to high-risk sexually violent offenders who have committed hands-on offenses and who are generally divided into two subgroups, namely rapists and child sexual abusers (De Vogel, De Ruiter, Van Beek, & Mead, 2004). According to Wilson, Mouilso, Gentile, Calhoun, and Zeichner (2015), rapists commit more nonsexual offenses than child sexual abusers.

1.1.2 Prevalence of Violence

Studies on the prevalence of violence focus predominantly on interpersonal violence (IPV) or domestic violence against women by their partner. For instance, Alhabib, Nur, and Jones (2010) reviewed the worldwide evidence on the prevalence of domestic violence against women, but the majority of the studies were conducted in North America (41%) and Europe (20%). The prevalence of lifetime domestic violence appeared to vary from 1.9% in Washington DC to 70% in Hispanic Latinas in the Southeast of the United States. Results showed that violence against women has reached epidemic proportions in many societies.

Koss (2000) concluded in an overview of the literature on partner violence in the United States that women are eight times more likely than men to be assaulted by an intimate partner and that independent estimates of the percentage of women who report domestic assaults to police range from 7% to 14%. Among the fraction of incidents known to police, almost half (48%) of the women were judged to have insufficient evidence for filing or acceptance of charges. The majority of perpetrators violated protection orders in some way within 2 years, 29% with severe violence. Although many women felt that temporary restraining orders helped document that abuse had occurred, few thought their partner believed he had to obey the order. Between 1992 and 1998, in Massachusetts half of the perpetrators battered a new victim within 2 years of their last restraining order, and 23% of offenders had two or more restraining orders taken out against them by different women. Civil protection orders did not appear to protect women adequately from further abuse, and primary reliance on these measures must be seriously questioned (Koss, 2000).

More specifically, Cho (2012) studied the differences in the prevalence of IPV and associated factors in women among major racial groups in the United States, using a nationally representative dataset from adults. The results showed that Blacks were victimized the most, followed by Whites and Latinos, and Asians were victimized the least. Asians were the least likely to be victimized by IPV, even when controlling for sociodemographic variables. Women who perceived themselves as financially secure were less likely to be victimized than those who did not, and older women were less likely to be victimized than younger women. Employment, education, and social networks did not affect victimization, and also race did not appear to be a significant predictor of perpetration.

1.1.3 Prevalence of Physical and Sexual Violence

Wincentak, Connolly, and Card (2017) reviewed 101 international studies reporting prevalence rates of physical and sexual teen dating violence for youth aged 13–18. They found an overall prevalence of 20% (ranging from 1% to 61%) for physical and 9% (ranging from 1% to 54%) for sexual teen dating violence. Gender differences in physical teen dating violence were significant for perpetration (boys 13% vs. girls 25%) but not for victimization (21% boys and girls). A different pattern was observed for sexual teen dating violence with girls reporting lower rates of perpetration compared with boys (3% vs. 10%) and higher rates of victimization (14% vs. 8%). Higher rates were found for sexual teen dating violence among older teens and for physical teen dating violence among cultural minority girls and among teens from disadvantaged neighborhoods.

Krahé (2018) reported on a study by the World Health Organization (2013) of the lifetime prevalence rate of women's experience of physical and sexual victimization by an intimate partner from the age of 15 years based on 151 original population-based studies from 81 countries. Only women who had ever been in a relationship were included. Across all 81 countries, the mean rate of women experiencing physical assault, sexual assault, or both from an intimate partner was 30%. However, there was considerable variation by region. The report also compiled prevalence rates of non-partner sexual assault among women regardless of whether they had ever been in a relationship. Across all countries, 7.2% of women reported non-partner sexual assault, but again there was substantial variability between regions. The likelihood of being sexually assaulted by a man outside an intimate relationship appeared to be far lower than being sexually assaulted by a romantic or dating partner.

Stoltenborgh, Bakermans-Kranenburg, Alink, and Van IJzendoorn (2015) combined and compared the results of a series of meta-analyses on the prevalence of child sexual, physical, and emotional abuse, and physical and emotional neglect. Research on child maltreatment appeared to be dominated by a focus on sexual abuse, on studies in developed parts of the world and research using self-report measures. The overall estimated prevalence rates for self-report studies were 12.7% for sexual abuse (7.6% among boys and 18.0% among girls), 22.6% for physical abuse, 36.3% for emotional abuse, 16.3% for physical neglect, and 18.4% for emotional neglect. The researchers concluded that child maltreatment is a widespread, global phenomenon affecting the lives of millions of children all over the world.

1.1.4 Prevalence of Sexual Violence

Sexual offending has relatively high prevalence rates. The percentage of individuals who have ever become a victim of child sexual abuse is approximately 20% (Pereda, Guilera, Forns, & Gómez-Benito, 2009a, 2009b) and the prevalence of rape is about 15% (Kolivas & Gross, 2007). The exact scope of sexual offending, however, is difficult to determine. Studies regarding the occurrence of sexual offending are often based on official statistics, which are known to be subject to under-reporting. Especially sexual offenses for which the perpetrator is known to the victim (e.g., incest) are less likely to be reported to the authorities than sexual offenses committed by strangers under threat of physical violence such as rape (Chaffin, 2008). In case of sexual abuse reported to law enforcement in the USA, 93% of juvenile victims knew the perpetrator: 59% were acquaintances, 34% were family members, while 7% were strangers to the victim (Snyder, 2000).

Hawkins and Domoney (2012) concluded from the literature that in the United Kingdom the lifetime risk of sexual assault is 1 in 5 for women (15–25%) and 1 in 33 (3%) for men. In 2009 and 2010 15,000 rapes and 55,000 sexual assaults were reported to the police, but it was estimated that this was only 10% of the adult rapes that actually happened. Only 12% of assaults were by strangers, but 45% were by acquaintances and 43% by intimate partners. The incidence of child sexual abuse could not be established, but estimates were 5–30% for girls and 1–15% for boys. Only one in 20–50 assaults of children was known to supervising authorities and it was suggested that the prevalence was far higher than that reflected in numbers reported.

Lisak and Miller (2002) found that in a group of 1882 students at a commuter university in the United States, 120 men reported acts which met legal definitions of rape or attempted rape, but who were never prosecuted by criminal justice authorities. A majority of these undetected rapists were repeating rapists, and a majority also committed other acts of interpersonal violence. The repeat rapists averaged 5.8 rapes each. The 120 rapists were responsible for 1225 separate acts of interpersonal violence, including rape, battery, and child physical and sexual abuse.

A meta-analysis of the prevalence of unacknowledged rape among American college students was performed by Wilson and Miller (2016). Twenty-eight studies, containing 5917 female rape survivors of 14 years and older, met the inclusion criteria. The overall weighted mean percentage of unacknowledged rape turned out to be 60.4%, but there was a large amount of heterogeneity and inconsistency among the included studies. The researchers found that prevalence was significantly higher among college student participants compared to non-college participants. Also, the findings supported that over half of all female rape survivors did not acknowledge that they had been raped.

A study in Chinese populations by Ma (2018) revealed no significant difference in the prevalence of childhood sexual abuse between Chinese men (9.1%) and women (8.9%). However, the prevalence of childhood sexual abuse in studies from mainland areas was significantly higher than that of Hong Kong/Taiwan. Ma's study was based on a meta-analysis from 36 articles with a total of 131,734 participants.

1.1.5 Sexual Perpetration and Victimization

Krahé et al. (2015) presented on young people's sexual victimization and perpetration from 10 European countries (Austria, Belgium, Cyprus, Greece, Lithuania, the Netherlands, Poland, Portugal, Slovakia, and Spain) using a shared measurement tool ($N = 3480$ participants, aged between 18 and 27 years). Between 19.7% and 52.2% of female and between 10.1% and 55.8% of male respondents reported having experienced at least one incident of sexual victimization since the age of consent. In two countries, victimization rates were significantly higher for men than for women. Between 5.5% and 48.7% of male and 2.6% and 14.8% of female participants reported having engaged in at least one act of sexual aggression perpetration, with higher rates for men than for women in all countries. Victimization rates correlated negatively with sexual assertiveness and positively with alcohol use in sexual encounters. Perpetration rates correlated positively with attitudes condoning physical dating violence and with alcohol use in men, and negatively with sexual assertiveness in women. At the country level, lower gender equality in economic power and in the work domain was related to higher male perpetration rates. Lower gender equality in political power and higher sexual assertiveness in women relative to men were linked to higher male victimization rates.

Peterson, Beagley, McCallum, and Artime (2019) asked a sample of 268 community men to complete an online survey on their adult sexual assault perpetration, their adult sexual assault victimization history, and their experiences of child sexual abuse. They also completed measures of traumatic sexual beliefs, dysfunctional sexual behaviors, sexual avoidance, sexual preoccupation, and distorted sexual self-concept. A statistically significant overlap was found between men's perpetration and victimization of adult sexual assault. Compared with victims-only, perpetrators-only, and men with no adult sexual assault history, men with a history of both perpetration and victimization reported the highest rates of childhood sexual abuse and the highest levels of distorted sexual self-concepts.

1.1.6 Victimization

Much research has shown that the health consequences of violence are far broader than injuries or death. Victims of violence are at risk of psychological and behavioral problems, including depression, alcohol abuse, anxiety, and suicidal behavior, and reproductive or sexual health problems, such as sexually transmitted diseases, unwanted pregnancies, and sexual dysfunction (Krug et al., 2002).

Bacchus, Ranganathan, Watts, and Devries (2018) reviewed 35 cohort studies to determine the magnitude and temporal direction of the association between recent intimate partner violence (IPV) and a range of adverse health outcomes or health risk behaviors.

Eight studies showed evidence of a positive association between recent IPV and subsequent depressive symptoms, and five studies demonstrated a positive, statistically significant relationship between depressive symptoms and subsequent IPV. Recent IPV was also associated with increased symptoms of subsequent postpartum depression in five studies, although there was substantial heterogeneity. There was some evidence of a bidirectional relationship between recent IPV and hard drug use and marijuana use, although studies were limited. There was no evidence of an association between recent IPV and alcohol use or sexually transmitted infections (STIs), although there were few studies and inconsistent measurement of alcohol and STIs. They concluded that exposure to violence has significant impacts.

Sexual offending is related to several mental health problems in a large number of victims. Internalizing disorders such as anxiety, depression, and posttraumatic stress disorder (PTSD) are among the most frequently reported problems (Mason & Lodrick, 2013), but victims also report physical health consequences (Jina & Thomas, 2013), substance use (Ullman, Relyea, Peter-Hagene, & Vasquez, 2013), and self-blame (Peter-Hagene & Ullman, 2016). A meta-analysis of studies on the effects of child sexual abuse revealed that victims might suffer from PTSD, depression, suicide, sexual promiscuity, and problems in academic achievement (Paolucci, Genius, & Violato, 2001).

Dworkin, Menon, Bystrynski, and Allen (2017) conducted a meta-analytic review of the literature from 1970 to 2014 to understand the degree to which (a) sexual assault confers general risk for psychological dysfunction rather than specific risk for posttraumatic stress and (b) differences in studies and samples account for variation in observed effects. Results indicated that people who have been sexually assaulted report significantly worse psychopathology than unassaulted comparisons. Sexual assault was associated with increased risk for all forms of psychopathology assessed, and relatively stronger associations were observed for posttraumatic stress and suicidality.

They concluded that experiencing sexual assault is a major risk factor for multiple forms of psychological dysfunction across populations and assault types.

Dworkin (2018) reviewed 39 studies dated between 1970 and 2014 representing 88,539 individuals experiencing adolescent/adult and/or lifetime sexual abuse and unassaulted individuals. Results indicated that most psychiatric disorders were more prevalent in survivors of sexual assault with depressive disorders and posttraumatic stress disorder (PTSD) especially prevalent.

1.1.7 Costs of Violence

Thielen et al. (2016) investigated a representative sample of 7076 Dutch inhabitants aged between 18 and 65 years. Exposure rates in the sample ranged from 7% for sexual abuse to 25% for emotional neglect. The mean annual adjusted excess costs were found to range between € 869 and € 2893 per abused person, depending on the type of child maltreatment. Depending on the estimated exposure rates, the annual societal costs at population level ranged between € 88 million and € 395 million per one million individuals aged between 18 and 65 years.

The estimated lifetime costs of rape per victim in the United States were studied by Peterson, DeGue, Florence, and Lokey (2017) using data from previous studies and the National Intimate Partner and Sexual Violence Survey. Costs were defined as financial consequences because of attributable impaired health, lost productivity, and criminal justice costs from the societal perspective. The estimated lifetime cost of rape appeared to be $122,461 per victim, or a population economic burden of nearly $3.1 trillion United States dollars over victims' lifetimes, based on data indicating that more than 25 million adults have been raped. This estimate included $1.2 trillion (39% of total) in medical costs, $1.6 trillion (52%) in lost work productivity among victims and perpetrators, $234 billion (8%) in criminal justice activities, and $36 billion (1%) in other costs, including victim property loss or damage. Government sources pay an estimated $1 trillion (32%) of the lifetime economic burden. The authors concluded that preventing sexual violence could avoid substantial costs for victims, perpetrators, healthcare payers, employers, and government payers.

Based on previous research and available data, Letourneau, Brown, Fang, Hassan, and Mercy (2018) estimated the U.S. economic impact of child sexual abuse. Costs of child sexual abuse were measured from the societal perspective and include healthcare costs, productivity losses, child welfare costs, violence/crime costs, special education costs, and suicide death costs. All costs were estimated in U.S. dollars and adjusted to the reference year 2015. Estimating 20 new cases of child sexual abuse that occurred in 2015, the lifetime economic burden of child sexual abuse is approximately $9.3 billion, the lifetime cost for victims of fatal child sexual abuse per female and male victim is on average $1,128,334 and $1,482,933, respectively, and the average lifetime cost for victims of nonfatal child sexual abuse is of $282,734 per female victim. For male victims of nonfatal child sexual abuse, there was insufficient information on productivity losses, contributing to a lower average estimated lifetime cost of $74,691 per male victim.

Peterson et al. (2018) combined data from previous studies with 2012 U.S. National Intimate Partner and Sexual Violence Survey data. Costs included attributable impaired health, lost productivity, and criminal justice costs from the societal perspective. The estimated intimate partner violence lifetime cost was $103,767 per female victim and $23,414 per male victim, or a population economic burden of nearly $3.6 trillion (2014 U.S. dollars) over victims' lifetimes, based on 43 million U.S. adults with victimization history. This estimate included $2.1 trillion (59%) in medical costs, $1.3 trillion (37%) in lost productivity among victims and perpetrators, $73 billion (2%) in criminal justice activities, and $62 billion (2%) in other costs, including victim property loss or damage. Government sources pay an estimated $1.3 trillion (37%) of the lifetime economic burden.

1.1.8 Costs and Benefits of Treatment

There is a lack of studies on the economic costs and benefits of offender treatment programs, probably because one of the most challenging questions is how to estimate the economic value of nonmonetary costs and benefits (Cohen, 2001). Nonmonetary costs can be divided in tangible costs such as medical costs and loss of wages, and in intangible costs such as pain, suffering, and reduced quality of life. For the determination of costs and benefits of a treatment program, a number of issues needs to be addressed, namely (1) from whose perspective are these costs and benefits measured, (2) what are the fixed costs and incremental costs per participant, (3) what are short-term and long-term benefits from such a program and how can these benefits be expressed in monetary terms, and finally (4) is there a difference between the targeted group for this treatment and the group exposed to treatment in earlier studies and is there evidence from replication studies. All these issues might explain why the number of studies on costs and benefits of treatment programs for offenders is limited. However, Cohen (2001) emphasized that even when a treatment program has been shown to reduce recidivism, it is also essential to know at what cost and at what benefit.

Gold et al. (2011) described the great pitfalls and challenges that arise when calculating the costs of IPV for families, populations, and governments. They reviewed the current research from the United Kingdom and Australia and concluded that evidence was small but promising. Interventions that have been economically evaluated to date appear cost-effective, offering additional benefits at relatively low additional cost, offering additional benefits at no increase in cost, or even offering additional benefits at a reduction in costs. In their opinion, an economic evaluation should always be considered in the design of IPV intervention research.

To calculate the extent of savings and benefits, Shapiro and Hassett (2012) analyzed a broad range of costs associated with violent crime in eight American cities.

Regarded as direct costs were local spending on policing, prosecuting and incarcerating the perpetrators of those crimes. These costs also encompass out-of-pocket medical expenses borne by surviving victims of violent crime as well as the income those victims must forgo as a result of the crimes. They also include the lost incomes that would otherwise be earned by the perpetrators of violent crimes had they not been apprehended. Altogether, the annual costs appear to range from $90 million per year in Seattle to around $200 million per year in Boston, Jacksonville, and Milwaukee, to more than $700 million in Philadelphia and nearly $1.1 billion for Chicago. Shapiro and Hassett (2012) also examined certain intangible costs associated with violent crime, including the pain and suffering of the surviving victims of violent crime and the costs to the families of murder victims. Across the eight cities, the total annual costs of violent crimes, including these intangible costs, ranged from more than $300 million per year in Seattle to more than $900 million in Boston, to some $3.7 billion per year in Philadelphia and $5.3 billion for Chicago. Budgetary savings that each of the eight cities should expect to achieve if their rates of violent crime declined by either 10% or 25%, including lower expenditures on law enforcement and the justice system, as well as the additional revenues that each city might expect to collect from applying local taxes to the income earned by those who otherwise would have been victims or perpetrators of those crimes. The estimated savings for municipal budgets from a 25% reduction in violent crime range from $6 million per year in Seattle to $12 million per year in Boston and Milwaukee, to $42 million per year in Philadelphia and $59 million for Chicago. Remarkably, the most substantial economic benefits associated with reduced rates of violent crime would arise from the impact of lower rates of violent crime on the housing values in the eight cities.

According to Settumba, Chambers, Shanahan, Schofield, and Butler (2018), the total judicial expenditures that offenders place on society were for the USA (2013), the UK (2015), and Australia (2016), respectively, 265 billion, 12 billion, and 11.5 billion United States dollars. The additional financial burden of crime was estimated at 1.7 trillion and 50 billion United States dollars in the USA (2012) and Australia (2014), respectively. These researchers found 17 studies, from the USA, Australia, and the UK, of economic evaluations of behavioral interventions (cognitive behavior therapy or multi-systemic therapy) among offenders in prison or the community. Six studies concerned young offenders (Borduin & Dopp, 2015) and 11 adults (Barrett & Byford, 2012), while 11 studies were cost-effectiveness analyses (CEAs) and 6 were cost-benefit analyses (CBAs). Cost-effectiveness studies focus, for example, on the cost per successfully treated offender who does not recidivate, while cost-benefit studies address the monetary values of benefits of treatment programs in relation to costs. It appeared not possible to state which treatment programs were most cost-effective or yielded more economic benefit given the methodological variations between the studies. All six CBA studies were found to have a positive net benefit or a cost-benefit ratio less than one, which means that the evaluated treatment yielded higher incremental benefits than the incremental costs when compared with an alternative. Among the CEA studies it was found that 6 out of 11 studies were more cost-effective than the alternatives, but three studies showed that the investigated treatment programs were not cost-effective when compared to their alternatives. The authors concluded that given the huge economic burden that offenders place on society in terms of the resources required to police, prosecute, treat, and rehabilitate this group, and the societal cost of crime, it is worrisome that so little attention is paid to economic aspects of intervention and treatment programs. They recommend that a culture of robust economic evaluations be developed to ensure that the available resources are spent on the most cost-effective programs (Settumba et al., 2018).

1.1.9 Summary

In industrialized countries, a relatively large amount of research has been done into the prevalence of perpetrators and victims of violent crimes by both government institutions and researchers from private institutions. Although studies often concern different populations and different periods, their findings all point in the same direction, namely that the physical and psychological consequences for victims are serious, and the economic burden on society is considerable. The number of perpetrators is relatively small because many violent crimes are committed by the same perpetrator, most offenses are not reported to the police because the perpetrator is known by the victim, and a relatively small number of declarations lead to a conviction.

1.2 Concepts

In the literature, concepts such as hostility, anger, aggression, and violence are often used interchangeably without additional delineation (Eckhardt, Norlander, & Deffenbacher, 2004; Norlander & Eckhardt, 2005). Therefore, several definitions are provided for concepts that are frequently used in this book, without describing their various theoretical contexts. Hostility is defined as the propensity to negatively interpret the behaviors of others even when their intentions are nonthreatening (Blackburn, 1993). Anger is taken to reflect an emotion that is expressed in behaviors such as persistent, intense looking, loud talking, and standing close. State anger is an acute emotional-physiological reaction that ranges from mild irritation to intense fury and rage. Trait anger, by contrast, is a personality dimension that reflects the person's chronic tendency to experience the emotion of state anger with higher frequency, intensity, and duration than the average individual (Veenstra, Bushman, & Koole, 2018). Human aggression is defined as any behavior intended to harm another person who does not want to be harmed (Bushman, 2018) or who is motivated to avoid that harm (Allen, Anderson, & Bushman, 2018). Violence is seen as a specific form of aggressive behavior that mainly involves the infliction of physical harm (Allen & Anderson, 2017; Browne & Howells, 1996). Two types of aggression are often distinguished, namely reactive and proactive or instrumental aggression (Dodge, 1991). Dodge, Lochman, Harnish, Bates, and Pettit (1997) described reactive aggression as "emotional, defensive and hot-tempered" and proactive aggression as "calculating, offensive and cold-blooded" (p. 38). Also, the reactive versus proactive distinction emphasizes the goal of the aggressive behavior, namely hurting someone versus obtaining some other goal, and emphasizes how thoughtless versus thoughtful the behavior is. Finally, the reactive versus proactive distinction reflects whether the behavior occurs in response to a (perceived) provocation or without provocation. The term personality domain refers in this book to one of the Big Five personality traits (Allen & Anderson, 2017; Costa Jr. & McCrae, 1992). Psychopathy refers to "selfish, callous, and remorseless use of others" in combination with a "chronically unstable and antisocial lifestyle" (Harpur, Hare, & Hakstian, 1989, p. 6).

Criminogenic needs are internal and external risk factors that are associated with a person's criminal behavior (Andrews & Bonta, 2010). Internal or personal criminogenic needs are an individual's characteristics and may comprise criminal history, drug, and alcohol use, feeling miserable, lack of prosocial conduct, and positive attitudes regarding criminality. External or environmental criminogenic needs relate to the criminal's social context regarding problems with housing, education and employment, income, and social interactions. Another critical distinction is the differentiation between static and dynamic risk factors. Static factors, such as having an extensive criminal history or having been raised in a single-parent family, are difficult or even impossible to change. On the other hand, dynamic factors such as inadequate social skills and antisocial attitudes and associates are, in principle, amenable to change.

1.3 Theories of Aggressive Behavior

In 1939, Dollard, Doob, Miller, Mowrer, and Sears presented the frustration-aggression hypothesis, which suggests that the existence of frustration always leads to some form of aggression. In this context, frustration is specified as the thwarting of a goal response, which is the final reinforcer in an ongoing behavior sequence. However, frustration can refer not only to the process of blocking a person's attainment of a reinforcer but also to the reaction to such blocking. Consequently, being frustrated means both that somebody else thwarted the access to reinforcers and that the reaction to this thwarting is one of annoyance. A few years later, Miller (1941) modified this position, in the sense that aggression is always preceded by frustration, but frustration does not always lead to aggression. In his criticism of the frustration-aggression hypothesis, Berkowitz (1978) also challenged the first point of departure by arguing that aggression can sometimes be instrumental or proactive, that is, intended to achieve a particular goal, even if someone is hurt by it. Moreover, there are indications that cognitions can influence the frustration that leads to aggression. The aggressor's interpretation of his feelings and his beliefs regarding the cause of his arousal can influence the strength of his attacks on the available target. Nowadays, frustration is seen as a possible but not necessary condition for aggressive behavior (Allen, Anderson, & Bushman, 2018).

According to Bandura's (1973, 2001) social cognitive learning theory, people acquire aggressive responses the same way as they acquire other forms of social behavior, namely by direct experience or by observing others. The theory explains the acquisition of aggressive behaviors via observational learning processes, and provides concepts for understanding and describing the beliefs and expectations that guide social behavior. Key concepts regarding the development and change of expectations and how one construes the social world provides insight into the acquisition of aggressive behaviors and in explaining instrumental aggression (Anderson & Bushman, 2002).

A developmental model of aggressive behavior during early childhood was presented by Huesmann (1988, 2018). According to this model, aggressive behavior is always a product of personal predisposing factors and precipitating situational factors. The predisposing factors exert their influence by creating encoded social cognitions including schemas about the world, scripts for social behavior, and normative beliefs about what is appropriate. These social cognitions interact with situational primes to determine behavior and are acquired primarily through observational learning. Children and adolescents who are repeatedly exposed to violence will acquire social cognitions promoting aggression that last into adulthood. Thus, violence can be caused simply through its observation (Huesmann, 2018).

Dodge and colleagues (Coie & Dodge, 2000; Crick & Dodge, 1994) were strongly influenced by Bandura, Huesmann, and Berkowitz when they articulated the role that ongoing social-information processing plays in directing aggressive behavior. According to Dodge (2002), social-information processing not only includes cognitive processing and affective experiences, but also involves the setting of goals for responding to the social situation, accessing one or more possible behavioral responses, evaluating the accessed behavioral responses, and selecting one for enactment, and then translating a desire to perform an action into behavior. Dodge and Coie (1987) and Dodge et al. (1997) theorized that the distinct ways in which people process social information and differences in people's social goals both influence the likelihood that they will engage in one of two types of aggression.

The General Aggression Model (GAM) of Anderson and Bushman (2002) considers the role of social, cognitive, developmental, and biological factors on aggression. The GAM includes elements from many domain-specific theories of aggression, such as neoassociation theory (Berkowitz, 1993), social learning theory (Bandura, 1973), and script theory (Huesmann, 1988). By unifying these theories into one coherent whole, the GAM is supposed to provide a broad framework for understanding aggression in many contexts. All determinants of aggressive behavior are organized into three stages (Allen, Anderson, & Bushman, 2018), namely Inputs (person and situation), Routes (affect, cognition, and arousal), and Outcomes (appraisal and decision processes), resulting in thoughtful action or impulsive action.

In their behavioral model, Nietzel, Hasemann, and Lynam (1999) confine themselves to violent delinquents. They integrated various "multifactor behavioral models" with "other criminological perspectives" which resulted in a four-factor model comprising (1) distal antecedents, i.e., biological, psychological and social dispositions that facilitate the development of violent behavior, (2) indicators of aggressive behavior at a (very) young age, (3) social and individual factors that cause early behavioral problems to evolve into chronic antisocial behavior, and (4) perpetuating factors that support the maintenance and escalation of the violent behavior. According to Nietzel et al. (1999), their model underscores the necessity of early preventive measures to curb the development and escalation of violent behavior.

Finally, Andrews and Bonta (2010) presented their General Personality and Cognitive Social Learning (GPCSL) model of criminal conduct. According to these authors, there are many routes to crime, but some experiences in life are more influential than others. Within the GPCSL, the domains of education and employment, family, leisure, and substance abuse are referred to as the Moderate Four risk/need factors. The most proximal factors influencing criminal behavior are criminal history, procriminal companions, attitudes and cognitions supportive of criminal behavior, and antisocial personality pattern. The GPCSL model views these as significant determinants of criminality, and they are referred to as the Big Four risk/need factors. Together these eight factors are referred to as the "Central Eight."

Some meta-analytic reviews have found evidence for the primacy of the Big Four over the Moderate Four risk/need factors among general offenders (Andrews & Bonta, 2010; Andrews, Bonta, & Wormith, 2006; Gendreau, Little, & Goggin, 1996). In all of these reviews, indicators of psychological distress/dysfunction performed relatively poorly compared to the Central Eight. Traditional clinical variables such as anxiety, depression, mood, and major psychotic symptoms are therefore seen as minor risk factors. A meta-analysis by Bonta, Blais, and Wilson (2013) revealed that the GPCSL risk/need factors are just as relevant for mentally disordered offenders as they are for non-disordered offenders. However, they found no support for prioritizing the Big Four in the prediction of general recidivism and mild support in the prediction of violent recidivism. Also, analyses of the clinical variables showed that, except for antisocial personality or psychopathy, these factors were not predictive of recidivism.

1.4 Theories of Sexually Aggressive Behavior

In their overview of theories of sexually aggressive behavior, Ward, Polaschek, and Beech (2006) distinguish three types of theories on sexual offending, namely (1) single-factor theories, (2) multi-factor theories, and (3) descriptive models.

1.4.1 Single-Factor Theories

In *single-factor theories*, one risk factor is explored in depth. Examples are the theories of cognitive distortions, deviant sexual preferences, and pornography. Cognitive distortions were defined by Abel et al. (1984) as belief systems that justify having sexual contact with children, but also as justifications, perceptions, and judgments used by sex offenders to rationalize child abusing behavior or sexually assaulting/raping a woman (Abel et al., 1989). According to Ward's Implicit Theory Model (Ward, 2000), *cognitive distortions* may arise from underlying implicit theories of sexual offenses toward children or adult women. Specific offense-supporting cognitions allow offenders to justify their sexually offensive behavior as acceptable (for example: "Children as sexual beings" or "Women are sex objects"). The Multi-Mechanism Theory of Cognitive Distortions (MMT-CD) of Szumski, Bartels, Beech, and Fisher (2018) provided an updated theoretical account of cognitive distortions in males by adopting a dual-process perspective and incorporating the concept of motivated cognition and the effects of visceral factors. They proposed that cognitive distortions arise from three mechanisms, which can be identified in terms of their temporal occurrence to an offense. Mechanism 1 accounts for cognitive distortions that arise long before an offense is committed but serve to influence an individual's life-course and goals in a way that eventually brings them closer to sexually offending. Mechanism 2 accounts for distortions that arise in the lead up to or immediately before a sexual offense, thus, providing a justification for committing an offense. Finally, Mechanism 3 accounts for distortions that are formed post-offense as a result of the adversarial context of the individual's social environment.

Theories of deviant sexual preferences, such as McGuire, Carlisle, and Young's Sexual Deviation Theory (McGuire, Carlisle, & Young, 1965) or Laws and Marshall's Conditioning Theory (Laws & Marshall, 1990), propose that men who engage in *sexually deviant behavior* do so because they prefer it to socially and sexually acceptable behavior. According to the Diagnostic and Statistical Manual of Mental Disorders 5 (DSM 5; American Psychiatric Association, 2013), people suffering from a paraphilic disorder (1) feel personal distress about their interest, not merely distress resulting from society's disapproval or (2) have a sexual desire or behavior that involves another person's psychological distress, injury, or death, or a desire for sexual behaviors involving unwilling persons or persons unable to give legal consent.

The theory of the sociologist Russell (1988, 1998) is mainly focused on the role of *pornography* in the etiology of rape, in which pornography is defined as "material that combines sex and/or the exposure of the genitals with abuse or degradation in a manner that appears to endorse, condone, or encourage such behavior" (Russell, 1998, p. 3). The starting point of Russell's theory is the feminist idea that sexually aggressive behavior is the product of a patriarchal society that uses (the threat of) aggressive sexual behavior as a means to suppress women (Russell & Bolen, 2000). To this end, it is proposed that Western society socialize men to become persons with a high inclination to the rape of women. For instance, 25–60% of American men report thinking that they were not unlikely to rape a woman if they would have the guarantee that they would not get caught (Malamuth, 1981). Also, 25–30% of the American men get aroused of violent images of rape (Malamuth & Check, 1980). Russell's model implies that pornography increases the chance of rape by four main effects: (1) pornography predisposes some men to want to rape women or intensifies the likelihood in those men already predisposed to do so, (2) undermines some men's internal inhibitions against acting out their rape desires, (3) undermines some men's social inhibitions against the acting out, and (4) undermines a woman's resistance, which increases the chance of rape. Russell (1998) stated that her model is in accordance with the empirical literature, but recognized that the model as such has not yet been empirically tested. However, recent research showed that the effects of (violent) pornography on sexually violent behavior are controversial. For instance, Wright, Tokunaga, and Kraus (2016) found that watching (violent) pornography contributes to more sexually violent behavior, while Malamuth (2018) concluded that this contributes only to more sexually violent behavior in men who are already (highly) predisposed to sexually aggressive behavior.

1.4.2 Multi-Factor Theories

Multi-factor theories are characterized by considering together the different risk factors that someone may predispose to a sexual offense in a particular situation. Examples of multi-factor theories are Finkelhor's Precondition Model of child sexual abuse (Finkelhor, 1984), Marshall and Barbaree's Integrated Theory of sexual offending in general (Marshall & Barbaree, 1990), Hall and Hirschmann's Quadripartite Model of rape and child sexual abuse (Hall & Hirschman, 1991), Malamuths's Confluence Model of Sexual Aggression (Malamuth, 1996), Ward and Siegert's Pathways Model, which is an integration of the three former models (Ward & Siegert, 2002), Ward and Beech's Integrative Theory of Sexual Offending (Ward & Beech, 2006), Stinson and Becker's Multimodal Self-Regulation Theory (Stinson & Becker, 2013; Stinson, Becker, & Sales, 2008), and finally Seto's Motivation-Facilitation Model of sexual offending (Seto, 2019).

For example, the Integrated Theory of Marshall and Barbaree (1990) suggests that evolutionary inheritance confers on males the capacity to sexually aggress, which must be controlled by appropriate socialization to instill social inhibitions toward such behavior. Variations in hormonal functioning during puberty and the ensuing early years of adolescence may make this task more or less difficult. Poor parenting, particularly the use of inconsistent and harsh discipline in the absence of love, may mean that men fail to acquire these constraints or may facilitate the fusion of sex and aggression rather than separate these two tendencies. Sociocultural attitudes because of, for instance, the availability of pornography may negatively interact with poor parenting to enhance the likelihood of sexual offending if these cultural beliefs express traditional patriarchal views. For example, a young man whose childhood experiences have ill-prepared him for appropriate sexual relationships may readily accept these views to bolster his sense of masculinity. If such a man gets intoxicated, angry, or stressed, and he finds himself in circumstances where he is not known or thinks he can get away with offending, then this man is likely to offend sexually.

Based on his research, Malamuth (1996) suggested that coercive sexual behavior against women is the result of several factors that may be organized into the hostile-masculinity and the impersonal-promiscuity path. Sexual aggression is proposed to be the result of the confluence of these paths. Hostile-masculinity combines two interrelated components, namely a defensive and hostile-distrustful orientation toward women and gratification from controlling or dominating women. The impersonal-promiscuity path refers to a non-committal, game-playing orientation in sexual relations. Several studies yielded empirical support for the validity of the two paths (Hunter, Figueredo, & Malamuth, 2010; Malamuth, Linz, Heavey, Barnes, & Acker, 1995). In later publications, Malamuth placed his sexual coercion theory in an evolutionary psychological perspective (Huppin & Malamuth, 2017; Malamuth, Huppin, & Paul, 2005). In this way, he wanted to explain why the average man is more motivated to enter into sexual relationships with women than vice versa and why sex is for men easier to separate from intimate emotions than for women. Such differences could contribute to the use of coercion to overcome the unwillingness and resistance of women in conflict situations.

According to the Integrated Theory of Sexual Offending (ITSO) of Ward and Beech (2006), there are three groups of factors, namely biological, environmental, and neuropsychological factors, which play an essential role in sexual offending. They suggest that in all human beings, genes and environmental factors, such as learning through experiences in the social environment, manifest themselves in three neuropsychological systems, namely motivation, perception, and action selection. The clinical problems that are seen in sexual assaults, such as deviant arousal, emotional problems, cognitive impairment, and interpersonal problems, arise from the interaction between genetic predisposition, social learning, and neurobiological and neuropsychological systems. These clinical problems, in turn, lead to criminal offenses. The theory states further that the consequences of the sexual offense reinforce and therefore maintain this behavior. The sexual offender becomes socially isolated which further limits the chance of typical social contacts, or the social environment encourages further sexist behavior (Ward, Fisher, & Beech, 2016).

In his motivation-facilitation model of sexual offending, Seto (2019) identified the traits of paraphilia, high sex drive, and intense mating effort as primary motivations for sexual offenses, as well as trait (e.g., antisocial personality) and state (e.g., intoxication) factors that can facilitate acting on these motivations when opportunities exist. The model was initially developed to explain contact sexual offending against children, but it was subsequently extended as an explanation for child pornography offending and for online solicitations of young adolescents. Seto (2019) stated that his model has the potential to be expanded to explain other forms of sexual offending, including sexual assaults of adults and noncontact offenses involving exhibitionism or voyeurism.

1.4.3 Descriptive Models

Examples of *descriptive models* are Marlatt's Relapse Model (Marlatt, 1985a, 1985b) and the Pithers-Marques Relapse Model of Sexual Offending (Pithers, Marques, Gibat, & Marlatt, 1983). The Relapse Prevention Model stems from the substance abuse field, where maintenance of abstinence following treatment is often a challenge. The model is based on the notion that the identification of thoughts and actions that lead from a lapse (a temporary slip or return to a previous behavior that one is trying to control or quit) to a relapse (a full-blown return to a pattern of behavior that one has been trying to moderate or quit altogether) helps an individual to intervene before a relapse occurs. Treatment is meant to help individuals to develop better and wider-ranging coping skills, and improve their confidence in their ability to manage risky situations. A lack of effective coping strategies is proposed to decrease an individual's sense of self-efficacy, thus increasing the chance of relapse (Laws, Hudson, & Ward, 2000). Pithers et al. (1983) applied the Relapse Prevention Model to the treatment of sexual offenders, arguing that sexual reoffending could often be avoided if the individual could better cope with high-risk situations. In order to achieve this goal, sexual offenders have to acquire insight into their thoughts, feelings, and behaviors that may lead to criminal behavior, followed by training in social skills, anger management, and problem-solving skills.

1.5 Neurobiological Explanations of Sexual Aggression

1.5.1 Testosterone and Serotonin

In several studies, a positive relationship has been found between *testosterone* levels and an increased prevalence of violent sexual offenses (Briken, Hill, & Berner, 2006). For instance, in a study of 520 sex offenders, the level of testosterone in the blood at the entry to a treatment clinic was found to be positively correlated with the degree of violence of the committed offense (Studer, Aylwin, & Reddon, 2005). Also, recidivism risk within 9 years turned out to be positively related to initial testosterone levels. Therefore, testosterone level has been proposed to be a robust predictor of violent sexual behavior, as strong as most static risk factors reported by Hanson and Bussière (1998). In dropouts from the treatment program in a study by Studer et al. (2005), testosterone level predicted recidivism significantly stronger than most static risk factors. Therefore, the authors stated that testosterone should have a greater role in risk assessment and the risk management of sexually violent offenders. According to Gooren (2011), Androgen Deprivation Therapy that is focused on lowering the level of testosterone raises the threshold at which erotosexual imagery and sexual activity occur, and therefore it may have a place in the treatment of unacceptable sexual behavior. However, a meta-analysis of 42 studies by Archer, Graham-Kevan, and Davies (2005) showed a very low overall correlation between testosterone and aggression, with associations being greater for younger men and general offenders.

Similarly, a meta-analysis on the relationship between testosterone and sexual aggression by Wong and Gravel (2018) yielded no overall difference in testosterone level between sex offenders and non-sex offenders. Based on the literature, Carré and Archer (2018) have recently concluded that testosterone influences aggression mainly in high dominance men, and those with low cortisol levels.

Serotonin has been recognized as the main neurotransmitter associated with impaired behavior inhibition (Briken & Kafka, 2007). Alterations in the serotonin system especially influence patients with affective and anxiety disorders, who may use sexual stimulation as a coping strategy. Serotonin also inhibits sexual arousal and reduces orgasmic and ejaculatory capacity. Consequently, selective serotonin reuptake inhibitors (SSRIs) have been used to improve symptomatology in patients with paraphilia and compulsive sexual behavior (Beech & Mitchell, 2005). However, studies on the reduction of sexual fantasies and sexually deviant behavior using SSRIs in patients with various paraphilias, have often relied on rather small samples and short follow-up periods. They were also not placebo-controlled and did not use sexual recidivism as the outcome variable (Briken, Hill, & Berner, 2014).

1.5.2 Pedophilia

Neurobiological research of sexual offenders focuses mainly on the subgroup of child sexual abusers, probably because child sexual abuse is perceived by the general public as more emotionally disturbing and morally unacceptable. However, it should be noted that not every child sexual abuser is a pedophile and not every pedophile is a child sexual abuser. Two groups of child sexual abusers can be distinguished: (1) those who show no paraphilic disorder, but sexually abuse children mostly because of general traumatizing family constellations and a lack of the necessary social skills to develop and maintain emotional and sexual relationships with appropriately aged peers and (2) those who do display a paraphilic disorder, namely pedophilia (i.e., the ongoing sexual preference for prepubescent minors) and/or hebephilia (i.e., the ongoing sexual preference for pubescent minors). In both cases, the consequences for the victimized children are huge (Tenbergen et al., 2015).

1.5.3 Neuropsychological Factors Related to Pedophilia

There are indications that pedophiles are characterized by neuropsychological *deficits in executive functions*, which may be the result of a prenatal or perinatal developmental disorder (Blanchard et al., 2003). A study by Suchy, Whittaker, Strassberg, and Eastvold (2009) compared pedophilic and non-pedophilic child sexual abusers with matched non-offender controls on semantic knowledge, executive functioning, processing speed, motor speed, auditory memory, and visual memory. Results indicated that the pedophilic child sexual abusers exhibited slower processing speed, non-pedophilic child molesters exhibited poorer semantic knowledge, and both child sexual abuser groups exhibited executive weaknesses as compared to non-offender controls. In a later study, Eastvold, Suchy, and Strassberg (2011) assessed executive functioning among pedophilic and non-pedophilic child sexual abusers, relative to non-sex offenders. Results revealed that (a) pedophilic child sexual abusers had an overall executive functioning profile that was different from that of non-sex offenders, but not different from non-pedophilic child sexual abusers, (b) child sexual abusers on the whole performed better than non-sex offenders on abstract reasoning and more poorly on inhibition, and (c) pedophilic child sexual abusers performed better on planning and exhibited better overall performance accuracy relative to non-pedophilic child sex offenders. These results suggest that pedophilic child sexual abusers exhibit a more deliberate, planful response style, characterized by greater self-monitoring, whereas non-pedophilic child sexual abusers appear to respond more impulsively. A similar study was conducted by Schiffer and Vonlaufen (2011). Their data suggested that non-pedophilic child sexual abusers showed more severe cognitive deficits than pedophilic child sexual abusers. However, the deficits in response inhibition were observed in both groups of child sexual abusers. A study by Suchy, Eastvold, Strassberg, and Franchow (2014) showed that pedophilic men were characterized by a distinct neurocognitive weakness, performing worse than controls on measures of behavioral inhibition and information processing but did not have a more planning-oriented response style. All these results suggest that convicted pedophilic child sexual abusers do show deficits in executive functioning, although these might be due to mental disturbances and not to the sexual preference for children (Tenbergen et al., 2015).

Several researchers have found a relation between socio-emotional problems in sex offenders and disorders in *social attachment* during infancy (Craissati, McClurg, & Browne, 2002). Consequently, child sexual abusers are supposed to be less able to have interpersonal relationships with peers and therefore are trying to have sexual relations with children (Ward & Siegert, 2002). Research showed that insecure attachment styles affect chemical processes in the brain. The neuropeptides of oxytocin and vasopressin play a crucial role in the neural processes underlying social attachment (Carter, 1998). Oxytocin mainly regulates care behavior, whereas vasopressin is more involved in aggressive sexual behavior. Beech and Mitchell (2005) argue that stressful experiences, partly through the effects on the serotonergic neurotransmitter system, can change the sensitivity of the oxytocin system for a long time and thereby the mechanisms that form the basis for social approach and attachment. Therefore, the knowledge on the biological basis of social attachment may guide the application of pharmacological treatment of sex offenders in which offensive behavior is associated with disorders in social attachment styles (Beech & Mitchell, 2005). Selective serotonin reuptake inhibitors (SSRIs) are sometimes prescribed for sex offenders because they may reduce sexual interest (Briken & Kafka, 2007), but they may also stimulate a positive social approach by increasing serotonin levels. Prolonged administration of SSRIs may also lead to increased plasticity of the brain and thus make the offender readier for therapy (Beech & Mitchell, 2005). The exploration by Beech and Mitchell on the role of psychoneurological deficiencies related to attachment problems in pedophilia is intriguing, but it is an area where there is still little empirical evidence available.

1.5.4 Neurobiology of Pedophilia

According to Seto (2009), three major neurobiological theories on pedophilia can be distinguished. Firstly, the "frontal lobe theory" refers to orbitofrontal and left and right dorsolateral prefrontal cortex differences that are often seen in pedophilic men. As the orbitofrontal cortex is responsible for behavior control, especially inhibiting sexual behavior, volume differences or dysfunction in this area may explain the sexual behavior disorder associated with pedophilia. For instance, in a fMRI study of pedophiles, Cantor et al. (2007) reported that abnormalities were found in two major fiber bundles of the brain, namely the superior frontal-occipital fasciculus and the right arcuate fasciculus, which could indicate a possible lack of connectivity within the circuit for the recognition of relevant sexual stimuli. Secondly, the "temporal lobe theory" refers to reports of hypersexuality accompanying pedophilia. Studies have shown that disturbances of the temporal lobes can result in an increase in pedophilic behaviors or an increase in the breadth of deviant sexual interests. These disturbances include temporal lesions and hippocampal sclerosis. Differential temporal lobe activations in pedophilic men that highlight a hypersexuality-specific activation profile supports the role of the temporal lobe in the expression of hypersexuality that is often seen with sexual behavior disorders. A third major neurobiological theory holds that differences in the sex dimorphic brain structures affected by the masculinization of the male brain would more strongly affect pedophilia development. These differences are supposed to be influenced by testosterone exposure. Furthermore, there is an additional theory (Seto, 2009) that combines the frontal and temporal lobe theories. It states that the frontal and temporal lobes affect pedophilic sexual preference expression and its associated behaviors differently, with the frontal lobe (orbitofrontal and dorsolateral prefrontal cortices) accounting for committing sexual offenses against children and the temporal lobe (amygdala and hippocampus) accounting for the sexual preoccupation with children often seen in pedophilic men. However, it should be noted that all these theories on pedophilia have shortcomings. They may explain the sexual behavior associated with pedophilia but not the deviant sexual preference. Also, they are based on studies with pedophiles who have other psychological disorder diagnoses, are incarcerated or otherwise legally sanctioned, or are not sufficiently diagnostically classified (Tenbergen et al., 2015).

1.5.5 Brain Alterations

In recent years, an increasing number of studies have been conducted on the structure and function of the pedophilic brain using neuroimaging techniques, such as functional and structural magnetic resonance imaging (fMRI, sMRI). Mohnke et al. (2014) reviewed the literature on this topic and concluded that child sexual abusers might suffer from frontal and temporal abnormalities that may be associated with impaired impulse inhibition. Furthermore, structural neuroimaging investigations show a smaller amygdala in pedophiles (Tenbergen et al., 2015). They concluded that support for a neurodevelopmental pathway comes from research investigating epigenetic dysregulation of sexual development in general, physical characteristics, and functional as well as structural brain differences in pedophilia. The push for neurobiological research has resulted in the aforementioned major theoretical developments, namely the frontal lobe theory, the temporal lobe theory, and the theory that the masculinization of the male brain would more strongly affect pedophilia development, which is all attempting to explain various aspects of pedophilia (Tenbergen et al., 2015). The finding in pedophilic child sexual abusers of noticeable structural and functional differences in size and function of the left and right dorsolateral prefrontal and orbitofrontal cortex has supported the frontal lobe theory. In several studies that highlight temporal and amygdalar lesions or functional activation differences support was found for the temporal-limbic theory, namely that pedophilia is related to structural and functional differences in the temporal lobes resulting in misattributed emotional salience and valence toward children (Tenbergen et al., 2015).

Altogether, it can be concluded that there is an increasing insight into the structure and function of the pedophile's brain. However, findings are not always unequivocal, among others because of methodological problems that make a comparison between studies difficult. There can be differences in age, legal status, intelligence, and comorbidity of the studied pedophiles and most studies were performed in incarcerated child sexual abusers.

1.6 Personality Theories

The five-factor model (Costa Jr. & McCrae, 1992) is a prominent theory of personality domains. The *agreeableness* domain describes to what extent people are directed toward interpersonal relationships and the needs of others, and *neuroticism* is characterized by a tendency to experience negative affectivity and psychological distress. *Openness to experience* refers to an active imagination (fantasy), aesthetic sensitivity, attentiveness to inner feelings, preference for variety, and intellectual curiosity, while *conscientiousness* is associated with the desire to do a task well, to take obligations to others seriously, to be efficient, and to be organized. Finally, individuals high in *extraversion* are likely to value achievement and stimulation, and unlikely to value tradition or conformity. Extraverts are often assertive, active, and sociable, shunning self-denial in favor of excitement and pleasure. Researchers who studied the relation between aggression and domains of the five-factor model (Gleason, Jensen-Campbell, & Richardson, 2004; Miller, Lynam, & Leukefeld, 2003) found that the neuroticism and agreeableness domains appeared to be especially associated with aggression. Hornsveld and De Kruyk (2005) studied a sample of 105 Dutch sexually violent and a sample of 69 nonsexually violent *outpatients*. They found that the sexually violent outpatients scored significantly higher on the domain neuroticism and significantly lower on the domains of agreeableness and conscientiousness than a norm group. When the sexually violent outpatients were compared with the nonsexually violent outpatients, the sexually violent outpatients were found to score significantly higher than the nonsexually violent patients on the neuroticism and agreeableness domains. A sample of 136 Dutch nonsexually and sexually violent forensic psychiatric *inpatients* were found to score significantly higher on the domain neuroticism and significantly lower on the domain agreeableness than a norm group (Hornsveld, Nijman, & Kraaimaat, 2008). Jones, Miller, and Lynam (2011) concluded after a meta-analytic review of the literature that aggressive behavior is related not only to the domains of neuroticism and agreeableness but also to the domain of conscientiousness. In our opinion, assessment of personality domains is not only important for the validation of the scores on other measures but especially relevant for therapists who want to know whether a certain problem behavior is situation-specific or occurs in several, more or less similar situations. In the latter case, special attention must be paid to the generalization of particular treatment results.

The link between psychopathy as measured with the Psychopathy Checklist-Revised (PCL-R; Hare, 1991, 2003) and different forms of aggressive behavior has been the topic of multiple studies. Several authors have demonstrated that violent patients with a relatively low score on psychopathy mainly show reactive aggression, whereas those with a relatively high score tend to be both reactively and proactively aggressive (Cima & Raine, 2009; Cornell et al., 1996; Woodworth & Porter, 2002). These two forms of aggression are probably related to different dynamic criminogenic needs and consequently require a different treatment approach (Andrews & Bonta, 2010; Woodworth & Porter, 2002). From a meta-analysis of Lynam and Derefinko (2006), psychopathy appeared to be related mainly to the agreeableness and conscientiousness domain and less to the neuroticism domain. With regard to sexual offending, several studies have found that the combination of psychopathy and sexual deviance is especially dangerous, such that sexual offenders who are both psychopathic and have deviant sexual interests are much more likely to sexually recidivate than sexual offenders who are psychopathic but without deviant sexual interests, or have deviant sexual interests but are not psychopathic (Harris et al., 2003; Hawes, Boccaccini, & Murrie, 2013; Hildebrand, De Ruiter, & De Vogel, 2004; Olver & Wong, 2006; Rice & Harris, 1997).

1.7 Treatment Theories

The Risk-Need-Responsivity model (RNR; Andrews, Bonta, & Hodge, 1990; Andrews & Bonta, 2010; Bonta & Andrews, 2007) is generally regarded as a leading guideline for the assessment and treatment of (sexual) offenders (Ward, Mesler, & Yates, 2007). The risk principle states that the intensity of treatment interventions should be matched to the offender's recidivism risk: offenders with a high risk of recidivism should receive more intensive treatment than offenders with a low risk of recidivism. Although static risk factors (i.e., historical/highly stable risk factors), such as prior (sexual) offenses, stranger victims, and antisocial personality disorder, are generally regarded as the best predictors of sexual recidivism (Hanson & Bussière, 1998; Hanson, Harris, Scott, & Helmus, 2007), static risk factors are unchangeable and therefore cannot be targeted during treatment. As a consequence, the need principle states that, in order to reduce the risk of (sexual) recidivism, treatment interventions should focus on criminogenic needs (i.e., changeable/dynamic risk factors), such as antisocial cognitions, personality features, and interpersonal skills (Andrews & Bonta, 2010). Finally, the responsivity principle states that treatment interventions are most effective when they are adapted to the abilities, skills, and learning styles of the offender.

The Good Lives Model of offender rehabilitation (GLM; Ward, 2002; Ward & Stewart, 2003; Ward & Gannon, 2006; Ward & Willis, 2016; Willis, Ward, & Levenson, 2014) was developed several years ago as a complementary approach for interventions that mainly focus on the reduction of risk factors (i.e., the RNR-principles). This strength-based treatment framework is based on the belief that people offend because they are trying to obtain primary human goods. According to the GLM-approach, sexual offending is merely an inadequate, inappropriate attempt to obtain these human goods. It goes onto argue that improving the capabilities and strengths of offenders by teaching them to obtain their life goals in socially acceptable, personally satisfying, and sustainable ways will reduce the risk of reoffending. Within this treatment framework, offenders formulate their life goals within several areas (i.e., life, knowledge, excellence in play, excellence in work, excellence in an agency, inner peace, relatedness, community, spirituality, pleasure, and creativity). All obstacles and steps toward the fulfillment of these life goals become treatment targets, which involve not only reducing risk factors (i.e., criminogenic needs) but also improving protective factors. To date, there has been not much empirical research on the effectiveness of GLM-based treatment interventions (Marshall & Marshall, 2014), although there seems to be consensus on a balanced treatment approach which focuses on both negative risk and positive protective behaviors (Marshall et al., 2005; Olver, Marshall, Marshall, & Nicholaichuk, 2018; Willis et al., 2014).

1.8 Forensic Psychiatric Patients: Legal Aspects

Forensic psychiatric patients differ from offenders in having a psychiatric disorder that according to a judge has contributed to committing the offense and which untreated complicates efforts to decrease recidivism risk to a socially acceptable level. Countries with a legal system that requires criminals to participate in treatment employ different criteria to this end. This may well reflect differing views of the role of government in the life of the individual (Beck, 1996). In *Canada*, forensic psychiatric patients are people who are under the care of the forensic mental health system, such as those who, due to mental disorder, have been judged unfit to stand trial or not criminally responsible (for more information see Pozzulo, Bennell, & Forth, 2018). "Fitness to stand trial" refers to whether a mental illness impairs an accused person's ability to understand and participate in his or her defense at any point during the trial proceedings. "Not criminally responsible" refers to whether a mental illness impaired one's volition and understanding to render him or her not legally culpable for the act. Court-ordered assessments of fitness and criminal responsibility must be conducted by a medical doctor. Once in the forensic mental health system, ongoing assessments inform placement, conditions, and disposition. For example, if found unfit to stand trial, the accused may be placed in a secure forensic psychiatric hospital and treated until he or she is judged fit, at which point the trial would resume. If found not criminally responsible, decisions about whether the person would be detained in a forensic psychiatric hospital and the conditions of detention, supervision, or discharge would be determined by a Review Board.

In *England and Wales*, forensic psychiatric patients are those people who are cared for in the forensic mental health system (either in a hospital or the community) as a result of not being fit to stand trial (*fitness to plead*) or not being *criminally responsible* for the act that they committed. *Fitness to plead* refers to whether an individual has the mental capacity to enter a plea, understand the proceedings of the trial, instruct a lawyer, challenge a juror, and understand the evidence presented. Judges decide as to whether an individual is unfit to plead from written or oral evidence from at least two registered medical practitioners. Criminal responsibility (or *men's rea*) refers to whether the individual knew at the time of the offense that the act was illegal; if it can be proved that he or she did not know this, then they can be found "not guilty" because they are not criminally responsible. If a defendant is found unfit to plead, then they are expected to have treatment either in a hospital or in the community, with the trial resuming once they have recovered. If an individual is found not guilty due on the ground of not being criminally responsible, they may be detained in a forensic mental health setting (high-security hospital, medium/low secure unit) or supervised by a community forensic mental health team, where they will be assessed and treated by a forensic/clinical team. Specific legislation exists that covers all aspects of mentally disordered offenders and their care with separate, although similar, legislation for England and Wales, Scotland, and Northern Ireland.

In *the Netherlands,* forensic psychiatric patients are offenders for whom the judge has found a connection between a psychiatric disorder and the offense committed, and offenders have committed an offense for which imprisonment of more than 4 years applies, such as severe assault, manslaughter, or murder. The decision of the judge is based on an assessment conducted by a psychiatrist or psychologist (Canton, Cosyns, & Van Kordelaar, 2015; Van Marle, 2000). Forensic psychiatric outpatients are offenders who have committed a violent offense, such as assault, robbery with violence, or serious threat of violence. They can be required to undergo the treatment as (a) an added condition for offenses to which maximum imprisonment for 3 years or less applies, (b) an alternative to prison for offenses to which maximum imprisonment for 6 months or less applies, (c) a condition for suspension of detention while awaiting trial, (d) part of a Penal Program, or (e) a supervision element for a protection agency. Sexually violent forensic psychiatric patients are often classified as child sex abusers or rapists (De Vogel et al., 2004).

Child sexual abuse is defined as sexual contact with victims under the age of 16 years, whereas rape concerns non-consensual sexual contact with a person of 16 years or above. Child sexual abuse is often divided into intrafamilial and extrafamilial child sexual abuse (Robertiello & Terry, 2007).

In *Belgium,* "internment" is a punitive replacement measure of indefinite duration. Internment is possible for delinquents who are both fully or partially accountable for their criminal acts. Unlike in the Netherlands, in Belgium it is not possible to impose detention as an additional penalty measure (Canton et al., 2015).

In the *United States,* law and practice often reflect a skepticism and mistrust of the role of government. The government's authority to interfere with an individual's autonomous decision-making or liberty interest is sharply restricted by statute and case law. Therefore, there is statutory authority for pre-trial psychiatric evaluations only if there is a question of competence to stand trial (fitness to plead), criminal responsibility or need for civil commitment. The defendant has a right to have counsel present during any psychiatric evaluation. If a defendant is found incompetent to stand trial (unfit to plead), then the criminal justice process stops until the defendant is restored to competency. An American psychiatrist is allowed to examine the defendant's attitude toward the crime, but not before adjudication. The one exception is a criminal responsibility evaluation (Beck, 1996). The bail reform act of the United States Supreme Court (1987) requires federal courts to detain prior to trial arrestees charged with certain serious felonies if the court concludes that no release conditions "will reasonably assure … the safety of any other person and the community." This new act raised judicial concerns about assessments of dangerousness.

A committee of the judiciary composed of judges and mental health professionals concluded that judges should not routinely ask mental health professionals to evaluate these cases, because these cases seldom involved mental disorder. The committee noted that mental health professionals have no expertise in evaluating potential violence independent of mental disorder (Beck, 1996). The practice of forensic psychiatry in the United States involves evaluation only, except in forensic hospitals or prisons. An integrated forensic psychiatric care system such as those in the United Kingdom or the Netherlands is lacking. Major problems are the absence of adequate primary healthcare for many forensic patients, the fragmentation of forensic healthcare services, the absence of specialized community forensic treatment services, and absence of any effective law to authorize and enforce involuntary community treatment for mentally ill patients who have committed criminal acts of serious violence. Outpatient commitment laws may serve this latter function in a few jurisdictions (Beck, 1996).

The DSM-classification definition of forensic psychiatric patients differs from country to country. In Dutch forensic psychiatric institutions about 67% of the admitted offenders has a cluster B personality disorder as their main diagnosis (Nagtegaal, Goethals, & Meynen, 2016), whereas in the United States (Silver, 1995) and Canada (Quinsey, Harris, Rice, & Cormier, 2006) most forensic psychiatric patients are primarily diagnosed with a psychotic disorder.

1.9 Conclusions and Recommendations

Aggressive behavior is more and more regarded as complex behavior that is multifactorial determined. Psychological, biological, and social factors all contribute to the development and maintenance of aggressive behavior. Consequently, theories about aggressive behavior can be formulated from all these perspectives. Also, the major problem is that these theories often relate to different populations. For example, The General Aggression Model (GAM) of Anderson and Bushman (2002) mainly focuses on aggression in adults, while Dodge and colleagues (Coie & Dodge, 2000; Crick & Dodge, 1994) developed their model for aggressive children. The confluence (mediational) theory of Malamuth (Malamuth, 1996; Malamuth & Hald, 2016) and the sociological theory of Russell (1998) pertain to the raping of adult women, but the motivation-facilitation model of sexual offending of Seto (2019) was initially limited to children. Theories on sexual aggression may differentiate between rapists and child sexual abusers, but a further distinction of the latter group into intrafamilial child sexual abusers and extrafamilial child sexual abusers is usually not made. The more crucial problem is that except for Malamuth's confluence model and its variants, no theoretical model has been tested empirically (Abbey, Jacques-Tiura, & LeBreton, 2011; Gijs, 2002; Knight & Sims-Knight, 2016).

In recent years, knowledge about neurobiological factors implicated in (sexual) aggressive behavior has increased considerably, but most knowledge relates to the structure and function of some regions of the brain that play an important role in (sexual) aggression but which, at least at this moment, cannot be influenced by medical interventions. Although it is often suggested that serotonin and testosterone are risk factors for (sexual) aggression, it has now become clear that these relations are complicated and that contextual factors are also involved.

Whether theories of aggression refer to all human beings or focus on one or several determinants of aggressive behavior, they are helpful for the formulation of individual treatment plans from functional analyses of risk and protective behaviors (Sturmey, 2008). These plans have to serve as the basis for the composition of group treatment programs, because they provide insight into the problem behaviors that a group of offenders has in common (for instance: lack of social skills for intimate relationships) and the problem behaviors that can be better treated with individual therapy (for example, a specific troublesome relationship with a certain family member).

In our opinion, the Risk-Need-Responsivity Model and the Good Lives Model are beneficial for the composition of treatment programs, but these models seem to be mainly relevant to the application of fundamental cognitive-behavioral principles to a specific target group, namely offenders. Characteristic of this approach is the emphasis on actual problem behaviors, empirically based treatment methods, and robust treatment evaluation. Initially, cognitive-behavioral treatment was focused on negative problem behaviors, but under the influence of Motivational Interviewing (Miller & Rollnick, 2002) and Positive Psychology (Peterson & Seligman, 2004) positive protective behaviors and specific wishes from clients or patients can now be part of an individual treatment plan, for instance in the form of Solution-Focused Therapy (Bannink, 2012). In any case, it should be noted that treatment plans for offenders have to serve two clients: the offender and the society which has to be protected against his or her potential future criminal behavior.

References

Abbey, A., Jacques-Tiura, A. J., & LeBreton, J. M. (2011). Risk factors for sexual aggression in young men: An expansion of the confluence model. *Aggressive Behavior, 37*, 450–464. https://doi.org/10.1002/ab.20399

Abel, G. G., Becker, J. V., & Cunningham-Rathner, J. (1984). Complications, consent, and cognitions in sex between children and adults. *International Journal of Law and Psychiatry, 7*, 89–103.

Abel, G. G., Gore, D. K., Holland, C. L., Camp, N., Becker, J. V., & Rathner, J. (1989). The measurement of cognitive distortions of child molesters. *Annals of Sex Research, 2*, 135–153.

Alhabib, S., Nur, U., & Jones, R. (2010). Domestic violence against women: Systematic review of prevalence studies. *Journal of Family Violence, 25*, 369–382. https://doi.org/10.1007/s10896-009-9298-4

Allen, J. J., & Anderson, C. A. (2017). Aggression and violence: Definitions and distinctions, Chapter 1. In P. Sturmey (Ed.), *The Wiley handbook of violence and aggression*. Chichester: Wiley-Blackwell. https://doi.org/10.1002/9781119057574

Allen, J. J., Anderson, C. A., & Bushman, B. J. (2018). The general aggression model. *Current Opinion in Psychology, 19*, 75–80. https://doi.org/10.1016/j.copsyc.2017.03.034

American Psychiatric Association. (2013). *Diagnostic and statistical manual of mental disorders 5 (DSM-5)*. Washington, DC: Author.

Anderson, C. A., & Bushman, B. J. (2002). Human aggression. *Annual Review of Psychology, 53*, 27–51.

Andrews, D. A., & Bonta, J. (2010). *The psychology of criminal conduct* (5th ed.). New Providence, NJ: Matthew Bender & Company.

Andrews, D. A., Bonta, J., & Hodge, R. D. (1990). Classification for effective rehabilitation: Rediscovering psychology. *Criminal Justice and Behavior, 17*, 19–52. https://doi.org/10.1177/0093854890017001004

Andrews, D. A., Bonta, J., & Wormith, J. S. (2006). The recent past and near future of risk/need assessment. *Crime and Delinquency, 52*, 7–27.

Archer, J., Graham-Kevan, N., & Davies, M. (2005). Testosterone and aggression: A reanalysis of Book, Starzyk, and Quinsey's (2001) study. *Aggression and Violent Behavior, 10*, 241–261.

Bacchus, L. J., Ranganathan, M., Watts, C., & Devries, K. (2018). Recent intimate partner violence against women and health: A systematic review and meta-analysis of cohort studies. *BMJ Open, 8*, e019995. https://doi.org/10.1136/bmjopen-2017-019995

Bandura, A. (1973). *Aggression: A social learning analysis*. Englewood Cliffs, NJ: Prentice Hall.

Bandura, A. (2001). Social cognitive theory: An agentic perspective. *Annual Review of Psychology, 52*, 1–26.

Bannink, F. (2012). *Practicing positive CBT. From reducing distress to building success*. Chichester: Wiley.

Barrett, B., & Byford, S. (2012). Costs and outcomes of an intervention programme for offenders with personality disorders. *The British Journal of Psychiatry, 200*, 336–341.

Beck, J. C. (1996). Forensic psychiatry in the USA and the UK: A clinician's view. *Criminal Behaviour and Mental Health, 6*, 11–127.

Beech, A. R., & Mitchell, I. J. (2005). A neurobiological perspective on attachment problems in sexual offenders and the role of selective serotonin reuptake inhibitors in the treatment of such problems. *Clinical Psychology Review, 25*, 153–182.

Berkowitz, L. (1978). Whatever happened to the frustration-aggression hypothesis? *American Behavioral Scientist, 21*, 691–708.

Berkowitz, L. (1993). *Aggression: Its causes, consequences, and control*. New York: McGraw-Hill.

Blackburn, R. (1993). *The psychology of criminal conduct: Theory, research, and practice*. Chichester: Wiley.

Blanchard, R., Kuban, M. E., Klassen, P., Dickey, R., Christensen, B. K., Cantor, J. M., et al. (2003). Self-reported head injuries before and after age 13 in pedophilic and nonpedophilic men referred for clinical assessment. *Archives of Sexual Behavior, 32*, 573–581. https://doi.org/10.1023/A:1026093612434

Bonta, J., & Andrews, D. A. (2007). *Risk-need responsivity model for offender assessment and rehabilitation*. Ottawa: Public Safety Canada.

Bonta, J., Blais, J., & Wilson, H. A. (2013). The prediction of risk for mentally disordered offenders: A quantitative synthesis. Corrections Research. User Report. www.publicsafety.gc.ca

Borduin, C. M., & Dopp, A. R. (2015). Economic impact of multisystemic therapy with juvenile sexual offenders. *Journal of Family Psychology, 29*, 687–696. https://doi.org/10.1037/fam0000113

Briken, P., Hill, A., & Berner, W. (2006). Paraphilien und Sexualdelinquenz: Neurobiologische und neuropsychologische Aspekte. Eine Uebersicht. *Zeitschrift für Sexualforschung, 19*, 295–314.

Briken, P., Hill, A., & Berner, W. (2014). Pharmacotherapy of sexual offenders and men who are at risk of sexual offending. In D. P. Boer, R. Eher, L. A. Craig, M. H. Miner, & F. Pfäfflin (Eds.), *International perspectives on the assessment and treatment of sexual offenders* (pp. 437–449). Chichester: Wiley-Blackwell.

Briken, P., & Kafka, M. P. (2007). Pharmacological treatments for paraphilic patients and sexual offenders. *Current Opinion in Psychiatry, 20*, 609–613.

Browne, K., & Howells, K. (1996). Violent offenders. In C. R. Hollin (Ed.), *Working with offenders. Psychological practice in offender rehabilitation* (pp. 188–210). Chichester: Wiley.

Bushman, B. J. (2018). Editorial overview: Aggression and violence. *Current Opinion in Psychology, 19*, iv–vi. https://doi.org/10.1016/j.copsyc.2017.12.001

Canton, W., Cosyns, P., & Van Kordelaar, W. (2015). Onderzoek en rapportage pro Justitia [Assessment and Pro Justitia reports]. In W. Canton, D. van Beek, L. Claes, L. Gijs, I. Jeandarme, & E. K. Haneveld (Eds.), *Handboek psychopathie en de antisociale persoonlijkheidsstoornis [Handbook psychopathy and the antisocial personality disorder]* (pp. 181–190). Utrecht: De Tijdstroom.

Cantor, J. M., Kabani, N., Christensen, B. K., Zipursky, R. B., Barbaree, H. E., Dickey, R., et al. (2007). Cerebral white matter deficiencies in pedophilic men. *Journal of Psychiatric Research, 42*, 167–183.

Carré, J. M., & Archer, J. (2018). Testosterone and human behavior: The role of individual and contextual variables. *Current Opinion in Psychology, 19*, 149–153.

Carter, C. S. (1998). Neuroendocrine perspectives on social attachment and love. *Psychoneuroendocrinology, 23*, 779–818.

Chaffin, M. (2008). Our minds are made up—Don't confuse us with the facts: Commentary on policies concerning children with sexual behavior problems and juvenile sex offenders. *Child Maltreatment, 13*, 110–121. https://doi.org/10.1177/1077559508314510

Cho, H. (2012). Racial differences in the prevalence of intimate partner violence against women and associated factors. *Journal of Interpersonal Violence, 27*, 344–363. https://doi.org/10.1177/0886260511416469

Cima, M., & Raine, A. (2009). Distinct characteristics of psychopathy relate to different subtypes of aggression. *Personality and Individual Differences, 47*, 835–840. https://doi.org/10.1016/j.paid.2009.06.031

Cohen, M. A. (2001). To treat or not to treat? A financial perspective. In C. R. Hollin (Ed.), *Handbook of offender assessment and treatment* (pp. 35–49). Chichester: Wiley.

Coie, J. D., & Dodge, K. A. (2000). Aggression and antisocial behavior. In W. Damon (Series Ed.) & N. Eisenberg (Vol. Ed.), *Handbook of child psychology. Social, emotional, and personality development* (Vol. 3, 5th ed., pp. 779–862). New York: Wiley.

Cornell, D. G., Warren, J., Hawk, G., Stafford, E., Oram, G., & Pine, D. (1996). Psychopathy in instrumental and reactive offenders. *Journal of Consulting and Clinical Psychology, 64*, 783–790. https://doi.org/10.1037/0022-006X.64.4.783

Costa Jr., P. T., & McCrae, R. R. (1992). *Revised NEO Personality Inventory (NEO-PI-R) and NEO Five-Factor Inventory (NEO-FFI): Professional manual*. Odessa, FL: Psychological Assessment Resources.

Craissati, J., McClurg, G., & Browne, K. (2002). The parental bonding experiences of sex offenders: A comparison between child molesters and rapists. *Child Abuse & Neglect, 26*, 909–921. https://doi.org/10.1016/S0145-2134(02)00361-7

Crick, N. R., & Dodge, K. A. (1994). A review and reformulation of social information-processing mechanisms in children's social adjustment. *Psychological Bulletin, 115*, 74–101.

De Vogel, V., De Ruiter, C., Van Beek, D., & Mead, G. (2004). Predictive validity of the SVR-20 and Static-99 in a Dutch sample of treated sex offenders. *Law and Human Behavior, 28*, 235–251.

Dodge, K. A. (1991). The structure and function of reactive and proactive aggression. In D. J. Pepler & K. H. Rubin (Eds.), *The development and treatment of childhood aggression* (pp. 201–218). Hillsdale, NJ: Erlbaum.

Dodge, K. A. (2002). Mediation, moderation, and mechanisms in how parenting affects children's aggressive behavior. In J. G. Borkowski, S. L. Ramey, & M. Bristol-Power (Eds.), *Parenting and the child's world: Influences on academic, intellectual, and social-emotional development* (pp. 215–229). Mahwah, NJ: Erlbaum.

Dodge, K. A., & Coie, J. D. (1987). Social-information-processing factors in reactive and proactive aggression in children's peer groups. *Journal of Personality and Social Psychology, 53*, 1146–1158.

Dodge, K. A., Lochman, J. E., Harnish, J. D., Bates, J. E., & Pettit, G. S. (1997). Reactive and proactive aggression in school children and psychiatrically impaired chronically assaultive youth. *Journal of Abnormal Psychology, 106*, 37–51.

Dollard, J., Doob, L. W., Miller, N. E., Mowrer, O. H., & Sears, R. R. (1939). *Frustration and aggression*. New Haven, CT: Yale University Press.

Dworkin, E. R. (2018). Risk for mental disorders associated with sexual assault: A meta-analysis. *Trauma, Violence, & Abuse*. https://doi.org/10.1177/1524838018813198

Dworkin, E. R., Menon, S. V., Bystrynski, J., & Allen, N. E. (2017). Sexual assault vicitimization and psychopathology: A review and meta-analysis. *Clinical Psychology Review, 56*, 65–81.

Eastvold, A., Suchy, Y., & Strassberg, D. (2011). Executive function profiles of pedophilic and nonpedophilic child molesters. *Journal of the International Neuropsychological Society, 17*, 295–307. https://doi.org/10.1017/S1355617710001669

Eckhardt, C., Norlander, B., & Deffenbacher, J. (2004). The assessment of anger and hostility: A critical review. *Aggression and Violent Behavior, 9*, 17–43. https://doi.org/10.1016/S1359-1789(02)001167

Finkelhor, D. (1984). *Child sexual abuse: New theory and research*. New York: Free Press.

Gendreau, P., Little, T., & Goggin, C. (1996). A meta-analysis of the predictors of adult offender recidivism: What works! *Criminology, 34*, 575–607.

Gijs, L. (2002). Etiologische theorieën over seksueel agressief gedrag: Een inleidend overzicht [Etiological theories about sexually aggressive behavior: An introductory overview]. *Tijdschrift voor Seksuologie [Dutch Journal of Sexology], 26*, 9–25.

Gleason, K. A., Jensen-Campbell, L. A., & Richardson, D. S. (2004). Agreeableness as a predictor of aggression in adolescence. *Aggressive Behavior, 30*, 43–61. https://doi.org/10.1002/ab.20002

Gold, L., Norman, R., Devine, A., Feder, G., Taft, A. J., & Hegarty, K. L. (2011). Cost-effectiveness of health care interventions to address intimate partner violence: What do we know and what else should we look for? *Violence Against Women, 17*, 389–403. https://doi.org/10.1177/1077801211398639

Gooren, L. J. (2011). Ethical and medical considerations of Androgen Deprivation Treatment of sex offenders. *Journal of Clinical Endocrinology & Metabolism, 96*, 3628–3637. https://doi.org/10.1210/jc.2011-1540

Hall, G. C. N., & Hirschman, R. (1991). Towards a theory of sexual aggression: A quadripartite model. *Journal of Consulting and Clinical Psychology, 59*, 662–669.

Hanson, R. K., & Bussière, M. T. (1998). Predicting relapse: A meta-analysis of sexual offender recidivism studies. *Journal of Consulting and Clinical Psychology, 66*, 348–362. https://doi.org/10.1037/0022-006X.66.2.348

Hanson, R. K., Harris, A. J. R., Scott, T., & Helmus, L. (2007). *Assessing the risk of sexual offenders on community supervision: The Dynamic Supervision Project*. Corrections Research User Report No. 2007-05. Ottawa: Public Safety Canada.

Hare, R. D. (1991). *The Hare psychopathy checklist-revised*. Toronto: Multi-Health Systems.

Hare, R. D. (2003). *Hare psychopathy checklist-revised (PCL-R)* (2nd ed.). Toronto: Multi-Health Systems.

Harpur, T. J., Hare, R. D., & Hakstian, A. R. (1989). Two-factor conceptualization of psychopathy: Construct validity and assessment implications. *Psychological Assessment, 1*, 6–17.

Harris, G. T., Rice, M. E., Quinsey, V. L., Lalumière, M. L., Boer, D., & Lang, C. (2003). A multisite comparison of actuarial risk instruments for sex offenders. *Psychological Assessment, 15*, 413–425.

Hawes, S. W., Boccaccini, M. T., & Murrie, D. C. (2013). Psychopathy and the combination of psychopathy and sexual deviance as predictors of sexual recidivism: Meta-analytic findings using the Psychopathy Checklist-Revised. *Psychological Assessment, 25*, 233–243.

Hawkins, A. P., & Domoney, C. (2012). Sexual assault and rape. *Obstetrics, Gynaecology and Reproductive Medicine, 22*, 199–204.

Hildebrand, M., De Ruiter, C., & De Vogel, V. (2004). Psychopathy and sexual deviance in treated rapists: Association with sexual and nonsexual recidivism. *Sexual Abuse: A Journal of Research and Treatment, 16*, 1–24. https://doi.org/10.1177/107906320401600101

Hornsveld, R. H. J., & De Kruyk, C. (2005). Forensic psychiatric outpatients with sexual offenses: Personality characteristics, aggression, and social competence. *Psychology, Crime & Law, 11*, 479–488.

Hornsveld, R. H. J., Nijman, H. L. I., & Kraaimaat, F. W. (2008). Aggression Control Therapy for violent forensic psychiatric patients: First results. *Psychology, Crime & Law, 14*, 1–18. https://doi.org/10.1080/10683160701340569

Huesmann, L. R. (1988). An information-processing model for the development of aggression. *Aggressive Behavior, 14*, 13–24.

Huesmann, L. R. (2018). An integrative theoretical understanding of aggression: A brief exposition. *Current Opinion in Psychology, 19*, 119–124.

Hunter, J., Figueredo, A., & Malamuth, N. (2010). Developmental pathways into social and sexual deviance. *Journal of Family Violence, 25*, 141–148. https://doi.org/10.1007/s10896-009-9277-9

Huppin, M., & Malamuth, N. M. (2017). Aggression for sexual access. In T. K. Shackelford & V. Weekes-Shackelford (Eds.), *Encyclopedia of evolutionary psychological science* (pp. 1–11). Basel: Springer. https://doi.org/10.1007/978-3-319-16999-6_1681-1

Jina, R., & Thomas, L. S. (2013). Health consequences of sexual violence against women. *Best Practice & Research Clinical Obstetrics and Gynaecology, 27*, 15–26. https://doi.org/10.1016/j.bpobgyn.2012.08.012

Jones, S. E., Miller, J. D., & Lynam, D. R. (2011). Personality, antisocial behavior, and aggression: A meta-analytic review. *Journal of Criminal Justice, 39*, 329–337.

Knight, R. A., & Sims-Knight, J. E. (2016). A theoretical integration of aetiological and typological models of rape. In D. P. Boer, A. R. Beech, & T. Ward (Eds.), *The Wiley handbook on the theories, assessment, and treatment of sexual offending* (Theories) (Vol. I, pp. 73–102). Chichester: Wiley-Blackwell.

Kolivas, E. D., & Gross, A. M. (2007). Assessing sexual aggression: Addressing the gap between rape victimization and perpetration prevalence rates. *Aggression and Violent Behavior, 12*, 315–328. https://doi.org/10.1016/j.avb.2006.10.002

Koss, M. P. (2000). Blame, shame, and community: Justice responses to violence against women. *American Psychologist, 55*, 1332–1343. https://doi.org/10.1037/0003-066X.55.11.1332

Krahé, B. (2018). Violence against women. *Current Opinion in Psychology, 19*, 6–10. https://doi.org/10.1016/j.copsyc.2017.03.017

Krahé, B., Berger, A., Vanwesenbeeck, I., Bianchi, G., Chliaoutakis, J., Fernández-Fuertes, A., et al. (2015). Prevalence and correlates of young people's sexual aggression perpetration and victimisation in 10 European countries. A multilevel analysis. *Culture, Health, & Sexuality, 17*, 682–699. https://doi.org/10.1080/13691058.2014.989265

Krug, E. G., Mercy, J. A., Dahlberg, L. L., Mercy, J. A., & Zwi, A. B. (2002). World report on violence and health. *The Lancet, 360*, 1083–1088.

Laws, D. R., Hudson, S. M., & Ward, T. (2000). In D. R. Laws, S. M. Hudson, & T. Ward (Eds.), *Remaking relapse prevention with sex offenders: A sourcebook The original model of relapse prevention with sex offenders: Promises unfulfilled* (pp. 3–24). Newbury Park, CA: Sage.

Laws, D. R., & Marshall, W. L. (1990). A conditioning theory of the etiology and maintenance of deviant sexual preference and behavior. In W. L. Marshall, D. R. Laws, & H. E. Barbaree (Eds.), *Handbook of Sexual Assault* (pp. 209–229). Boston, MA: Springer.

Letourneau, E. J., Brown, D. S., Fang, X., Hassan, A., & Mercy, J. A. (2018). The economic burden of child sexual abuse in the United States. *Child Abuse & Neglect, 79*, 413–422. https://doi.org/10.1016/j.chiabu.2018.02.020

Lisak, D., & Miller, P. M. (2002). Repeat rape and multiple offending among undetected rapists. *Violence and Victims, 17*, 73–84. https://doi.org/10.1891/vivi.17.1.73.33638

Lynam, D. R., & Derefinko, K. J. (2006). Psychopathy and personality. In C. J. Patrick (Ed.), *Handbook of psychopathy* (pp. 133–155). New York: Guilford.

Ma, Y. (2018). Prevalence of childhood sexual abuse in China: A meta-analysis. *Journal of Child Sexual Abuse, 27*, 107–121. https://doi.org/10.1080/10538712.2018.1425944

Malamuth, N. M. (1981). Rape proclivity among males. *Journal of Social Issues, 37*, 138–157.

Malamuth, N. M. (1996). The confluence model of sexual aggression: Feminist and evolutionary perspectives. In D. M. Buss & N. M. Malamuth (Eds.), *Sex, power, conflict: Evolutionary and feminist perspectives* (pp. 269–295). New York: Oxford University Press.

Malamuth, N. M. (2018). "Adding fuel to the fire"? Does exposure to non-consenting adult or to child pornography increase risk of sexual aggression? *Aggression and Violent Behavior, 41*, 74–89. https://doi.org/10.1016/j.avb.2018.02.013

Malamuth, N. M., & Check, J. V. P. (1980). Penile tumescence and perceptual responses to rape as a function of the victim's perceived reactions. *Journal of Applied Social Psychology, 10*, 528–547.

Malamuth, N. M., & Hald, G. M. (2016). The Confluence Mediational Model of sexual aggression. In D. P. Boer, A. R. Beech, & T. Ward (Eds.), *The Wiley handbook on the theories, assessment, and treatment of sexual offending* (Theories) (Vol. I, pp. 53–71). Chichester: Wiley-Blackwell. https://doi.org/10.1002/9781118574003.wattso003

Malamuth, N. M., Huppin, M., & Paul, B. (2005). Sexual coercion. In D. M. Buss (Ed.), *The handbook of evolutionary psychology* (pp. 394–418). Hoboke, NJ: Wiley.

Malamuth, N. M., Linz, D., Heavey, C. L., Barnes, G., & Acker, M. (1995). Using the confluence model of sexual aggression to predict men's conflict with women: A 10-year follow-up study. *Journal of Personality & Social Psychology, 69*, 353–369.

Marlatt, G. A. (1985a). Relapse prevention: Theoretical rationale and overview of the model. In G. A. Marlatt & J. R. Gordon (Eds.), *Relapse prevention: Maintenance strategies in the treatment of addictive behaviors* (pp. 3–70). New York: Guilford.

Marlatt, G. A. (1985b). Situational determinants of relapse and skill-training interventions. In G. A. Marlatt & J. R. Gordon (Eds.), *Relapse prevention: Maintenance strategies in the treatment of addictive behaviors* (pp. 71–127). New York: Guilford.

Marshall, W. L., & Barbaree, H. E. (1990). An integrated theory of the etiology of sexual offending. In W. L. Marshall, D. R. Laws, & H. E. Barbaree (Eds.), *Handbook of sexual assault: Issues, theories, and treatment of the offender* (pp. 257–275). New York: Plenum.

Marshall, W. L., & Marshall, L. E. (2014). The future of sexual offender treatment programs. In D. P. Boer, R. Eher, L. A. Craig, M. H. Miner, & F. Pfäfflin (Eds.), *International perspectives on the assessment and treatment of sexual offenders* (pp. 707–740). Chichester: Wiley-Blackwell.

Marshall, W. L., Ward, T., Mann, R. E., Moulden, H., Fernandez, Y. M., Serran, G., et al. (2005). Working positively with sexual offenders: Maximizing the effectiveness of treatment. *Journal of Interpersonal Violence, 20*, 1096–1114. https://doi.org/10.1177/0886260505278514

Mason, F., & Lodrick, Z. (2013). Psychological consequences of sexual assault. *Best Practice & Research Clinical Obstetrics and Gynaecology, 27*, 27–37. https://doi.org/10.1016/j.bpobgyn.2012.08.015

McGuire, R. J., Carlisle, J. M., & Young, B. G. (1965). Sexual deviations as conditioned behavior: A hypothesis. *Behaviour Research and Therapy, 2*, 185–190.

Miller, J. D., Lynam, D., & Leukefeld, C. (2003). Examining antisocial behavior through the five-factor model of personality. *Aggressive Behavior, 29*, 497–514.

Miller, N. E. (1941). The frustration-aggression hypothesis. *Psychological Review, 48*, 337–342.

Miller, W. R., & Rollnick, S. (2002). *Motivational interviewing. Preparing people for change* (2nd ed.). New York: Guilford.

Mohnke, S., Muller, S., Amelung, T., Kruger, T. H., Ponseti, J., Schiffer, B., et al. (2014). Brain alterations in paedophilia: A critical review. *Progress in Neurobiology, 122C*, 1–23. https://doi.org/10.1016/j.pneurobio.2014.07.005

Nagtegaal, M. H., Goethals, K., & Meynen, G. (2016). Mandatory treatment of forensic psychiatric patients in the Netherlands: Costs and benefits in perspective. *Dutch Journal of Psychiatry, 58*, 739–745.

Nietzel, M. T., Hasemann, D. M., & Lynam, D. R. (1999). Behavioral perspectives on violent behavior. In V. B. Van Hasselt & M. Hersen (Eds.), *Handbook of psychological approaches with violent offenders: Contemporary strategies and issues* (pp. 39–66). New York: Kluwer Academic/Plenum.

Norlander, B., & Eckhardt, C. (2005). Anger, hostility, and male perpetrators of intimate partner violence: A meta-analytic review. *Clinical Psychology Review, 25*, 119–152.

Olver, M. E., Marshall, L. E., Marshall, W. L., & Nicholaichuk, T. P. (2018). A long-term outcome assessment of the effects on subsequent reoffense rates of a prison-based CBT/RNR sex offender treatment program with strength-based elements. *Sexual Abuse*. https://doi.org/10.1177/1079063218807486

Olver, M. E., & Wong, S. C. P. (2006). Psychopathy, sexual deviance, and recidivism among sex offenders. *Sexual Abuse: A Journal of Research and Treatment, 18*, 65–82.

Pereda, N., Guilera, G., Forns, M., & Gómez-Benito, J. (2009a). The international epidemiology of child sexual abuse: A continuation of Finkelhor (1994). *Child Abuse & Neglect, 33*, 331–342. https://doi.org/10.1016/j.chiabu.2008.07.007

Paolucci, E. O., Genuis, M. L., & Violato, C. (2001). A meta-analysis of the published research on the effects of child sexual abuse. *Journal of Psychology, 135*, 17–36. https://doi.org/10.1080/00223980109603677

Pereda, N., Guilera, G., Forns, M., & Gómez-Benito, J. (2009b). The prevalence of child sexual abuse in community and student samples: A meta-analysis. *Clinical Psychology Review, 29*, 328–338. https://doi.org/10.1016/j.cpr.2009.02.007

Peter-Hagene, L. C., & Ullman, S. E. (2016). Longitudinal effects of sexual assault victims' drinking and self-blame on posttraumatic stress disorder. *Journal of Interpersonal Violence, 31*, 1074–1094. https://doi.org/10.1177/0886260514564069

Peterson, C., DeGue, S., Florence, C., & Lokey, C. N. (2017). Lifetime economic burden of rape among U.S. adults. *American Journal of Preventive Medicine, 52*, 691–701.

Peterson, C., Kearns, M. C., McIntosh, W. L., Estefan, L. F., Nicolaidis, C., McCollister, K. E., et al. (2018). Lifetime economic burden of intimate partner violence among U.S. adults. *American Journal of Preventive Medicine, 55*, 433–444. https://doi.org/10.1016/j.amepre.2018.04.049

Peterson, C., & Seligman, M. E. P. (2004). *Character strength and virtues. A handbook and classification*. Oxford: Oxford University Press.

Peterson, Z. D., Beagley, M. C., McCallum, E. B., & Artime, T. M. (2019). Sexual attitudes and behaviors among men who are victims, perpetrators, or both victims and perpetrators of adult sexual assault. *Psychology of Violence, 9*, 221–234. https://doi.org/10.1037/vio0000187

Pithers, W. D., Marques, J. K., Gibat, C. C., & Marlatt, G. A. (1983). Relapse prevention with sexual aggressiveness: A self-control model of treatment and maintenance of change. In J. G. Greer & I. R. Stuart (Eds.), *The sexual aggressor: Current perspectives on treatment* (pp. 214–239). New York: Van Nostrand Reinhold.

Pozzulo, J., Bennell, C., & Forth, A. (2018). *Forensic psychology* (5th ed.). Don Mills: Pearson.

Quinsey, V. L., Harris, G. T., Rice, M. E., & Cormier, C. (2006). *Violent offenders: Appraising and managing risk* (2nd ed.). Washington, DC: American Psychological Association.

Ramsey-Klawsnik, H. (2003). Elder sexual abuse within the family. *Journal of Elder Abuse and Neglect, 15*, 43–58.

Rice, M. E., & Harris, G. T. (1997). Cross-validation and extension of the Violence Risk Appraisal Guide or child molesters and rapists. *Law and Human Behavior, 21*, 231–241.

Robertiello, G., & Terry, K. J. (2007). Can we profile sex offenders? A review of sex offender typologies. *Aggression and Violent Behavior, 12*, 508–518. https://doi.org/10.1016/j.avb.2007.02.010

Russell, D. E. H. (1988). Pornography and rape: A causal model. *Political Psychology, 9*, 41–73.

Russell, D. E. H. (1998). *Dangerous relationships: Pornography, misogyny, and rape*. Thousand Oaks, CA: Sage.

Russell, D. E. H., & Bolen, R. M. (2000). *The epidemic of rape and child sexual abuse in the United States*. Thousand Oaks, CA: Sage.

Schiffer, B., & Vonlaufen, C. (2011). Executive dysfunctions in pedophilic and non-pedophilic child molesters. *Journal of Sexual Medicine, 8*, 1975–1984. https://doi.org/10.1111/j.1743-6109.2010.02140.x

Seto, M. C. (2009). Pedophilia. *Annual Review of Clinical Psychology, 5*, 391–407. https://doi.org/10.1146/annurev.clinpsy.032408.153618

Seto, M. C. (2019). The motivation-facilitation model of sexual offending. *Sexual Abuse: A Journal of Research and Treatment, 31*, 3–24. https://doi.org/10.1177/1079063217720919

Settumba, S. N., Chambers, G. M., Shanahan, M., Schofield, P., & Butler, T. (2018). Are we getting value for money from behavioral interventions for offenders? A research note reviewing the economic evaluation literature. *American Journal of Criminal Justice, 43*, 411–431. https://doi.org/10.1007/s12103-017-9399-1

Shapiro, R. J., & Hassett, K. A. (2012). *The economic benefits of reducing violent crime: A case study of 8 American cities*. Washington, DC: National Criminal Justice Reference Service.

Silver, E. (1995). Punishment or treatment? Comparing the lengths of confinement of successful and unsuccessful insanity defendants. *Law and Human Behavior, 19*, 375–388.

Snyder, H. N. (2000). *Sexual assault of young children as reported to law enforcement: Victim, incident, and offender characteristics*. Washington, DC: U.S. Department of Justice, Office of Justice Programs, Bureau of Justice Statistics.

Stinson, J. D., & Becker, J. V. (2013). *Treating sex offenders. An evidence-based manual*. New York: Guilford.

Stinson, J. D., Becker, J. V., & Sales, B. D. (2008). Self-regulation and the etiology of sexual deviance: Evaluating causal theory. *Violence and Victims, 23*, 35–51. https://doi.org/10.1891/0886-6708.23.1.35

Stoltenborgh, M., Bakermans-Kranenburg, M. J., Alink, L. R. A., & Van IJzendoorn, M. H. (2015). The prevalence of child maltreatment across the globe: Review of a series of meta-analyses. *Child Abuse Review, 24*, 37–50. https://doi.org/10.1002/car.2353

Studer, L. H., Aylwin, A. S., & Reddon, J. (2005). Testosterone, sexual offense recidivism, and treatment effect among adult male sex offenders. *Sexual Abuse: A Journal of Research and Treatment, 17*, 171–181.

Sturmey, P. (2008). *Behavioral case formulation and intervention*. New York: Wiley.

Suchy, Y., Eastvold, A. D., Strassberg, D. S., & Franchow, E. I. (2014). Understanding processing speed weaknesses among pedophilic child molesters: Response style vs. neuropathology. *Journal of Abnormal Psychology, 123*, 273–285. https://doi.org/10.1037/a0035812

Suchy, Y., Whittaker, J. W., Strassberg, D. S., & Eastvold, A. (2009). Neurocognitive differences between pedophilic and nonpedophilic child molesters. *Journal of the International Neuropsychological Society, 15*, 248–257. https://doi.org/10.1017/S1355617709090353

Szumski, F., Bartels, R. M., Beech, A. R., & Fisher, D. (2018). Distorted cognition related to male sexual offending: The multi-mechanism theory of cognitive distortions (MMT-CD). *Aggression and Violent Behavior, 39*, 139–151. https://doi.org/10.1016/j.avb.2018.02.001

Tenbergen, G., Wittfoth, M., Frieling, H., Ponseti, J., Walter, M., Walter, H., et al. (2015). The neurobiology and psychology of pedophilia: Recent advances and challenges. *Frontiers in Human Neuroscience, 9*, 344. https://doi.org/10.3389/fnhum.2015.00344

Thielen, F. W., Ten Have, M., De Graaf, R., Cuijpers, P., Beekman, A., Evers, S., et al. (2016). Long-term economic consequences of child maltreatment: A population- based study. *European Child & Adolescent Psychiatry, 25*, 1297–1305. https://doi.org/10.1007/s00787-016-0850-5

Ullman, S. E., Relyea, M., Peter-Hagene, L., & Vasquez, A. L. (2013). Trauma histories, substance use coping, PTSD, and problem substance use among sexual assault victims. *Addictive Behaviors, 38*, 2219–2223. https://doi.org/10.1016/j.addbeh.2013.01.027

Van Marle, H. J. C. (2000). Forensic services in the Netherlands. *International Journal of Law and Psychiatry, 23*, 515–531. https://doi.org/10.1016/S0160-2527(00)00049-2

Veenstra, L., Bushman, B. J., & Koole, S. L. (2018). The facts on the furious: A brief review of the psychology of trait anger. *Current Opinion in Psychology, 19*, 98–103. https://doi.org/10.1016/j.copsyc.2017.03.014

Ward, T. (2000). Sexual offenders' cognitive distortions as implicit theories. *Aggression and Violent Behavior, 5*, 491–507.

Ward, T. (2002). Good lives and the rehabilitation of offenders: Promises and problems. *Aggression and Violent Behavior, 7*, 513–528. https://doi.org/10.1016/S1359-1789(01)00076-3

Ward, T., & Beech, A. (2006). An integrated theory of sexual offending. *Aggression and Violent Behavior, 11*, 44–63.

Ward, T., Fisher, S., & Beech, A. (2016). An integrated theory of sexual offending. In A. Phenix & H. M. Hoberman (Eds.), *Sexual offending: Predisposing antecedents, assessments and management* (pp. 1–11). New York: Springer.

Ward, T., & Gannon, T. A. (2006). Rehabilitation, etiology, and self-regulation: The comprehensive good lives model of treatment for sex offenders. *Aggression and Violent Behavior, 11*, 77–94. https://doi.org/10.1016/j.avb.2005.06.001

Ward, T., Mesler, J., & Yates, P. M. (2007). Reconstructing the risk-need-responsivity model: A theoretical elaboration and evaluation. *Aggression and Violent Behavior, 12*, 208–228. https://doi.org/10.1016/j.avb.2006.07.001

Ward, T., Polaschek, D. L. L., & Beech, A. R. (2006). *Theories of sexual offending*. Chichester: Wiley.

Ward, T., & Siegert, R. J. (2002). Toward a comprehensive theory of child sexual abuse: A theory knitting perspective. *Psychology, Crime & Law, 9*, 219–224.

Ward, T., & Stewart, C. (2003). Criminogenic needs and human needs: A theoretical model. *Psychology, Crime & Law, 9*, 125–143. https://doi.org/10.1080/1068316031000116247

Ward, T., & Willis, G. (2016). Dynamic risk factors and offender rehabilitation: A comparison of the Good Lives Model and the Risk-Need-Responsivity model. In D. R. Laws & W. O'Donohue (Eds.), *Treatment of sex offenders: Strengths and weaknesses in assessment and intervention* (pp. 175–190). New York: Springer.

Willis, G. M., Ward, T., & Levenson, J. S. (2014). The Good Lives Model (GLM): An evaluation of GLM operationalization in North American treatment programs. *Sexual Abuse: A Journal of Research and Treatment, 26*, 58–81.

Wilson, L., Mouilso, E., Gentile, B., Calhoun, K., & Zeichner, A. (2015). How is sexual aggression related to nonsexual aggression? A meta-analytic review. *Aggression and Violent Behavior, 24*, 199–213. https://doi.org/10.1016/j.avb.2015.04.010

Wilson, L. C., & Miller, K. E. (2016). Meta-analysis of the prevalence of unacknowledged rape. *Trauma, Violence, & Abuse, 17*, 149–159. https://doi.org/10.1177/1524838015576391

Wincentak, K., Connolly, J., & Card, N. (2017). Teen dating violence: A meta-analytic review of prevalence rates. *Psychology of Violence, 7*, 224–241. https://doi.org/10.1037/a0040194
Wong, J. S., & Gravel, J. (2018). Do sex offenders have higher levels of testosterone? Results from a meta-analysis. *Sexual Abuse: A Journal of Research and Treatment, 30*, 147–168. https://doi.org/10.1177/1079063216637857
Woodworth, M., & Porter, S. (2002). In cold blood: Characteristics of criminal homicides as a function of psychopathy. *Journal of Abnormal Psychology, 111*, 436–445.
World Health Organization. (2013). Global and regional estimates of violence against women: Prevalence and health effects of intimate partner violence and non-partner sexual violence. Retrieved from http://www.who.int/iris/bitstream/10665/85239/1/9789241564625_eng.pdf
Wright, P. J., Tokunaga, S., & Kraus, S. (2016). A meta-analysis of pornography consumption and actual acts of sexual aggression in general population studies. *Journal of Communication, 66*, 183–205. https://doi.org/10.1111/jcom.12201

Chapter 2
Dynamic Risk Factors of Violent and Sexually Violent Offenders

Ruud H. J. Hornsveld, Floris W. Kraaimaat, Kevin L. Nunes, and Emma J. Palmer

2.1 Introduction

Based on empirical research, Andrews and Bonta (2010) formulated eight factors, the Central Eight that are associated with general recidivism. (See Chap. 1 for a discussion of the Central Eight.) The Central Eight factors can be divided into static (not or hardly changeable) factors such as a history of antisocial behavior and antisocial personality pattern, and dynamic (changeable) factors such as school/work or leisure/recreation. These dynamic risk factors vary from individual characteristics (e.g., antisocial cognition) to broad domains or areas of interest (e.g., education/work). The latter requires functional analyses (Hart, Sturmey, Logan, & McMurran, 2011) for the determination of the various problem behaviors that have to be targets of an individual treatment plan (Chap. 4).

R. H. J. Hornsveld (✉)
Erasmus University Medical Center, Rotterdam, The Netherlands
e-mail: ruud.hornsveld@ziggo.nl

F. W. Kraaimaat
Radboud University Nijmegen, Nijmegen, The Netherlands

K. L. Nunes
Carleton University, Ottawa, Canada

E. J. Palmer
University of Leicester, Leicester, UK

R. H. J. Hornsveld et al. (eds.), *Assessment and Obligatory Treatment of Violent and Sexually Violent Offenders*, Advances in Preventing and Treating Violence and Aggression, https://doi.org/10.1007/978-3-030-27840-3_2

2.2 Violent Offenders

2.2.1 Dynamic Risk Factors

According to Morgan, Kroner, and Mills (2012), several studies have demonstrated that dynamic risk variables are important proximal antecedents in the prediction of criminal behavior. For example, Quinsey, Jones, Book, and Barr (2006) studied the *Dynamic Risk Appraisal Scale* (DRAS, Quinsey, Harris, Rice, & Cormier, 2006) in a sample of 568 Canadian forensic psychiatric patients, partly institutionalized, partly living in the community. The DRAS contains 23 items for general risk and a subscale with ten items for violence risk, which have to be completed by the patient's or client's caregiver. The authors found that over an average period of 33 months, the scale differentiated patients who had incidents of a violent or sexual nature from those who did not. Using a revised version of the *Problem Identification Checklist* (PIC-R; Ostapiuk, Stringer, & Craig, 2000), Nagi, Ostapiuk, Craig, Hacker, and Beech (2009) found in a sample of 25 British psychiatric (mostly psychotic) inpatients and 24 outpatients preliminary validation for the predictive accuracy of the PIC-R for violence. Additionally, the findings suggested that short-term risk of violence within a population of mostly psychotic patients may be more related to dynamic and clinical risk variables rather than to static ones. More or less comparable results were found by De Vries Robbé, De Vogel, and Douglas (2013) in a sample of 188 Dutch patients discharged from forensic psychiatric treatment with a history of violent or sexual offending. The combined evaluation of risk- and protective factors from the HCR-20 (De Vogel & De Ruiter, 2006) and the SAPROF (De Vries Robbé, De Vogel, Koster, & Bogaerts, 2015) appeared to have good predictive validity for violent recidivism after treatment. Protective factors were found to provide incremental predictive validity over the use of risk factors alone. However, in a study of Philipse, Koeter, Van der Staak, and Van den Brink (2006), data on static and dynamic risk factors were collected for 151 patients discharged from Dutch forensic psychiatric hospitals. They concluded that a small set of static predictors yielded a good estimate of future reconvictions and that inclusion of dynamic predictors did not add predictive power.

Although research on the relationship between recidivism risk and certain personality traits or specific problem behaviors is scarce, several authors have studied the relationship between individual characteristics of violent offenders and aggressive behavior. Regarding personality traits, Jones, Miller, and Lynam (2011) found in a meta-analysis of 53 studies that aggression seems to be positively correlated to the Big Five domain of Neuroticism, and negatively to the domains Agreeableness and Conscientiousness. Porter and Woodworth (2006) concluded from several studies that "there is a clear relation between psychopathy and aggressive behavior" (p. 490). A review of the research from the last decade by Porter, Woodworth, and Black (2018) supported this conclusion.

When it comes to moral reasoning, several studies have found support for a relationship between moral reasoning and offending. Moral reasoning refers to how individuals reason about and justify their behavior to moral issues, with a focus on social perspective-taking (Gibbs, 2003; Kohlberg, 1969, 1984). For example, Stams et al. (2006) conducted a meta-analysis of 50 studies and concluded that offenders had on average a lower level of moral maturity than non-offenders. Van Vugt et al. (2011) also performed a meta-analysis of 19 studies and found that less mature stages of moral development were related to a higher recidivism risk.

Other authors have reported that violent offenders with a relatively low score on psychopathy mainly show reactive aggression, whereas those with a relatively high score tend to show both reactive and proactive aggression (Cima & Raine, 2009; Cornell et al., 1996; Woodworth & Porter, 2002). Social anxiety may mainly play a role in reactive and not so much in proactive aggression because offenders with a relatively high score on psychopathy usually do not experience anxiety when they want to reach their goal. Andrews and Bonta (2010) suggested that the two forms of aggression require a different treatment approach because they seem to be related to different dynamic criminogenic needs. When not managed adequately, these risk factors may result in aggressive or violent behavior (Berkowitz, 2013; Novaco, 2013).

More specifically, Hornsveld, Nijman, and Kraaimaat (2008) compared a sample of 136 Dutch forensic psychiatric inpatients and 200 forensic psychiatric outpatients with norm groups of nonclinical volunteers. Both the outpatients and the inpatients had higher scores for self-reported neuroticism and lower scores for agreeableness than the norms. The outpatients also had lower scores for openness and conscientiousness and higher scores for disposition to anger than the norms, and the inpatients had lower scores for self-reported social anxiety and higher scores for social skills. Both the inpatients and the outpatients reported less anxiety and more social skills in social situations such as giving criticism. However, they avoided behavior such as providing a compliment because of social anxiety. The outpatients had lower scores for psychopathy but higher scores for self-reported aggressive behavior than the inpatients. Probably, outpatients may find themselves in an environment where aggressive behavior is more often permitted and reinforced. Inpatients, however, stay in a highly structured institution in which aggressive behavior is not tolerated (Nijman, De Kruyk, & Van Nieuwenhuizen, 2004). Hornsveld, Nijman, and Kraaimaat (2008) also found that self-reported aggression in Dutch male violent forensic psychiatric patients is significantly correlated to self-reported neuroticism, trait and state anger, and social anxiety in situations involving criticism. In their study, self-reported aggressive behavior was found to be positively correlated to the old factor 2 ("chronically unstable and antisocial lifestyle") of the Psychopathy Checklist-Revised (Hare, 1991), and negatively to self-reported agreeableness and social skills in situations where a compliment can be given.

Hornsveld et al. (2016) compared the personality traits and problem behaviors in 59 Dutch female offenders (outpatients and detainees) with those in 170 male offenders (outpatients and detainees) who were all convicted of a violent crime. The violent female offenders scored significantly higher on neuroticism and trait anger and significantly lower on hostility than the male offenders. A subgroup of female forensic psychiatric outpatients did not differ from a subgroup of male outpatients on all measures, whereas a subgroup of female detainees scored significantly higher on anger and aggression, but lower on hostility and psychopathy than did a subgroup of male detainees. However, all effect sizes were small.

2.2.2 *Differences Between Violent Detainees and Violent Forensic Psychiatric Inpatients*

A study by Hornsveld, Bulten, De Vries, and Kraaimaat (2008) indicated that, compared with the average male Dutch person, violent Dutch detainees and forensic psychiatric inpatients (males) scored significantly lower on self-reported agreeableness. Inpatients also had significantly higher scores on questionnaires for the measurement of neuroticism and the disposition to anger. Both groups reported less social anxiety when criticism is given, and they appeared to exhibit this behavior more frequently than the norm group. In situations where somebody can be complimented, both groups reported more social anxiety and less frequently exhibited such skills. When both groups were compared with each other, inpatients had higher scores for antisocial lifestyle, neuroticism, and disposition to anger. Male detainees seem to be, in particular, characterized by an antisocial attitude and inadequate social skills, whereas inpatients distinguish themselves more from the average Dutch male by impulsivity, antisocial attitudes, a tendency to experience anger, and inadequate social skills. Altogether, differences between detainees and inpatients seem to be limited. Although the number of interviewed detainees in this study was rather small ($n = 50$), scores on some PCL-R items seems to indicate provisionally that a rather high percentage was suffering from an antisocial personality disorder (82%). Fazel and Danesh (2002) found among male prisoners a prevalence of antisocial personality disorder ranging from 28% to 65%, but they did not report upon the seriousness of the crimes for which the prisoners were convicted or the length of imprisonment. Given the fact that the detainees in the study of Hornsveld et al. (2008) were convicted of severe violent crimes and sentenced to imprisonment of at least four years, we considered our preliminary finding as not surprising. Therefore, violent detainees may, just as violent inpatients, benefit from a treatment program that focuses on anger management, prosocial skills (in intimate relations), and prosocial norms and values.

2.2.3 *Conclusions*

Based on the literature, our research, and our clinical experience, treatment programs for violent offenders should focus on state anger, hostility, social anxiety, social skills, and moral reasoning. Traits that are important for the treatment of both violent offenders and violent forensic psychiatric patients (responsivity issues) are

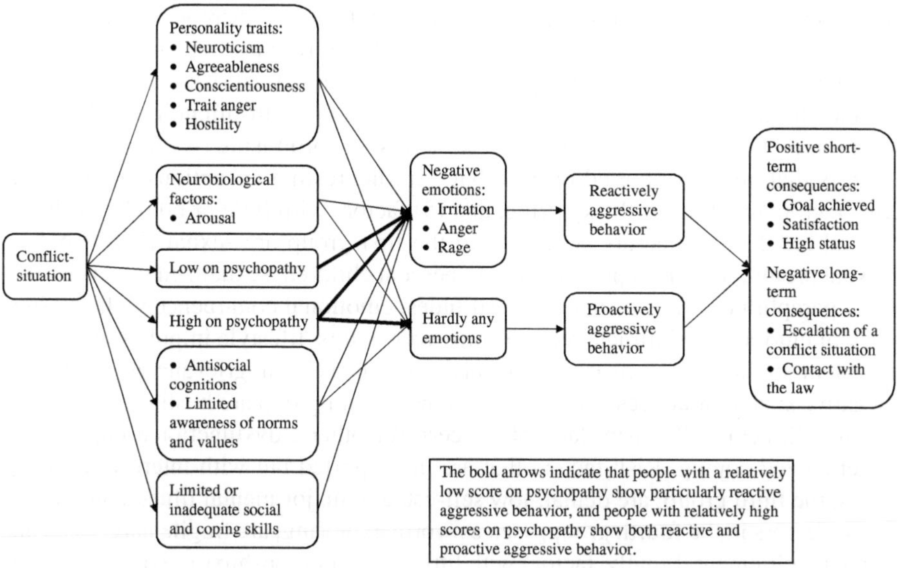

Fig. 2.1. A heuristic model for the maintenance of aggressive behavior in male violent offenders

neuroticism, agreeableness, conscientiousness, trait anger, and psychopathy. Consequently, we postulated the following preliminary heuristic model for the maintenance of aggressive behavior in male violent offenders (Fig. 2.1).

2.3 Sexually Violent Offenders

2.3.1 Dynamic Risk Factors

A meta-analysis of 82 studies of 29,450 sex offenders that was conducted by Hanson and Morton-Bourgon (2005) showed that the major predictors of general and violent recidivism were variables related to antisocial orientation, such as antisocial personality, antisocial traits, and a history of rule violation. Sexual deviancy and antisocial orientation were the major predictors of sexual recidivism for both adult and adolescent sexual offenders. For the general categories of deviant sexual attitudes and intimacy deficits, some of the individual variables were related to sexual recidivism (e.g., emotional identification with children, conflicts in intimate relationships) and some were not (e.g., loneliness). The results also suggested that the factors that initiate sexual offending may not be the same as the factors associated with persistence. Negative family backgrounds and internalization of psychological problems are common among sexual offenders, but these factors were unrelated to sexual recidivism. However, there is some evidence that sex offenders are more likely than other groups to respond to stress through sexual acts and deviant fantasies, thereby creating discrete periods where they are at increased risk of sexual recidivism.

Mann, Hanson, and Thornton (2010) categorized potential risk factors according to the strength of the evidence for their relationship with offending and divided them into (1) empirically supported risk factors, (2) promising risk factors, (3) risk factors that are unsupported overall, but with interesting exceptions, (4) potential risk factors that are worth exploring, and (5) factors with little or no relationship to sexual recidivism. Factors belonging to the first group are sexual preoccupation, sexual preference for prepubescent or pubescent children, sexualized violence, multiple paraphilias, offense-supportive attitudes, emotional congruence with children, lack of emotionally intimate relationships with adults, lifestyle impulsiveness, poor problem-solving skills, resistance to rules and supervision, grievance/hostility, and negative social influences. Risk factors in the second group are hostile beliefs about women, Machiavellianism, lack of concern for others, dysfunctional coping, and externalized coping. Risk factors that are unsupported but with interesting exceptions, the third group, are denial, low self-esteem, major mental illness, and loneliness. Factors in the fourth group, seen as worth exploring, are fragile narcissism and sexual entitlement. Finally, factors with little or no relationship to sexual recidivism are depression, general social skills deficits, poor victim empathy, and lack of motivation for treatment.

Kraanen and Emmelkamp (2017) reviewed the literature on substance abuse among sex offenders. Their review showed that about a third to half of the sex offenders have a history of any substance abuse, a third to half of the sex offenders have a history of alcohol misuse and that about a fifth to a quarter of the sex offenders has a history of drug misuse. Furthermore, about a quarter to third of the sex offenders appeared to be intoxicated at the time of the offense, but the researchers did not distinguish between rapists and child sexual abusers.

Unfortunately, the number of empirical studies is limited where the dynamic risk factors of a sample of sex offenders was compared to a norm group or where subsamples of sexual offenders were compared with each other. For example, a study by Dennison, Stough, and Birgden (2001) with the NEO Personality Inventory-Revised (Costa Jr. & McCrae, 1992) revealed that 32 child sexual abusers scored lower on extraversion than 33 nonclinical volunteers, but not lower on agreeableness. Serin, Malcolm, Khanna, and Barbaree (1994) found in 33 rapists a significantly higher score on the Psychopathy Checklist-Revised (PCL-R, Vertommen, Verheul, De Ruiter, & Hildebrand, 2002), a predictor of violent recidivism (Hare & Neumann, 2009), than in 32 child sexual abusers. Also, in later studies, rapists were found to have higher psychopathy scores than child sexual abusers (Porter et al., 2000). Seidman, Marshall, Hudson, and Robertson (1994) used the Disposition scale of the State-Trait Anger Expression Inventory (Spielberger, 1988) in 15 child abusers, 17 rapists, 15 domestic offenders, and 33 nonclinical volunteers. They found that both groups of sex offenders were not more disposed to anger than nonsexually violent offenders and a nonclinical control group.

Several studies have used implicit association test (IAT, Greenwald, McGhee, & Schwartz, 1998) measures to assess implicit sexual interest in child abusers.

From these studies, it became apparent that child sexual abusers associate children more strongly with sex than do other types of offenders (Babchishin, Nunes, & Hermann, 2013). Hornsveld, Gerritsma, Kanters, Zwets, and Roozen-Vlachos (2014) investigated 16 child sexual abusers, 22 rapists, and 59 nonsexually violent offenders using the Sexual Violence Risk-20 (SVR-20; Hildebrand, De Ruiter, & Van Beek, 2001), the PCL-R (Vertommen et al., 2002), self-report questionnaires, and an IAT developed for their research. In this IAT, participants had to put stimuli like pictures or words into the correct category (for example, "child," "adult," "sex," or "non-sex") as quickly as possible. They found respectively with the PCL-R, self-report questionnaires, and the IAT that the child abusers scored lower on psychopathy and aggressive behavior than the rapists and associated submissiveness relatively more often with sexual attraction. Ciardha and Gormley (2012) used another instrument to measure implicit cognitions, namely a modified version of the Stroop task, in a group of 24 child abusers and a group of nonclinical subjects. The sexual interest of the (extra- and intrafamilial) child sexual abusers resulted in shorter response times in children's pictures compared with those in adult pictures.

2.3.2 Endocrinological Risk Factors

As we have discussed in Chap. 1, the relationship between deviant sexuality and endocrine functions has not been well established (Briken, Hill, & Berner, 2006; Briken & Kafka, 2007). Nevertheless, in sex offenders, various pharmacological interventions are used to influence the endocrinological determinants of sexual behavior. Based on their research, Studer, Aylwin, and Reddon (2005) stated that testosterone should be more involved in the risk assessment and the risk management of sexually violent offenders.

Selective serotonin reuptake inhibitors (SSRIs) are not only effective in reducing irritability, impulsivity, and aggression but have also been used to improve symptomatology in patients with paraphilias and sexual compulsive or addictive-like behaviors. Possible effects of SSRIs are general inhibition of sexual activity, reduction of impulsiveness, relief of depressive symptoms or anxiety disorders, and an indirect reduction of testosterone levels (Briken, Hill, & Berner, 2014). However, as we already mentioned in Chap. 1, these effects are ascertained in non-random control studies with small samples that did not use recidivism as an outcome measure.

Although studies in sex offenders do not support a hypothesis of relatively increased testosterone levels associated with paraphilic behavior or sexual offending, antiandrogen treatments such as CPA (cyproterone acetate) or MPA (medroxyprogesterone), and LHRHs (luteinizing hormone-releasing hormone agonists) are used particularly in sexual offenders with paraphilias (Gooren, 2011). However, it should be noted that the studies on the effects of antiandrogen treatments are not based on controlled, double-blind studies. Also, all antiandrogenic treatments carry the risk of severe side effects such as thromboembolism, osteoporosis, diabetes, hypertension, obesity, and liver dysfunctions (Briken et al., 2014).

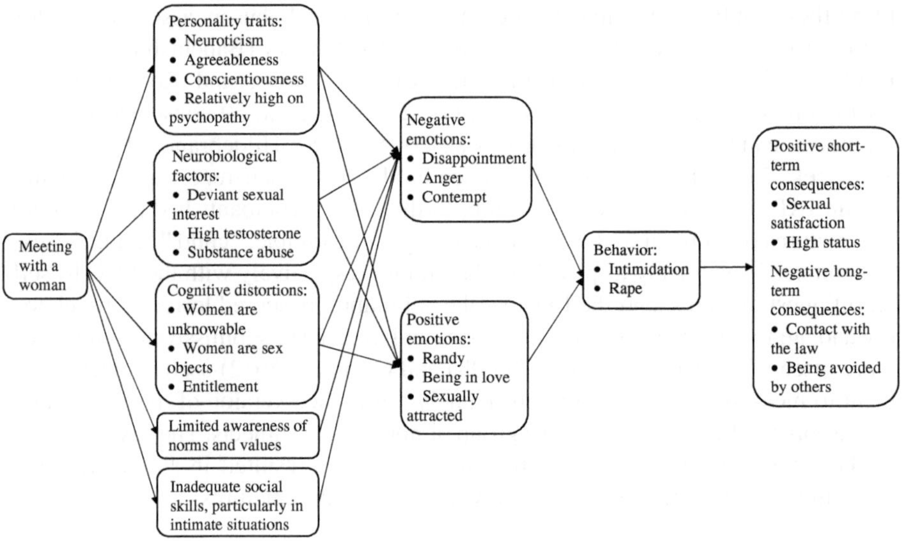

Fig. 2.2 A heuristic model for the maintenance of sexually aggressive behavior in rapists

2.3.3 Conclusions

Based on the literature, our research, and our clinical experience, treatment programs for sexually violent offenders should focus on deviant sexual interest (possibly associated with an increased testosterone level or lowered serotonin level), hostility toward women, distorted cognitions, social skills in intimate relations, moral awareness, and substance abuse. Traits that are important for the treatment of both populations (responsivity issues) are neuroticism, agreeableness, conscientiousness, anger, and psychopathy. On the basis of these factors, a preliminary heuristic model was postulated for the maintenance of aggressive behavior in both rapists (Fig. 2.2) and child sexual abusers (Fig. 2.3).

2.4 General Conclusions and Recommendations

Although the research discussed in this chapter provides an insight into most risk factors of violent and sexually violent offenders, an important limitation is the lack of their specificity, for instance, between domestically violent offenders and non-domestically violent offenders. Only in the case of sex offenders is a division sometimes made between rapists and child sexual abusers. In part, this lack of specificity has to do with the sometimes small numbers in specific subgroups of offenders. In our model for child sexual abusers, we included the testosterone and serotonin variables, despite the various results of assessment studies (see Chap. 1).

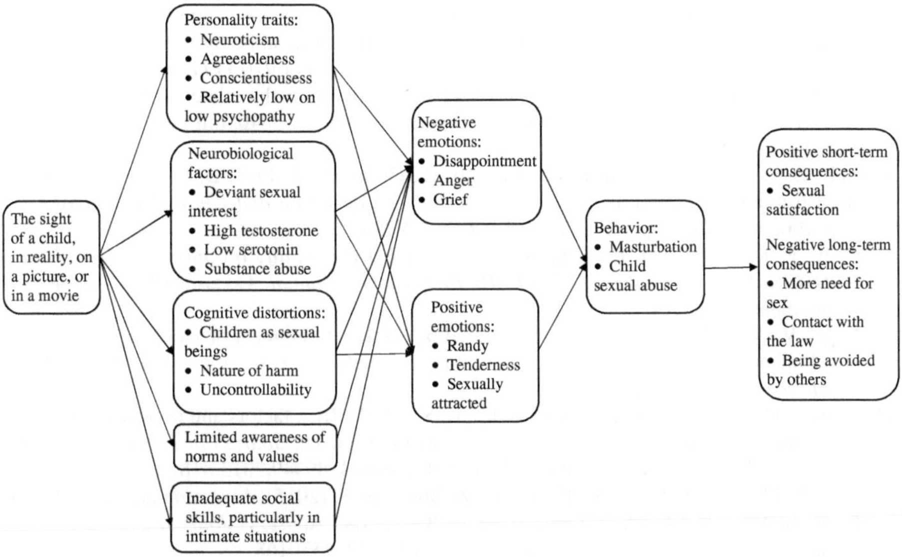

Fig. 2.3 A heuristic model for the maintenance of sexually aggressive behavior in child sexual abusers

Nevertheless, the dynamic factors described can be used to develop broad treatment programs for the benefit of violent offenders and sexually violent offenders, but further research is needed for the development of programs for very specific subgroups of violent and sexually violent offenders.

References

Andrews, D. A., & Bonta, J. (2010). *The psychology of criminal conduct* (5th ed.). New Providence, NJ: Matthew Bender & Company.

Babchishin, K. M., Nunes, K. L., & Hermann, C. A. (2013). The validity of implicit association test (IAT) measures of sexual attraction to children: A meta-analysis. *Archives of Sexual Behavior, 42*, 487–499. https://doi.org/10.1007/s10508-012-0022-8

Berkowitz, L. (2013). A different view of anger: The cognitive-neoassociation conception of the relation of anger to aggression. *Aggressive Behavior, 38*, 322–333. https://doi.org/10.1002/ab.21432

Briken, P., Hill, A., & Berner, W. (2006). Paraphilien und Sexualdelinquenz: Neurobiologische und neuropsychologische Aspekte. Eine Uebersicht. *Zeitschrift für Sexualforschung, 19*, 295–314.

Briken, P., Hill, A., & Berner, W. (2014). Pharmacotherapy of sexual offenders and men who are at risk of sexual offending. In D. P. Boer, R. Eher, L. A. Craig, M. H. Miner, & F. Pfäfflin (Eds.), *International perspectives on the assessment and treatment of sexual offenders* (pp. 437–449). Chichester: Wiley-Blackwell.

Briken, P., & Kafka, M. P. (2007). Pharmacological treatments for paraphilic patients and sexual offenders. *Current Opinion in Psychiatry, 20*, 609–613.

Ciardha, C. Ó., & Gormley, M. (2012). Sexual offenders against children using a pictorial modified Stroop task to explore the sexual interests of sexual offenders against children. *Sexual Abuse: A Journal of Research and Treatment, 24*, 175–197. https://doi.org/10.1177/1079063211407079

Cima, M., & Raine, A. (2009). Distinct characteristics of psychopathy relate to different subtypes of aggression. *Personality and Individual Differences, 47*, 835–840. https://doi.org/10.1016/j.paid.2009.06.031

Cornell, D. G., Warren, J., Hawk, G., Stafford, E., Oram, G., & Pine, D. (1996). Psychopathy in instrumental and reactive offenders. *Journal of Consulting and Clinical Psychology, 64*, 783–790. https://doi.org/10.1037/0022-006X.64.4.783

Costa Jr., P. T., & McCrae, R. R. (1992). *Revised NEO Personality Inventory (NEO-PI-R) and NEO Five-Factor Inventory (NEO-FFI): Professional manual.* Odessa, FL: Psychological Assessment Resources.

De Vogel, V., & De Ruiter, C. (2006). Structured professional judgment of violence risk in forensic clinical practice: A prospective study into the predictive validity of the Dutch HCR-20. *Psychology, Crime & Law, 12*, 321–336.

De Vries Robbé, M., De Vogel, V., & Douglas, K. S. (2013). Risk factors and protective factors: A two-sided dynamic approach to violence risk assessment. *The Journal of Forensic Psychiatry and Psychology, 24*, 440–457. https://doi.org/10.1080/14789949.2013.818162

De Vries Robbé, M., de Vogel, V., Koster, K., & Bogaerts, S. (2015). Assessing protective factors for sexually violent offending with the SAPROF. *Sexual Abuse: A Journal of Research and Treatment, 27*, 51–70. https://doi.org/10.1177/1079063214550168

Dennison, S. M., Stough, C., & Birgden, A. (2001). The big 5-dimensional personality approach to understanding sex offenders. *Psychology, Crime & Law, 7*, 243–261. https://doi.org/10.1080/10683160108401796

Fazel, S., & Danesh, J. (2002). Serious mental disorder in 23000 prisoners: a systematic review of 62 surveys. *The Lancet, 359*, 545–550.

Gibbs, J. C. (2003). *Moral development and reality: Beyond the theories of Kohlberg and Hoffman.* Thousand Oaks, CA: Sage.

Gooren, L. J. (2011). Ethical and medical considerations of Androgen Deprivation Treatment of sex offenders. *Journal of Clinical Endocrinology & Metabolism, 96*, 3628–3637. https://doi.org/10.1210/jc.2011-1540

Greenwald, A. G., McGhee, D. E., & Schwartz, J. L. K. (1998). Measuring individual differences in implicit cognition: The implicit association test. *Journal of Personality and Social Psychology, 85*, 1464–1480. https://doi.org/10.1037/0022-3514.74.6.1464

Hanson, R. K., & Morton-Bourgon, K. E. (2005). The characteristics of persistent sexual offenders: A meta-analysis of recidivism studies. *Journal of Consulting and Clinical Psychology, 73*, 1153–1163. https://doi.org/10.1037/0022-006X.73.6.1154

Hare, R. D. (1991). *The hare psychopathy checklist-revised.* Toronto: Multi-Health Systems.

Hare, R. D., & Neumann, C. S. (2009). Psychopathy: Assessment and forensic implications. *The Canadian Journal of Psychiatry, 54*, 791–802. https://doi.org/10.1093/med/9780199551637.003

Hart, S., Sturmey, P., Logan, C., & McMurran, M. (2011). Forensic case formulation. *International Journal of Forensic Mental Health, 10*, 118–126. https://doi.org/10.1080/14999013.2011.577137

Hildebrand, M., De Ruiter, C., & Van Beek, D. (2001). *SVR-20. Richtlijnen voor het Beoordelen van het risico van seksueel gewelddadig gedrag [SVR-20. Guidelines for the assessment of the risk of sexual violence].* Utrecht: Forum Educatief.

Hornsveld, R. H., Bulten, B. H., de Vries, E. T., & Kraaimaat, F. W. (2008). Violent forensic psychiatric inpatients and violent detainees in the Netherlands. *Journal of Forensic Psychiatry and Psychology, 19*, 407–419. https://doi.org/10.1080/14789940802190145

Hornsveld, R. H. J., Gerritsma, C. H. S., Kanters, T., Zwets, A. J., & Roozen-Vlachos, S. (2014). Criminogene factoren van seksueel gewelddadige terbeschikkinggestelden [Criminogenic factors of sexually violent offenders detained by hospital order]. *Tijdschrift voor Psychiatrie [Dutch Journal of Psychiatry], 56*, 430–438.

Hornsveld, R. H. J., Nijman, H. L. I., & Kraaimaat, F. W. (2008). Aggression Control Therapy for violent forensic psychiatric patients: First results. *Psychology, Crime & Law, 14*, 1–18. https://doi.org/10.1080/10683160701340569

Hornsveld, R. H. J., Zwets, A. J., Leenaars, P. E. M., Kraaimaat, F. W., Bout, R., Lagro-Janssen, A. L. M., et al. (2018). Violent female offenders compared with violent male offenders on psychological determinants of aggressive behavior. *International Journal of Offender Therapy and Comparative Criminology, 62*, 450–467. https://doi.org/10.1177/0306624X16648109

Jones, S. E., Miller, J. D., & Lynam, D. R. (2011). Personality, antisocial behavior, and aggression: A meta-analytic review. *Journal of Criminal Justice, 39*, 329–337.

Kohlberg, L. (1969). Stage and sequence: The cognitive-developmental approach to socialization. In D. A. Goslin (Ed.), *Handbook of socialization theory and research* (pp. 347–480). Chicago, IL: Rand McNally.

Kohlberg, L. (1984). *Essays on moral development: The psychology of moral development*. San Francisco, CA: Harper and Row.

Kraanen, F. L., & Emmelkamp, P. M. G. (2017). Alcohol and drugs in relation to sexual offending. In T. Sanders (Ed.), *The Oxford handbook of sex offences and sex offenders* (pp. 143–162). New York: Oxford University Press.

Mann, R. E., Hanson, R. K., & Thornton, D. (2010). Assessing risk sexual recidivism: Some proposals on the nature of psychologically meaningful risk factors. *Sexual Abuse: A Journal of Research and Treatment, 22*, 191–217. https://doi.org/10.1177/1079063210366039

Morgan, R. D., Kroner, D. G., & Mills, J. F. (2012). *Re-entry: Dynamic risk assessment*. Rockville, MD: National Institute of Justice/NCJRS. https://www.ncjrs.gov/pdffiles1/nij/grants/238075.pdf

Nagi, C., Ostapiuk, E. B., Craig, L. A., Hacker, D., & Beech, A. R. (2009). Using the revised Problem Identification Checklist to predict inpatient and community violence: A pilot study. *British Journal of Forensic Practice, 11*, 4–13.

Nijman, H., De Kruyk, C., & Van Nieuwenhuizen, C. (2004). Behavioral changes during forensic psychiatric (TBS) treatment in the Netherlands. *International Journal of Law and Psychiatry, 27*, 79–85. https://doi.org/10.1016/j.ijlp.2003.12.001

Novaco, R. W. (2013). Reducing anger-related offending: What works. In L. A. Craig, L. Dixon, & T. A. Gannon (Eds.), *What works in offender rehabilitation. An evidence-based approach to assessment and treatment* (pp. 211–236). Wiley-Blackwell: Chichester.

Ostapiuk, E., Stringer, I., & Craig, L. A. (2000). *Some modifications and revisions to the Problem Identification Checklist*. Unpublished manuscript, Forensic Psychology Practice Ltd., Sutton and Coldfield.

Philipse, M. W. G., Koeter, M. W. J., Van der Staak, C. P. F., & Van den Brink, W. (2006). Reliability and discriminant validity of dynamic reoffending risk indicators in forensic clinical practice. *Criminal Justice and Behavior, 32*, 643–664.

Porter, S., Fairweather, D., Drugge, J., Hervé, H., Birt, A., & Boer, D. P. (2000). Profiles of psychopathy in incarcerated sexual offenders. *Criminal Justice and Behavior, 27*, 216–233.

Porter, S., & Woodworth, M. (2006). Psychopathy and aggression. In C. J. Patrick (Ed.), *Handbook of psychopathy* (pp. 481–494). New York: Guilford.

Porter, S., Woodworth, M. T., & Black, P. J. (2018). Psychopathy and aggression. In C. J. Patrick (Ed.), *Handbook of psychopathy* (2nd ed., pp. 611–634). New York: Guilford.

Quinsey, V. L., Harris, G. T., Rice, M. E., & Cormier, C. (2006). *Violent offenders: Appraising and managing risk* (2nd ed.). Washington, DC: American Psychological Association.

Quinsey, V. L., Jones, G. B., Book, A. S., & Barr, K. N. (2006). The dynamic prediction of antisocial behavior among forensic psychiatric patients. A prospective field study. *Journal of Interpersonal Violence, 21*, 1539–1565. https://doi.org/10.1177/0886260506294238

Seidman, B. T., Marshall, W. L., Hudson, S. M., & Robertson, P. J. (1994). An examination of intimacy and loneliness in sex offenders. *Journal of Interpersonal Violence, 9*, 518–534.

Serin, R. C., Malcolm, B., Khanna, A., & Barbaree, H. E. (1994). Psychopathy and deviant sexual arousal in incarcerated sexual offenders. *Journal of Interpersonal Violence, 9*, 3–11.

Spielberger, C. D. (1988). *State-Trait-Anger-Expression-Inventory*. Palo Alto, CA: Consulting Psychologist Press.

Stams, G. J., Brugman, D., Dekovic, M., van Rosmalen, L., van der Laan, P., & Gibbs, J. C. (2006). The moral judgment of juvenile delinquents: A meta-analysis. *Journal of Abnormal Child Psychology, 24*, 697–713. https://doi.org/10.1007/s10802-006-9056-5

Studer, L. H., Aylwin, A. S., & Reddon, J. (2005). Testosterone, sexual offense recidivism, and treatment effect among adult male sex offenders. *Sexual Abuse: A Journal of Research and Treatment, 17*, 171–181.

Van Vugt, E., Gibbs, J., Stams, G. J., Bijleveld, C., Hendriks, J., & Van der Laan, P. (2011). Moral development and recidivism: A meta-analysis. *International Journal of Offender Therapy and Comparative Criminology, 55*, 1234–1250. https://doi.org/10.1177/0306624X10396441

Vertommen, H., Verheul, R., de Ruiter, C., & Hildebrand, M. (2002). *De herziene versie van Hare's Psychopathie Checklist (PCL-R) [The revised version of Hare's Psychopathy Checklist (PCL-R)]*. Lisse: Swets Test Publishers.

Woodworth, M., & Porter, S. (2002). In cold blood: Characteristics of criminal homicides as a function of psychopathy. *Journal of Abnormal Psychology, 111*, 436–445.

Chapter 3
The Use of Self-Report Questionnaires

Ruud H. J. Hornsveld, Floris W. Kraaimaat, Henk L. I. Nijman, Sabine J. Roza, Kevin L. Nunes, and Emma J. Palmer

3.1 Introduction

Self-report questionnaires are widely used in the forensic field, both for the assessment of individual offenders and for the evaluation of treatment programs. However, the validity of such questionnaires in this population is controversial. This chapter provides an overview of the internal and external factors that may affect the responding on these scales in various forensic populations. Internal factors refer to factors that relate to individual respondent characteristics, such as the tendency to socially desirable responding, insight into one's behavior, and moral awareness. External factors relate to the circumstances in which the questionnaires are completed, such as the presence or absence of an assessor, the format and content of the questionnaires, and the setting in which the respondent resides.

R. H. J. Hornsveld (✉)
Erasmus University Medical Center, Rotterdam, The Netherlands
e-mail: ruud.hornsveld@ziggo.nl

F. W. Kraaimaat
Radboud University Nijmegen, Nijmegen, The Netherlands

H. L. I. Nijman
Radboud University, Nijmegen, The Netherlands

S. J. Roza
Erasmus University Medical Center, Rotterdam, The Netherlands

K. L. Nunes
Carleton University, Ottawa, Canada

E. J. Palmer
University of Leicester, Leicester, UK

R. H. J. Hornsveld et al. (eds.), *Assessment and Obligatory Treatment of Violent and Sexually Violent Offenders*, Advances in Preventing and Treating Violence and Aggression, https://doi.org/10.1007/978-3-030-27840-3_3

3.2 Internal Factors

3.2.1 Socially Desirable Responding

Socially Desirable responding (SDR) is usually defined as the inclination of respondents to place themselves in a favorable light (Paulhus, 2002). Research into the influence of SDR typically uses two instruments, namely the Marlow-Crowne Social Desirability Scale (MC-SDS, Crowne & Marlowe, 1960) and the Balanced Inventory of Desirable Responding (BIDR; Paulhus, 1984, 1988). The MC-SDS consists of 33 items, of which 15 are negative (e.g., "I am sometimes irritated by people who ask favors of me.") and 18 are positive (e.g., "I never hesitate to go out of my way to help someone in trouble."). The answer options are "true" or "not true." A socially desirable answer gets the score 1. Otherwise, the score is 0. The minimum score is therefore 0 and the maximum score of 33. Andrews and Meyer (2003) investigated the original MC-SDS with 33 items and the short version with 13 Items (MC-C) in 1,096 people suspected of an offense. These individuals scored significantly higher on both versions of the MC-SDS than the non-offenders from several other studies. The authors, therefore, concluded that both versions could be used to measure self-deception as part of a forensic assessment.

The BIDR has 40 items that are stated as propositions. The items belong to two scales of 20 items each, namely Self-Deception (tends to report honest but positively colored responses, e.g., "I rarely appreciate criticism.") and Impression Management (intentionally making a positive impression on others, e.g., "I always declare everything at customs."). The Self-Deception scale was later subdivided into two subscales, namely "Self-Deceptive Enhancement" (e.g., "My first impressions always turn out to be right.") and Self-Deceptive Denial (e.g., "I have never thought about killing someone."). Respondents rate their agreement with the statement on a seven-point scale. The scoring key is balanced. After reversing the negatively keyed items, one point is added for each extreme response (6 or 7). Hence, all scores on the SD- and IM subscale can range from 0 to 20. All 40 items may be summed to yield an overall measure of SDR. The higher the item score, the more socially desirable it has been answered. In a study by Paulhus (1988), the total score on the BIDR correlated 0.71 with the total score on the MC-SDS.

3.2.2 Socially Desirable Responding in University Students

There has been a good amount of research into the influence of SDR on the scores of self-reporting questionnaires for personality traits in university students. Holden (2007) found that the task of responding to the most favorable response had a great influence on the validity criterion (in this case a personality trait), but Holden and Passey (2010) noted that this was not true when there was little at stake for the participants. Finally, Holden and Book (2012) concluded that the relationship between

SDR and self-reporting of personality characteristics is related to a number of factors, namely (a) the way in which SDR is operationalized, (b) the investigation procedure (SDR is implicit or is experimentally induced), (c) the importance of the results for the participants, and (d) the psychometric properties of the personality questionnaire used. A fifth factor that possibly plays a role is the subject of a questionnaire (Hendriks, 2011). For example, Davis, Thake, and Vilhena (2010) investigated the alcohol consumption of 568 university students using, inter alia, the Balanced Inventory of Desirable Responding (BIDR; Paulhus, 2002) and questionnaires about alcohol abuse. Their research showed that students who scored high on the subscale Impression Management reported 20–33% less alcohol consumption and reported about 50% less drunkenness than the students who scored low on that subscale. No significant connection was found between the subscale Self-Deception and alcohol consumption. The authors concluded that in people with high scores on Impression Management, the validity of self-reported use of alcohol with associated risks might be limited because alcohol abuse by respondents is considered to be socially abusive behavior. The use of self-reporting questionnaires for such individuals may, according to the researchers, lead to an underestimation of harmful and risky alcohol consumption.

3.2.3 Socially Desirable Responding in Offenders

Offenders are often assumed to complete self-report questionnaires in a socially desirable way because they would think that a favorable score has a positive impact on their legal status (Kalmus & Beech, 2005). In the literature, several studies have investigated this issue. For example, Mills, Loza, and Kroner (2003) found in their survey of 124 male delinquents that the Self-Appraisal Questionnaire (SAQ, Loza, 1996), a self-report risk assessment measure predictive of general and violent recidivism, was significantly negatively related to both BIDR subscales. However, in a follow-up study (Mills & Kroner, 2006) of 172 male offenders on the validity of the Measure of Criminal Attitudes and Associates (MCAA; Mills & Kroner, 1999), a self-report questionnaire on antisocial attitudes, offenders scoring highly on the subscale Impression Management of the BIDR unexpectedly reported less antisocial attitudes. High scores on Impression Management were significantly negatively related to recidivism risk. Similar results were also found in other studies (Davis et al., 2010; Mathie & Wakeling, 2011; Mills & Kroner, 2005); namely, those who scored low on SDR and thus had relatively fair responses, had a higher recidivism risk. Based on a meta-analysis of 31 independent samples, Gray and Mills (2011) concluded that offenders are scoring lower on measures of SDR, particularly Impression Management, and were significantly more criminally oriented in comparison to offenders who scored higher on measures of SDR. Their finding indicates that the measurement of SDR within forensic assessment is confounded by risk-related content and may, therefore, lead to a potential systematic bias.

3.2.4 Socially Desirable Responding in Sex Offenders

In the sex offender population, specific factors can contribute to SDR, such as wanting to make a macho impression or to avoid a diagnosis of being "sexually deviant" (Kroner & Weekes, 1996). Bumby (1996) developed the MOLEST scale and the RAPE scale for the assessment of cognitive distortions in child sexual abusers and rapists of adult women, respectively. He found that both scales were not significantly correlated with the MC-SDS. Arkowitz and Vess (2003), however, considered that the MOLEST scale and the RAPE scale are too sensitive to SDR for use in sex offenders who should undergo compulsory treatment, although they did not investigate this assumption. Mathie and Wakeling (2011) studied the association between SDR and several other measurement instruments used to identify treatment need in 1730 male sexual offenders. SDR was measured with the BIDR (Paulhus, 1984), social functioning with nine questionnaires such as the Self-Esteem Questionnaire (Webster, Mann, Thornton, & Wakeling, 2006), offense-specific factors with seven questionnaires such as Hypermasculinity Inventory (Mosher & Sirken, 1984), and the sexual recidivism risk with the Risk Matrix 2000/s (Thornton et al., 2003), a checklist with seven items that assesses past demographic and criminal history in order to predict sexual recidivism. The results of the study suggested that the degree of SDR and its impact on self-assessment questionnaires were fairly low. Correlations between SDR and the offense-specific measurement instruments ranged from −0.34 to 0.36 for the Self-Deception subscale, and from −0.26 to 0.20 for the Impression Management subscale. Again, lower risk offenders appeared to employ socially desirable responding to a greater extent than higher risk offenders. According to Mathie and Wakeling (2011), their study demonstrated that the extent of socially desirable responding among a sample of incarcerated sexual offenders was smaller than assumed. Furthermore, the impact of socially desirable responding on self-report measures is lower than expected, providing some evidence that self-report questionnaires used with forensic populations can be accurate and valid.

3.2.5 Understanding of Own Behavior and Moral Awareness

When it concerns SDR, relatively little attention has been given to the issue of the extent to which respondents have insight into their behavior and the moral standards of the society in which they live. A questionnaire can only be completed honestly if the respondent has a good understanding of how he or she behaves in a particular situation. If the respondent wishes to answer in a socially desirable way, then he or she must be aware of the behaviors that are considered normal by a majority of people.

Research on insight into one's behavior has been conducted primarily in psychiatric patients, such as individuals with schizophrenia (Bell, Fiszdon, Richardson, Lysaker, & Bryson, 2007), manic patients (Adida et al., 2008), and adolescents with psychiatric disorders (Salbach-Andrae, Klinkowski, Lenz, & Lehmkuhl, 2009).

However, insufficient research has been conducted to date on insight into personal behavior of offenders and nonclinical adults with a low level of education and low socioeconomic status.

3.3 External Factors

3.3.1 Attendance or Absence of a Researcher

In recent years, the digital completion of questionnaires has increased sharply. Campos, Zucoloto, Bonafé, Jordani, and Maroco (2011) compared three electronic self-report questionnaires on burnout with a written format and concluded that electronic questionnaires are a user-friendly and reasonably reliable way to collect data. They suggest that a particular advantage is the fact that there is a much-reduced level of influence from the researcher during or after the completion of the questionnaire.

Among offenders, however, in our opinion, it is advisable to complete the questionnaires in the presence of a researcher. Many offenders have a low level of education and sometimes do not understand certain words or phrases (for example: "What's a poem?"). Also, a researcher can see how the questionnaires are completed, ranging from excessive attention and effort to rushed. In our experience, offenders relatively often have to be motivated to continue completing questionnaires because they get bored or discouraged easily. If questionnaires are completed in the context of scientific research, it is essential to let the respondents know that the results are not included in their official files and will have no influence on their treatment or legal status (Drenth & Sijtsma, 2006).

3.3.2 Free-Answers or Choice-Answers

Several authors have recommended the use of "production tools" instead of multiple-choice "recognition tools" with offenders (Gavaghan, Arnold, & Gibbs, 1983; Stams et al., 2006; Van Vugt et al., 2011), with Drenth and Sijtsma (2006) calling for free-answer tests versus choice-response tests. For free-answer questionnaires, respondents are asked to write their responses to questions, after which those comments are scored by an independent reviewer. These written responses might then give more direct information about the behavior of respondents because they do not have to consider what a "correct" or "best" score is on the Likert scale, as with choice-answers questionnaires. However, the disadvantage of the free-answer questionnaires is that assessing and categorizing the answers to the researcher is a time-consuming issue (Drenth & Sijtsma, 2006). Also, when using these free-answer questionnaires, adequate inter-rater reliability can be difficult to ensure.

3.3.3 Setting

In the literature, relatively little attention had been paid to the possible influence of the setting in which the respondent resides (admitted or detained versus in outpatient treatment or on leave versus nonclinical volunteer) when answering questionnaires. For example, Olver, Kingston, Nicholaichuk, and Wong (2014) found in 392 detained sex offenders that they did not score in a particularly pathological manner on a battery of psychometric measures. Kelsey, Rogers, and Robinson (2015) administered the Psychopathic Personality Inventory-Revised (PPI-R; Lilienfeld & Widows, 2005), a self-assessment questionnaire with 154 items for the measurement of psychopathy, in a sample of 86 detainees. The detainees were found to score lower on the questionnaire than students and other nonclinical volunteers. Kanters et al. (2016) compared 28 inpatient child sex abusers with 61 outpatient child sexual abusers at a forensic psychiatric outpatient clinic. Compared to the inpatients, the outpatients showed a significantly lower risk of recidivism, as measured by the Sexual Violence Risk-20 (SVR-20; Boer, Wilson, Gauthier, & Hart, 1997). However, on the self-report questionnaires for aggression, hostility, and social anxiety, outpatient child sexual abusers scored significantly higher than inpatient child sexual abusers. Also, the outpatients showed significantly more positive self-esteem than the inpatients. A possible explanation for these striking differences may be that the supervision and structure of prison or forensic psychiatric institution have a dampening effect on negative behavior (Hornsveld, Kraaimaat, Bouwmeester, Polak, & Zwets, 2014) and that as a consequence, detainees and inpatients completed the questionnaires more truthfully. The striking differences in scores on questionnaires between detainees or forensic psychiatric inpatients, on the one hand, and forensic psychiatric outpatients or offenders on parole, on the other hand, require further investigation.

3.4 Questionnaires for Non-English-Speaking Countries

The majority of questionnaires used in forensic populations were developed in Anglo-Saxon and English-speaking countries. To achieve construct equivalence of these questionnaires in non-English-speaking countries requires at least two steps. First, the text has to be translated and cultural words or idioms sometimes need to be adjusted to ensure they capture the same concepts. Second, a psychometric investigation has to be performed on the reliability and validity of the questionnaire. In the case of satisfactory reliability and validity, norms have to be calculated for relevant populations (e.g., average population, detainees, forensic in- and outpatients). The necessity of these steps is illustrated by some examples of research with the Aggression Questionnaire (AQ) and the Novaco Anger Scale-Provocation Inventory (NAS-PI).

The psychometric properties of the Aggression Questionnaire (AQ; Buss & Perry, 1992) and the Aggression Questionnaire-Short Form (AQ-SF; Bryant & Smith, 2001) have been studied in nonclinical samples of various non-English-speaking countries. All these studies confirmed the four-factor structure (Physical Aggression, Verbal Aggression, Hostility, and Anger) of the two questionnaires in nonclinical, mostly well-educated samples (children, adolescents, and adults) from countries, such as Argentina (Reyna, Ivacevich, Sanchez, and Brussino (2011), France (Genoud & Zimmermann, 2009), Germany (Von Collani & Werner, 2005), Italy (Fossati, Maffei, Acquarini, & Di Ceglie, 2003), Japan (Nakano, 2001), Pakistan (Iftikhar & Malik, 2014), and Spain (Santisteban, Alvarado, and Recio (2007). These results support the construct validity of both versions in nonclinical samples. Also, all these studies demonstrated that the internal consistency of the subscales was satisfactory, although none of these studies investigated, for instance, the test-retest reliability or a possible difference in scores between aggressive and nonaggressive volunteers.

However, studies on the factor structure of the AQ and its short version AQ-SF in samples of offenders or forensic psychiatric patients have yielded different results. For instance, Williams, Boyd, Cascardi, and Poythress (1996) found that a confirmatory factor analysis of the AQ in 200 offenders (females and males) yielded a poor fit for the four-factor model, and the internal consistency of the Verbal Aggression subscale was below acceptable limits. Offenders with aggressive offenses did not display significantly higher AQ scores than offenders with nonaggressive offenses, which questions the discriminatory validity of the scale. Diamond, Wang, and Buffington-Vollum (2005) analyzed the factor structure of the AQ and AQ-SF in a sample of 786 male, mentally ill prisoners and concluded that the four factors of the 12-item AQ-SF produced the best fit. In a second study, Diamond and Magaletta (2006) found that a confirmatory factor analysis supported the four-factor structure of the AQ-SF across both genders in a sample of 916 male and 355 female offenders. The internal consistency coefficients of the subscales varied from sufficient to good. Hornsveld, Muris, Kraaimaat, and Meesters (2009) found in 344 Dutch violent forensic psychiatric patients (male in- and outpatients) as well as in 160 secondary vocational students (males) that the psychometric properties of the AQ (Dutch version) was less satisfactory than previously observed in populations of Dutch college or university students (females and males). For instance, the four-factor structure could not be confirmed in both samples, and the internal consistency, inter-item correlations, and item-scale correlations of the Verbal Aggression scale were found to be unsatisfactory in the subsample of inpatients and students. On the contrary, the psychometric properties of the AQ-SF (Bryant & Smith, 2001) were better than those of the original full-length version. Furthermore, the construct validity of the AQ and AQ-SF was sufficiently demonstrated by meaningful patterns of correlations with other measures of aggression, anger, and hostility. Inpatients scored lower on the AQ and AQ-SF than the students, when controlling for age differences across samples. Pettersen, Nunes, and Cortoni (2018) found some support for the four-factor structure with the AQ-SF, but not with the AQ in their confirmatory factor analyses with a sample of 271 Canadian incarcerated male violent offenders. In another study with 293 Canadian incarcerated male sexual offenders,

Pettersen, Nunes, and Cortoni (2016) did not find support for the four-factor structure for either the AQ or AQ-SF. However, higher scores on the Physical Aggression subscale for both the AQ and AQ-SF were moderately associated with higher risk of sexual recidivism ($r = 0.36$ and 0.33, respectively), as measured by the Static 99, an actuarial risk assessment instrument (Hanson & Thornton, 2000).

Another instrument that is frequently used in the forensic field is the Novaco Anger Scale-Provocation Inventory (NAS-PI; Novaco, 2003). An initial investigation of the NAS-PI in three California state hospitals showed that the internal consistency of both NAS-PI scales was excellent and the test-retest reliability was good, as was the predictive validity (Novaco, 1994). Since this study, the psychometric properties of successive versions (an intermediate 1998 version and the formally published 2003 version) have been examined in various offender populations. For instance, Mills, Kroner, and Forth (1998) found in a sample of 102 violent offenders and 102 nonviolent offenders that internal consistency and test-retest reliability were good and convergent validity was demonstrated. However, the violent offenders had significantly lower scores on the NAS-PI than did the nonviolent offenders. On the other hand, a study by Jones, Thomas-Peter, and Trout (1999) in a sample of 58 males, who were referred to a clinical facility for anger management training, and a sample of 79 male and 133 female employees of National Health Service in the United Kingdom showed that the clinical sample scored significantly higher on the NAS-PI than the nonclinical sample.

Research on the factor structure of the NAS-PI (1994 version) was carried out by Jones, Thomas-Peter, and Gangstad (2003) in a sample of 354 British outpatients referred for an anger management training and a sample of 212 healthcare employees. Exploratory factor analysis of the data from the combined clinical and nonclinical sample yielded three factors, which were not consistent with the domains (Cognitive, Arousal, and Behavior) initially defined by Novaco (1994). Another exploratory factor analysis of the 1994 version of the NAS was published in the manual for the final version of the NAS-PI (Novaco, 2003). This analysis was performed in a sample of 1101 civil commitment inpatients with severe mental disorders. Results did not yield a factor structure that was following the original subscales of the instrument. A similar result was obtained in the 2003 NAS standardization sample of 1546 nonclinical, multi-ethnic individuals in four geographic regions of the United States (Novaco, 2003). Finally, the three subscales structure was also not supported in a study by Baker, Van Hasselt, and Sellers (2008) in a sample of 1308 adult incarcerated offenders (959 men, 349 women), arrested for domestic violence or drug-related offenses.

A Swedish translation of the 1998 version of the NAS-PI was evaluated by Lindqvist, Dåderman, and Hellström (2005) in a sample of 95 violent male prisoners (some of them with diagnosed personality disorders). The questionnaire appeared to have good internal consistency, and convergent validity appeared to be excellent. The factor structure of this version the NAS-PI (1998 version) was investigated in a sample of 100 undergraduate male students by Lindqvist, Dåderman, and Hellström (2003). Again, the results did not yield a factor structure that was in accordance with the original subscales of the instrument. Hornsveld, Muris, and Kraaimaat (2011) investigated the 1994 version of the NAS-PI in 336 Dutch violent forensic psychiatric patients (male in- and outpatients) and 320 Dutch secondary vocational students (females and males) and found that the three-subscale structure of the original NAS could not be confirmed. However, the internal consistency of the NAS and the PI was excellent, and the test-retest reliability of the NAS was good. The validity of the NAS and the PI was supported by a meaningful pattern of correlations with alternative measures of anger and personality traits. Forensic psychiatric outpatients displayed higher NAS scores than secondary vocational students, but inpatients scored even lower than this nonclinical control group.

To summarize, self-report questionnaires that yield an acceptable fit of their factor or subscale structure in a nonclinical population do not necessarily do so in populations of violent offenders, violent forensic psychiatric patients, or secondary vocational students. One of the reasons might be that most investigated nonclinical populations have higher levels of education. In general, considering internal consistency and convergent validity, the translated versions of the AQ and NAS-PI show comparable results with the original English version in nonclinical volunteers, offenders, and forensic psychiatric patients. However, studies in nonclinical populations often lack a comparison between aggressive and nonaggressive participants.

3.5 Conclusions and Recommendations

In this chapter, three issues have been considered on the use of self-report questionnaires among offenders, namely (a) the influence of internal factors such as SDR, insight, and moral awareness, (b) the influence of external factors such as the presence or absence of a researcher, the questionnaire form and content, and the setting in which the respondent resides, and (c) the psychometric properties of two commonly used self-report questionnaires. Based on literature and clinical experience, we draw the following conclusions.

Research from different populations reveals that socially desirable responses seem to be associated with factors such as (a) the extent to which the self-report responses will be used to make decisions relevant to the respondent (e.g., whether or not to grant early release from a secure hospital or prison), (b) the theme of the questionnaire (personal characteristics versus socially or legally proscribed behavior), (c) the investigation procedure (SDR is unwittingly or is experimentally induced), and (d) the psychometric properties of the questionnaire used. It was also noted that the MC-SDS and the BIDR have the limitation that they were developed using samples of university students and that the assumed factor structure has not been investigated in non-American offenders or forensic psychiatric patients. Unfortunately, research is also lacking in the relationship between SDR on the one hand and insight into own behavior and moral awareness on the other hand.

Among offenders, it may be advisable to use, as far as possible, free-answer questionnaires, in which respondents formulate a comment on an item instead of ticking an appropriate response. Unfortunately, so far, there has been little research into differences in validity between free-answer and choice-answer questionnaires for adult offenders or forensic psychiatric patients. The presence of a person to monitor and assist with the completion has the advantage that it may motivate offenders to fill in the questionnaires entirely and that he or she can answer questions about difficult words. The influence of the setting on answering questionnaires may also be important. Differences in scores on questionnaires between detainees or forensic psychiatric inpatients on the one hand and outpatients or nonclinical volunteers, on the other hand, deserve further investigation. Can these differences be explained by the structure and the supervision of the forensic psychiatric institution or do other factors play a role too, such as differences in psychopathology? Alternatively, are detainees in prison or patients in a forensic psychiatric institution better "trained" in masking their problem behaviors than outpatients, offenders in the community, or nonclinical volunteers?

An essential problem with the use of self-report questionnaires among offenders is that for most the psychometric properties have not sufficiently been investigated in their target group and that relevant norms are lacking. The use of subscale scores is not advisable when the subscales are not supported by further psychometric research. Norms of nonclinical volunteers may be of importance to outpatients or offenders living in the community, but less to inpatients or detainees. When using self-report questionnaires among offenders, it should always be taken into consideration that respondents may be able to complete the questionnaires in a socially desirable way and that their insight into their behavior and their moral maturity may be limited. This is especially important when the questionnaire scores are used for decisions at an individual level, and there is much at stake for the respondent.

Various researchers (for example, Andrews & Bonta, 2010) have argued for the use of a combination of different ways of measurement instruments, such as structured interviews, observation scales, and recording of incidents. In our opinion, the use of several types of measures is necessary because each type has specific limitations. In a closed setting, a comparison of the score on a questionnaire with that on an observation scale can provide relevant information about a patient's insight into his or her behavior (Nijman, Bjørkly, Palmstierna, & Almvik, 2006). However, for each measurement type, an appraisal must always be made between the meaning of the information gathered on the one hand and the constraints of the instrument in question on the other (Drenth & Sijtsma, 2006).

In the context of scientific research, it seems less useful to compare the scores of inpatients or detainees to self-report questionnaires with those of outpatient patients or offenders in the community. Also, it is vital that the psychometric properties of the MC-SDS (33- and 13-item version) and the BIDR be investigated in (non-English-speaking) offender populations.

3.6 New Developments

There are indications that self-report questionnaires for dynamic factors can make a valuable contribution to the risk assessment of (sex) offenders (Douglas & Skeem, 2005; Van den Berg et al., 2018). Beech, Friendship, Erikson, and Hanson (2002) found, for example, in a sample of 140 child abusers that adding the questionnaire data on potentially dynamic risk factors resulted in a significant improvement in risk assessment based on static factors. However, it should be noted that the different studies into the added value of dynamic factors for risk assessment have been performed in samples of offenders; therefore, the results cannot be applied to individual offenders. According to Hart, Michie, and Cooke (2007), "actuarial risk assessments cannot yet be used to estimate the individual risk of future violence with some degree of reliability, and should, therefore, be used with caution" (p. 60).

For some dynamic (changeable) factors of recurrence risk, specific questionnaires have been developed, for example, to measure hostility (PSF-AV, Hornsveld, Nijman, Hollin, & Kraaimaat, 2007), moral maturity (SRM-AV, Hornsveld, Kraaimaat, & Zwets, 2012), and attitude towards women (HVL; Hornsveld, Timonen, Kraaimaat, Zwets, & Kanters, 2014). All three instruments are free-answer questionnaires. However, these three new questionnaires are still in the first stage, and further psychometric research is needed.

A second exciting development is the use of self-report questionnaires as a risk assessment instrument. Some researchers found that the predictive ability of some self-report questionnaires corresponded to that of commonly used actuarial instruments (Loza & Green, 2003; Walters, 2006). Here too, further research will have to show whether specific self-report questionnaires can be used to determine the recurrence risk at an individual level, especially because there may be major interests for a respondent.

All in all, in our opinion, there is currently no reason not to recommend self-report questionnaires from the forensic field. However, users should take account of the limitations of these types of measures discussed in this chapter.

References

Adida, M., Clark, L., Pomiettoa, P., Kaladjian, A., Besnier, N., Azorina, J., et al. (2008). Lack of insight may predict impaired decision making in manic patients. *Bipolar Disorders, 10*, 829–837.

Andrews, D. A., & Bonta, J. (2010). *The psychology of criminal conduct* (5th ed.). New Providence, NJ: Matthew Bender & Company.

Andrews, P., & Meyer, R. G. (2003). Marlow-Crowne Social Desirability Scale and short form C: Forensic norms. *Journal of Clinical Psychology, 59*, 483–492. https://doi.org/10.1002/jclp.10136

Arkowitz, S., & Vess, J. (2003). An evaluation of the Bumby RAPE and MOLEST scales as measures of cognitive distortions with civilly committed sexual offenders. *Sexual Abuse: A Journal of Research and Treatment, 15*, 237–249.

Baker, M. T., Van Hasselt, V. B., & Sellers, A. H. (2008). Validation of the Novaco Anger Scale in an incarcerated offender population. *Criminal Justice and Behavior, 35*, 741–754. https://doi.org/10.1177/0093854808316275

Beech, A., Friendship, C., Erikson, M., & Hanson, R. K. (2002). The relationship between static and dynamic risk factors and reconviction in a sample of U.K. child abusers. *Sexual Abuse: A Journal of Research and Treatment, 14*, 155–167.

Bell, M., Fiszdon, J., Richardson, R., Lysaker, P., & Bryson, G. (2007). Are self-reports valid for schizophrenia patients with poor insight? Relationship of unawareness of illness to psychological self-report instruments. *Psychiatry Research, 151*, 37–46.

Boer, D. P., Wilson, R. J., Gauthier, C. M., & Hart, S. D. (1997). Assessing risk for sexual violence: Guidelines for clinical practice. In C. D. Webster & M. A. Jackson (Eds.), *Impulsivity: Theory, assessment, and treatment* (pp. 326–342). New York: Guilford.

Bryant, F. B., & Smith, B. D. (2001). Refining the architecture of aggression: A measurement model for the Buss-Perry Aggression Questionnaire. *Journal of Research in Personality, 35*, 138–167.

Bumby, K. M. (1996). Assessing the cognitive distortions of child molesters and rapists: Development and validation of the MOLEST and RAPE Scales. *Sexual Abuse: A Journal of Research and Treatment, 8*, 37–54.

Buss, A. H., & Perry, M. (1992). The aggression questionnaire. *Journal of Personality and Social Psychology, 63*, 452–459.

Campos, J. A. D. B., Zucoloto, M. L., Bonafé, F. S. S., Jordani, P. C., & Maroco, J. (2011). Reliability and validity of self-reported burnout in college students: A cross randomized comparison of paper-and-pencil vs. online administration. *Computers in Human Behavior, 27*, 1875–1883. https://doi.org/10.1016/j.chb.2011.04.011

Crowne, D. P., & Marlowe, D. (1960). A new scale of social desirability independent of psychopathology. *Journal of Consulting Psychology, 24*, 349–354.

Davis, C. G., Thake, J., & Vilhena, N. (2010). Social desirability biases in self-reported alcohol consumption and harms. *Addictive Behaviors, 35*, 302–311. https://doi.org/10.1016/j.addbeh.2009.11.001

Diamond, P. M., & Magaletta, P. R. (2006). The short-form Buss-Perry Aggression Questionnaire (BPAQ-SF): A validation study with federal offenders. *Assessment, 13*, 227–240.

Diamond, P. M., Wang, E. W., & Buffington-Vollum, J. (2005). Factor structure of the Buss-Perry Aggression Questionnaire (BPAQ) with mentally ill male prisoners. *Criminal Justice and Behavior, 32*, 546–564.

Douglas, K. S., & Skeem, J. L. (2005). Violence risk assessment. Getting specific about being dynamic. *Psychology, Public Policy, and Law, 11*, 347–383. https://doi.org/10.1037/1076-8971.11.3.347

Drenth, P. J. D., & Sijtsma, K. (2006). *Testtheorie. Inleiding in de theorie van de psychologische test en zijn toepassingen [Testtheory. Introduction to the theory of the psychological test and its applications]*. Houten: Bohn Stafleu van Loghum.

Fossati, A., Maffei, C., Acquarini, E., & Di Ceglie, A. (2003). Multigroup confirmatory component and factor analyses of the Italian version of the Aggression Questionnaire. *European Journal of Psychological Assessment, 19*, 54–65.

Gavaghan, M. P., Arnold, K. D., & Gibbs, J. C. (1983). Moral judgment in delinquents and nondelinquents: Recognition versus production measures. *Journal of Psychology, 114*, 267–274. https://doi.org/10.1080/00223980.1983.9915424

Genoud, P. A., & Zimmermann, G. (2009). *French version of the 12-item Aggression Questionnaire: Preliminary psychometric properties*. 11th Congress of the Swiss Psychological Society, Neuchâtel.

Gray, A. L., & Mills, J. F. (2011). Measuring Socially Desirable Responding within a forensic context: Response style or criminal proclivity. *Crime Scene. Psychology Behind Bars and in Front of the Bench, 18*, 13–15.

Hanson, K. R., & Thornton, D. (2000). Improving risk assessments for sex offenders: A comparison of three actuarial scales. *Law and Human Behavior, 24*, 119–136. https://doi.org/10.1023/A:1005482921333

Hart, S. D., Michie, C., & Cooke, D. J. (2007). Precision of actuarial risk assessment instruments. Evaluating the 'margins of error' of group v. individual predictions of violence. *British Journal of Psychiatry, 190*(Suppl. 49), s60–s65. https://doi.org/10.1192/bjp.190.5s60

Hendriks, V. (2011). Meten en meetinstrumenten [Measuring and measurement instruments]. In I. Franken & W. Van den Brink (Eds.), *Handboek Verslaving [Handbook addiction]* (pp. 245–274). Utrecht: De Tijdstroom.

Holden, R. R. (2007). Socially desirable responding does moderate personality scale validity both in experimental and non-experimental contexts. *Canadian Journal of Behavioural Science, 39*, 184–201. https://doi.org/10.1037/cjbs2007015

Holden, R. R., & Book, A. S. (2012). Faking does distort self-report personality assessment. In M. Ziegler, C. MacCann, & R. D. Roberts (Eds.), *New perspectives on faking in personality assessment* (pp. 71–84). New York: Oxford University Press.

Holden, R. R., & Passey, J. (2010). Socially desirable responding in personality assessment: Not necessarily faking and not necessarily substance. *Personality and Individual Differences, 49*, 446–450. https://doi.org/10.1016/j.paid.2010.04.015

Hornsveld, R. H. J., Kraaimaat, F. W., Bouwmeester, S., Polak, M. A., & Zwets, A. J. (2014). Behavior on the ward of personality disordered inpatients and chronically psychotic inpatients during a three-year stay in a Dutch forensic psychiatric hospital. *The Journal of Forensic Psychiatry and Psychology, 25*, 684–704. https://doi.org/10.1080/14789949.2014.947308

Hornsveld, R. H. J., Kraaimaat, F. W., & Zwets, A. J. (2012). The Adapted Version of the Sociomoral Reflection Measure (SRM-AV) in Dutch forensic psychiatric patients. *International Journal of Forensic Mental Health, 11*, 1–9. https://doi.org/10.1080/14999013.2012.723667

Hornsveld, R. H. J., Muris, P., Kraaimaat, F. W., & Meesters, C. (2009). The Aggression Questionnaire in Dutch violent forensic psychiatric patients and secondary vocational students. *Assessment, 16*, 181–192.

Hornsveld, R. H. J., Muris, P. E. H. M., & Kraaimaat, F. W. (2011). The Novaco Anger Scale-Provocation Inventory (1994 version) in Dutch forensic psychiatric patients. *Psychological Assessment, 23*, 937–944. https://doi.org/10.1037/a0024018

Hornsveld, R. H. J., Timonen, B., Kraaimaat, F. W., Zwets, A. J., & Kanters, T. (2014). The Attitudes toward Women Inventory (AWI) in Dutch violent forensic psychiatric inpatients. *Journal of Forensic Psychology Practice, 14*, 383–397. https://doi.org/10.1080/15228932.2014.964105

Iftikhar, R., & Malik, F. (2014). Translation and validation of Aggression Questionnaire in a Pakistani children cohort. *Pakistan Journal of Social and Clinical Psychology, 12*, 39–45.

Jones, J., Thomas-Peter, B., & Gangstad, B. (2003). An investigation of the factor structure of the Novaco Anger Scale. *Behavioural and Cognitive Psychotherapy, 31*, 429–437.

Jones, J. P., Thomas-Peter, B. A., & Trout, A. (1999). Normative data for the Novaco Anger Scale from a non-clinical sample and implications for clinical use. *British Journal of Clinical Psychology, 38*, 417–424.

Kalmus, E., & Beech, A. R. (2005). Forensic assessment of sexual interest: A review. *Aggression and Violent Behavior, 10*, 193–218. https://doi.org/10.1016/j.avb.2003.12.002

Kanters, T., Hornsveld, R. H. J., Nunes, K. L., Zwets, A. J., Buck, N. M. L., Muris, P., & Van Marle, H. J. C. (2016). Aggression and social anxiety are associated with sexual offending against children. *International Journal of Forensic Mental Health, 15*, 265–273. https://doi.org/10.1080/14999013.2016.1193073.

Kelsey, K. R., Rogers, R., & Robinson, E. V. (2015). Self-report measures of psychopathy: What is their role in forensic assessments? *Journal of Psychopathology and Behavioral Assessment, 37*, 380–391. https://doi.org/10.1007/s10862-014-9475-5

Kroner, D. G., & Weekes, J. R. (1996). Balanced Inventory of Desirable Responding: Factor structure, reliability, and validity with an offender sample. *Personality and Individual Differences, 21*, 323–333.

Lilienfeld, S. O., & Widows, M. (2005). *Professional manual for the psychopathic personality inventory-revised (PPI-R)*. Lutz, FL: Psychological Assessment Resources.

Lindqvist, J. K., Dåderman, A. M., & Hellström, A. (2003). Swedish adaptations of the Novaco Anger Scale-1998, the Provocation Inventory, and the State-Trait Anger Expression Inventory-2. *Social Behavior and Personality, 31*, 773–788.

Lindqvist, J. K., Dåderman, A. M., & Hellström, A. (2005). Internal reliability and construct validity of the Novaco Anger Scale-1998-S in a sample of violent prison inmates in Sweden. *Psychology, Crime & Law, 11*, 223–237.

Loza, W. (1996) Self-Appraisal Questionnaire (SAQ): A tool for assessing violent and nonviolent recidivism. Unpublished manuscript.

Loza, W., & Green, K. (2003). The Self-Appraisal Questionnaire. A self-report measure for predicting recidivism versus clinician-administered measures: A 5-year follow-up study. *Journal of Interpersonal Violence, 18*, 781–797. https://doi.org/10.1177/0886260503253240

Mathie, N. L., & Wakeling, H. C. (2011). Assessing socially desirable responding and its impact on self-report measures among sexual offenders. *Psychology, Crime & Law, 17*, 215–237. https://doi.org/10.1080/10683160903113681

Mills, J. F., & Kroner, D. G. (1999). Measures of Criminal Attitudes and Associates (MCAA). Unpublished instrument and user's guide.

Mills, J. F., & Kroner, D. G. (2005). An investigation into the relationship between socially desirable responding and offender self-report. *Psychological Services, 2*, 70–80. https://doi.org/10.1037/1541-1559.2.1.70

Mills, J. F., & Kroner, D. G. (2006). Impression management and self-report among violent offenders. *Journal of Interpersonal Violence, 21*, 178–192. https://doi.org/10.1177/0886260505282288

Mills, J. F., Kroner, D. G., & Forth, A. E. (1998). Novaco Anger Scale: Reliability and validity within an adult criminal sample. *Assessment, 5*, 237–248.

Mills, J. F., Loza, W., & Kroner, D. G. (2003). Predictive validity despite social desirability: Evidence for the robustness of self-report among offenders. *Criminal Behaviour and Mental Health, 13*, 140–150.

Mosher, D. L., & Sirken, M. (1984). Measuring a Macho personality constellation. *Journal of Research in Personality, 18*, 150–163.

Nakano, K. (2001). Psychometric evaluation of the Japanese adaptation of the Aggression Questionnaire. *Behaviour Research and Therapy, 39*, 853–858.

Nijman, H., Bjørkly, S., Palmstierna, T., & Almvik, R. (2006). Assessing aggression of psychiatric patients: Methods of measurement and its prevalence. In D. Richter & R. Whittington (Eds.), *Violence in mental health settings. Causes, consequences, management* (pp. 11–23). New York: Springer.

Novaco, R. W. (1994). Anger as a risk factor for violence among the mentally disordered. In J. Monahan & H. J. Steadman (Eds.), *Violence and mental disorder* (pp. 21–59). Chicago, IL: University of Chicago Press.

Novaco, R. W. (2003). *The Novaco Anger Scale and Provocation Inventory: Manual*. Los Angeles, CA: Western Psychological Services.

Olver, M. E., Kingston, D. A., Nicholaichuk, T. P., & Wong, S. C. P. (2014). A psychometric examination of treatment change in a multisite sample of treated Canadian federal sexual offenders. *Law and Human Behavior, 38*, 544–559. https://doi.org/10.1037/lhb0000086

Paulhus, D. L. (1984). Two-component models of socially desirable responding. *Journal of Personality and Social Psychology, 46*, 598–609.

Paulhus, D. L. (1988). *Manual for the Balanced Inventory of Desirable Responding (BIDR-7)*. Toronto/Buffalo: Multi-Health Systems.

Paulhus, D. L. (2002). Socially desirable responding: The evolution of a construct. In H. I. Braun, D. N. Jackson, & D. E. Wiley (Eds.), *The role of constructs in psychological and educational measurement* (pp. 49–60). Mahwah, NJ: Erlbaum.

Pettersen, C., Nunes, K. L., & Cortoni, F. (2016). Does the factor structure of the Aggression Questionnaire hold for sexual offenders? *Criminal Justice and Behavior, 43*, 811–829. https://doi.org/10.1177/0093854815618692

Pettersen, C., Nunes, K. L., & Cortoni, F. (2018). The factor structure of the Aggression Questionnaire with violent offenders. *International Journal of Offender Therapy and Comparative Criminology*. Advance online publication.

Reyna, C., Ivacevich, M. G. L., Sanchez, A., & Brussino, S. (2011). The Buss-Perry Aggression Questionnaire: Construct validity and gender invariance among Argentinean adolescents. *International Journal of Psychological Research, 4*, 30–37.

Salbach-Andrae, H., Klinkowski, N., Lenz, K., & Lehmkuhl, U. (2009). Agreement between youth-reported and parent-reported psychopathology in a referred sample. *European Child & Adolescent Psychiatry, 18*, 136–143. https://doi.org/10.1007/s00787-008-0710-z

Santisteban, C., Alvarado, J. M., & Recio, P. (2007). Evaluation of a Spanish version of the Buss and Perry Aggression Questionnaire: Some personal and situational factors related to the aggression scores of young subjects. *Personality and Individual Differences, 42*, 1453–1465. https://doi.org/10.1016/j.paid.2006.10.019

Stams, G. J., Brugman, D., Dekovic, M., van Rosmalen, L., van der Laan, P., & Gibbs, J. C. (2006). The moral judgment of juvenile delinquents: A meta-analysis. *Journal of Abnormal Child Psychology, 24*, 697–713. https://doi.org/10.1007/s10802-006-9056-5

Thornton, D., Mann, R., Webster, S., Blud, L., Travers, R., Friendship, C., & Erikson, M. (2003). Distinguishing between and combining risks for sexual and violent recidivism. In R. A. Prentky, E. S. Janus, & M. C. Seton (Eds.), *Understanding and managing sexually coercive behavior. Annals of the New York Academy of Sciences, 989*, 223–235.

Van den Berg, J. W., Smid, W. J., Schepers, K., Wever, E. C., Van Beek, D. J., Janssen, E., et al. (2018). The predictive properties of dynamic sex offender risk assessment instruments: A meta-analysis. *Psychological Assessment, 30*, 179–191. https://doi.org/10.1037/pas0000454

Van Vugt, E., Gibbs, J., Stams, G. J., Bijleveld, C., Hendriks, J., & Van der Laan, P. (2011). Moral development and recidivism: A meta-analysis. *International Journal of Offender Therapy and Comparative Criminology, 55*, 1234–1250. https://doi.org/10.1177/0306624X10396441

Von Collani, G., & Werner, R. (2005). Self-related and motivational constructs as determinants of aggression. An analysis and validation of a German version of the Buss-Perry Aggression Questionnaire. *Personality and Individual Differences, 38*, 1631–1643. https://doi.org/10.1016/j.paid.2004.09.027

Walters, G. D. (2006). Risk-appraisal versus self-report in the prediction of criminal justice outcomes: A meta-analysis. *Criminal Justice and Behavior, 33*, 279–304. https://doi.org/10.1177/0093854805284409

Webster, S. D., Mann, R. E., Thornton, D., & Wakeling, H. C. (2006). Further validation of the short self-esteem scale with sexual offenders. *Legal and Criminological Psychology, 12*, 207–216.

Williams, T. Y., Boyd, J. C., Cascardi, M. A., & Poythress, N. (1996). Factor structure and convergent validity of the Aggression Questionnaire in an offender population. *Psychological Assessment, 8*, 398–403.

Chapter 4
Assessment of Violent and Sexually Violent Offenders

Ruud H. J. Hornsveld, Floris W. Kraaimaat, Kevin L. Nunes, and Emma J. Palmer

4.1 Introduction

Assessment of violent offenders has two functions. First, to identify treatment needs/risk factors at the point of assessment. Secondly, to evaluate changes that have occurred as a result of treatment and to see if this has resulted in a reduced risk of future violent behavior. Researchers such as Andrews and Bonta (2010) have argued that in the assessment of offenders a combination of different types of measuring instruments such as structured interviews, observation scales, self-report questionnaires, and incident recording has to be used because each type of instrument has its advantages and disadvantages. The collected information must therefore always be related to the limitations of the instrument in question (Drenth & Sijtsma, 2006). Diagnostics and researchers of detainees and forensic psychiatric patients should also realize that the controlled and structured environment of penitentiary institution or a forensic psychiatric institution can have a disruptive and often dampening effect on the behavior, whether measured with a self-report questionnaire, an observation scale, or a risk assessment instrument (Hornsveld, Kraaimaat,

R. H. J. Hornsveld (✉)
Erasmus University Medical Center, Rotterdam, The Netherlands
e-mail: ruud.hornsveld@ziggo.nl

F. W. Kraaimaat
Radboud University Nijmegen, Nijmegen, The Netherlands

K. L. Nunes
Carleton University, Ottawa, Canada

E. J. Palmer
University of Leicester, Leicester, UK

R. H. J. Hornsveld et al. (eds.), *Assessment and Obligatory Treatment of Violent and Sexually Violent Offenders*, Advances in Preventing and Treating Violence and Aggression, https://doi.org/10.1007/978-3-030-27840-3_4

Bouwmeester, Polak, & Zwets, 2014). There is also a chance that patients or detainees may show socially desirable behavior because they know that they are being observed (see Chap. 3).

4.2 Psychiatric evaluation

For the assessment of DSM-5 classifications (American Psychiatric Association, 2013), two versions of the Structured Clinical Interview can be used, namely the *SCID-5-CV* and the *SCID-5-DP.* The *Structured Clinical Interview for DSM-5 Disorders, Clinician Version* (SCID-5-CV; First, Williams, Karg, & Spitzer, 2015) is a semi-structured interview for the classification of formerly Axis I disorders and is divided into the following relatively independent modules: mood episodes and persistent depressive disorder, psychotic and related symptoms, differential diagnosis of psychotic disorders, differential diagnosis of mood disorders, disorders in the use of a drug, anxiety disorders, obsessive-compulsive disorder and post-traumatic stress disorder, attention deficit/hyperactivity disorder in adults, screening for other current disorders, and adaptation disorder. The *Structured Clinical Interview for DSM-5 Personality Disorders* (SCID-5-DP; First, Spitzer, Williams, & Benjamin, 2015) is a semi-structured interview for the assessment of the following personality disorders: paranoid, schizoid, schizotypal, antisocial, borderline, histrionic, narcissistic, avoidant, dependent, and obsessive-compulsive. Interviews are conducted by a clinician or qualified mental health care professional with knowledge and insight into the DSM-5 classification and the classification criteria. Freedman et al. (2013) found that the interrater reliability of 15 DSM-5 classifications varied from good to very good but was questionable for antisocial personality disorder and four other classifications. A study by Narrow et al. (2013) revealed that the test–retest reliabilities of DSM-5 symptoms were good or excellent.

When psychotic disorders are suspected, the *Positive and Negative Syndrome Scale* (PANSS; Kay, Fiszbein, & Opler, 1987) can be considered for assessment or further exploration. This scale has 30 items divided into three subscales: The Positive Scale (7 items), Negative Scale (7 items), and a General Psychopathology Scale (16 items). Each item on the PANSS is accompanied by a complete definition as well as detailed anchoring criteria for all seven rating points, which represent increasing levels of psychopathology: 1 = absent, 2 = minimal, 3 = mild, 4 = moderate, 5 = moderate-severe, 6 = severe, and 7 = extreme. In assigning ratings, the scorer first refers to the item definition to determine the presence of a symptom. The severity of an item, if present, is then judged by deciding which anchoring point best characterizes the patient's functioning, whether or not all elements of the description are observed. The highest applicable rating point is always assigned, even if the patient meets criteria for lower ratings as well. Kay, Opler, and Lindenmayer (1988) found in a sample of 82 acute and chronic schizophrenics that the interrater reliabilities were in the 0.80's, and significant correlations emerged with corresponding criterion measures. The PANSS positive and negative scales were inversely intercorrelated when general psychopathology had been partialed out.

Various later studies have questioned the reliability, the validity, and the subscale structure of the PANSS. For instance, Van der Gaag et al. (2006a, 2006b) could not confirm a five-factor structure, previously found in 25 earlier studies on the factor structure of the PANSS. Their factor-analytic study with a sample of 5,769 schizophrenic patients revealed a different solution with five factors, namely Positive symptoms, Negative symptoms, Disorganization symptoms, Excitement, and Emotional distress. This revised five-factor model covers all 30 items of the PANSS. Khan et al. (2013) examined the cross-cultural differences of the PANSS across six geo-cultural regions. Data were obtained for 1,169 raters from Eastern Asia, India, Northern Europe, Russia plus Ukraine, Southern Europe, and the United States. They concluded that there were significant differences in response to a number of items on the PANSS, possibly caused by a lack of equivalence between the original and translated versions, cultural differences among interpretation of items or scoring parameters. Finally, a study by Wu, Lan, Hu, Lee, and Liou (2015) on the validation of a Chinese-Mandarin version of the PANSS in a sample of 813 schizophrenic patients yielded a Cronbach's alpha of 0.928 and intra-class coefficient of 0.878. A confirmatory factor analysis of 17 items resulted in a good fit with five factors, namely Positive, Negative, Cognitive, Depressive, and Excitement.

4.3 Risk Assessment

Risk assessment is a method of determining the (statistical) probability that an offender will re-offend, which is needed to determine the intensity of treatment for offenders and the likelihood of reoffending after discharge (Bonta & Andrews, 2007; Prentky, Barbaree, & Janus, 2015). The available risk assessment methods can be categorized into two main approaches: clinical judgment and actuarial assessment (Hanson, 2000). The clinical judgment approach determines risk levels with clinical evaluations from forensic clinicians, which can be solely based on personal experience (unstructured clinical judgment) or guided by a list of relevant risk factors associated with sexual recidivism (structured professional judgment). In contrast with actuarial risk assessment, risk levels are determined by the presence/absence of empirically well-supported factors that differentiate (sexual) recidivists from non-recidivists. Risk assessment instruments can be distinguished between actuarial measures that use static (historical) factors such as age at first offense and prior criminal history, and those that use a combination of static and dynamic (changeable) risk factors such as substance abuse and unemployment. Risk assessment instruments with static and dynamic risk factors predict better than those with just static risk factors (Eher, Matthes, Schilling, Haubner-MacLean, & Rettenberger, 2012; Klepfisz, Daffern, & Day, 2016; Mann, Hanson, & Thornton, 2010).

Risk levels can be calculated by solely using a statistical scoring algorithm (pure actuarial approach), which can be adjusted afterwards based on essential considerations not addressed in the standardized assessment (adjusted actuarial approach).

Individual risk scores are compared to recidivism rates of large offender groups with similar risk levels, indicating the probable rate of (sexual) recidivism for that individual. Almost all risk assessment methods emphasize the use of various risk factors for determining recidivism, and there is consensus for the superiority of structured approaches over unstructured approaches (Grove, 2005; Hanson & Morton-Bourgon, 2009). Assessment, including risk assessment, is done before and after treatment intervention. To promote treatment motivation, the use of risk assessment instruments of so-called protective factors can be considered, although their contribution to the estimate of recidivism risk is unclear (Klein, Rettenberger, Yoon, Köhler, & Briken, 2014; Tharp et al., 2012; Thornton, Kelley, & Nelligan, 2017).

4.3.1 Violent Offenders

One of the most often used violent risk assessment instruments is the *Historical Clinical Risk Management-20, version 3* (HCR-20^{V3}; Douglas, Hart, Webster, Belfrage, & Guy, 2014; Hart, Webster, Belfrage, Guy, & Wilson, 2014). The HCR-20 is an instrument for assessing risk of violent behavior with 20 items divided into three subscales, namely a Historical scale (10 items, for example, item H5: Substance Use), a Clinical scale (5 items, for example, item C2: Violent Ideation or Intent), and a Risk Management scale (5 items, for example, R3: Personal Support). The items are evaluated for presence by using a seven-point scale (no / no + /partly – / partly / partly + / yes – / yes) and on relevance to a three-point scale (low/moderate/ high). Based on the scores on the scales a final judgment on violence, serious bodily injury or acute threatening weight fire using a five-point scale (low/low-moderate/ moderate/moderate-high/high).

Another frequently used risk assessment instrument is the *Level of Service Inventory-Revised* (LSI-R; Andrews & Bonta, 1995), which has 54 items divided into ten domains: Criminal History, Education/Employment, Financial, Family/ Marital, Accommodation, Leisure/Recreation, Companions, Alcohol/Drug Problems, Emotional/Personal, and Attitude/Orientation. Although the LSI-R is not designed to assess the risk of violent recidivism, there is a growing body of research supporting the use of the LSI-R to assess the risk of general recidivism for different offender groups, including violent offenders. The LSI-R has been revised into the LS/CMI (Andrews, Bonta, & Wormith, 2004) to include case management strategies (Craig, Beech, & Cortoni, 2013).

For the assessment of psychopathy, the most widely used instrument is the *Psychopathy Checklist-Revised* (PCL-R; Hare, 1991, 2003). The 2003 version of this list includes 20 items, with four facets: Interpersonal (e.g., grandiose self-worth), Affective (e.g., callous/Lack of empathy), Lifestyle (e.g., impulsivity), and Antisocial (e.g., juvenile delinquency). The items are scored using a three-point scale, with 0 = "not applicable," 1 = "slightly applicable," and 2 = "applicable." In the United States, a score of 30 is used as a cutoff score for psychopathy, but in Europe, a cutoff score of 25 is more commonly used (Lammers, Keulen-de Vos, De Groot, & Uzieblo, 2015). In a recent study by Zwets, Hornsveld, Neumann, Muris, and Van Marle (2015b), the four-facet structure could be confirmed in Dutch forensic psychiatric inpatients, with both a personality disorder and a chronic psychotic disorder as their main diagnosis.

4.3.2 Dynamic Risk Assessment

According to Morgan, Kroner, and Mills (2012), several studies have demonstrated that dynamic variables are important proximal antecedents in the prediction of criminal behavior. For example, Quinsey, Jones, Book, and Barr (2006) developed the *Dynamic Risk Appraisal Scale* (DRAS, Quinsey, Harris, Rice, & Cormier, 2005) using items from the Problem Identification Checklist (PIC; Rice, Harris, Quinsey, & Cyr, 1990) and the Proximal Risk Factor Scale (PRFS; Quinsey, Coleman, Jones, & Altrows, 1997). The DRAS contains 23 items for general risk and a subscale with ten items for violence risk, which have to be completed by the patient's or client's caregiver. The scale has been studied in a sample of 568 Canadian forensic psychiatric patients, partly institutionalized, partly living in the community, by completing it monthly for an average of 33 months. During the follow-up, there were 265 incidents, 86 of which were violent. The authors found that the average ratings on the scale differentiated patients who had incidents of a violent or sexual nature from those who did not. Also, changes in monthly staff ratings predicted the imminent occurrence of antisocial and violent behaviors.

Using a revised version of the *Problem Identification Checklist* (PIC-R; Ostapiuk, Stringer, & Craig, 2000), Nagi, Ostapiuk, Craig, Hacker, and Beech (2009) found in a sample of 25 British psychiatric inpatients and 24 outpatients preliminary validation for the predictive accuracy of the PIC-R for violence. Additionally, the findings suggested that short-term risk of violence within a population of mostly psychotic patients may be more related to dynamic and clinical risk variables rather than to static ones. However, in a study of Philipse, Koeter, Van der Staak, and Van den Brink (2006), data on static and dynamic risk factors were collected for 151 patients discharged from Dutch forensic psychiatric hospitals. They concluded that a small set of static predictors yielded a reasonable estimate of future reconvictions and that inclusion of dynamic predictors did not add predictive power.

4.3.3 Sexually Violent Offenders

For the assessment of sexually violent offenders, several specific instruments are available (Rettenberger, Matthes, Boer, & Eher, 2010), such as the *Sexual Violence Risk-20* (SVR-20; Boer, Wilson, Gauthier, & Hart, 1997). The SVR-20 is a checklist of 20 items that are classified into three subscales, namely Sexual Offenses (7 items about past sexual offenses), Psychosocial Adjustment (11 items about other relatively stable features and current functioning), and Future Plans (2 items about current and future functioning). For the (negative formulated) items there are the following scoring options: 0 = absent, 1 = possibly present, and 2 = clearly present. Item scores can be added together as a measure of the likelihood of sexual violence recidivism, but assessors also need to use their clinical judgment in attributing sex offenders to risk categories. A recent study by Kanters et al. (2017) showed that the structured professional judgment of the SVR-20 in Dutch forensic psychiatric inpatients was more predictive of sexual, violent, and general recidivism than its actuarial scoring method. However, this finding is in contrast with the overall superiority of actuarial measures for predicting recidivism. For instance, a study by Rettenberger, Boer, and Eher (2011) revealed that the SVR-20 total score yields moderate to good predictive accuracy for general criminal, violent, general sexual, and sexual hands-on recidivism after an average follow-up period of more than 4 years.

An alternative to the SVR-20 is the Static/Stable/Acute (SSA) group of measures, in which the Static-99R (Harris, Phenix, Hanson, & Thornton, 2003) is used to assess recidivism risk, the Stable-2007 (Fernandez, Harris, Hanson, & Sparks, 2012) is used to determine stable dynamic criminological factors, and the Acute-2007 (Hanson & Harris, 2012) is used for the measurement of acute dynamic risk factors. The *Static-99R* is a ten-point review tool, with most items scored on a two-point scale (for example, item 8: (unrelated victim): 0/1) and sometimes with a four-point scale (for example, item 5 (previous sexual offenses): 0/1/2/3). The total score is the sum of the items. The total score can be classified in a risk category, ranging from low through low-average to average-high to high. The *Stable 2007* contains 12 stable dynamic items, for example, item 3: emotional identification with children. Items are scored using response categories. There is an additional item for offenders with victims under 14 years. The total score can be assigned to the risk categories "low, moderate, or high." The *Acute 2007* contains seven acute dynamic risk factors, for example, item 3: sexual preoccupation. Items are also scored based on response categories. The total score may range from low to moderate to high.

4.4 Instruments for Problem Behaviors and Personality Domains

4.4.1 Self-Report Questionnaires for Problem Behaviors

While there are many measures that assess anger and aggression, there are three questionnaires which are recommended because translations are available in several non-English-speaking populations, namely the Novaco Anger Scale-Provocation Inventory (NAS-PI; Novaco, 1994, 2003), the Aggression Questionnaire (AQ; Buss & Perry, 1992; Buss & Warren, 2000), and the Aggression Questionnaire-Short Form (AQ-SF; Bryant & Smith, 2001)[1].

[1]Dutch versions, scoring, factors, and norms can be found in: Hornsveld, R. H. J. (2018), *Meetinstrumenten voor de forensische psychiatrie.* Rijswijk, NL: Challenger Press. Available at: https://www.agressiehanteringstherapie.nl/nl/menu/boeken

The *Novaco Anger Scale-Provocation Inventory* (NAS-PI; Novaco, 1994, 2003) is a two-part questionnaire to assess anger as a problem of psychological functioning. The original NAS-part contained 48 items in three interrelated subscales, namely Cognitive ("I feel like I am getting a raw deal out of life."), Arousal (e.g., "I feel agitated and unable to relax."), and Behavioral (e.g., "When someone yells at me, I yell back at them."). In 2003, Novaco added the fourth scale of Anger Regulation to the NAS that has 12 items (e.g., "If someone says something nasty, I can swallow my pride and let it go."). Items are rated on a three-point scale (1 = never true, 2 = sometimes true, 3 = always true). The PI-part has 25 items that refer to anger-eliciting situations (e.g., "Someone keeps making noise when you are trying to concentrate.") rated on a four-point scale (1 = not at all angry, 2 = a little angry, 3 = fairly angry, 4 = very angry). Translated versions of the NAS-PI have been used in the Netherlands (1994 version; Hornsveld, Muris, & Kraaimaat, 2011) and Sweden (1998 version; Lindqvist, Dåderman, & Hellström, 2005). More information on the psychometric properties of the NAS-PI is provided in Chap. 3.

The *Aggression Questionnaire* (AQ; Buss & Perry, 1992; Buss & Warren, 2000) originally had 29 items spread among four subscales, namely Physical Aggression (e.g., "I have threatened people I know"), Verbal Aggression (e.g., "My friends say I'm somewhat argumentative"), Anger (e.g., "I have trouble controlling my temper"), and Hostility (e.g., "Other people always seem to get the breaks"). Respondents answered the items on this version of the AQ using a five-point scale ranging from 1 = extremely uncharacteristic of me to 5 = extremely characteristic of me. In 2001, Buss and Warren published a new version of the AQ with 34 items, 27 (often reformulated) items of the original version and six new items in a fifth subscale Indirect Aggression. Items of this new version are scored using a scale ranging from 1 = not at all like me to 5 = completely like me. Translations of the original AQ have been used in countries including Argentina (Reyna, Ivacevich, Sanchez, & Brussino, 2011), France (Genoud & Zimmermann, 2009), Germany (Von Collani & Werner, 2005), Italy (Fossati, Maffei, Acquarini, & Di Ceglie, 2003), Japan (Nakano, 2001), the Netherlands (Hornsveld, Muris, Kraaimaat, & Meesters, 2009), Pakistan (Iftikhar & Malik, 2014), and Spain (Santisteban, Alvarado, and Recio (2007). For more information on the psychometric properties of the original AQ, see Chap. 3.

The *Aggression Questionnaire-Short Form* (AQ-SF; Bryant & Smith, 2001) is a shortened version of the Aggression Questionnaire of Buss and Perry (1992) with 12 items across the same four subscales as the full AQ. A translated version of the AQ-SF has been used, among others, in the Netherlands (Hornsveld et al., 2009). More information on the AQ-SF can be found in Chap. 3.

For the measurement of social anxiety and social skills, several instruments are available. The *Inventory of Interpersonal Situations* (IIS; Van Dam-Baggen & Kraaimaat, 1999) is recommended because it is a self-report questionnaire with both a Discomfort and a Frequency scale, each consisting of the same 35 items formulated as responses to specific social situations. The reliability and validity of the IIS have been investigated in several adult psychiatric and non-psychiatric samples. Factor analysis of the Discomfort scale yielded five components representing the following domains of social behavior: expressing criticism and opinion, giving compliments, initiating contacts, positive self-statements, and doing and refusing requests. The Frequency scale showed a rather clear structure of eight components that represent the following domains of social behavior: giving criticism, expressing an opinion, giving compliments, initiating contacts, positive self-statements, stand up for yourself, making a request, and refusing a request. The scales of Discomfort and Frequency showed stability over time. Cronbach's α's revealed a sufficiently high internal consistency on both scales, while the conceptual structure was shown to be rather invariant across socially anxious and non-socially anxious groups. The IIS scales were able to discriminate between socially anxious and non-socially anxious samples and showed significant relationships with independent measures of social anxiety. The IIS scales demonstrated high predictive validity for overt behavior in social situations. The IIS is currently available in both British and American English, Dutch, French, German, and Turkish versions (www.floriskraaimaat.nl)..

Other frequently used self-report questionnaires for social anxiety or social phobia are the Social Phobia and Anxiety Inventory (SPAI; Turner, Beidel, Dancu, & Stanley, 1989), the Social Phobia Scale (SPS; Mattick & Clarke, 1998), and the Social Interaction Anxiety Scale (SIAS; Mattick & Clarke, 1998). The SPAI assesses specific somatic symptoms, cognitions, and behavior across a range of potentially fear-producing situations. The SPS measures fears of being scrutinized or observed by others during routine activities (e.g., "I get nervous that people are staring at me as I walk down the street."), whereas the SIAS assesses anxiety related to interactions with others (e.g., "I find it difficult to disagree with another's point of view."). Both the SPS and SIAS were designed to measure the subtypes of nongeneralized and generalized social phobia according to the DSM-IIIR or DSM-IV criteria (American Psychiatric Association, 1987, 1994). Several studies have shown that these instruments have acceptable to excellent psychometric properties (Olivares, García-López, & Hidalgo, 2001) and are all able to make distinctions between social phobic patients and patients with other anxiety disorder diagnoses. However, the SPAI appeared to be a better predictor of social phobia group membership than the SPS and the SIAS (Peters, 2000). Spanish versions of the SPS and SIAS are available (Olivares et al., 2001).

4.4.2 Self-Report Questionnaires for Personality Domains

Several authors have provided evidence for the relation of Big Five personality traits with aggression and violence (Barlett & Anderson, 2012; Jones, Miller, & Lynam, 2011). For the measurement of these traits, the use of the *NEO Five-Factor Inventory* (NEO-FFI; Costa Jr. & McCrae, 1992) is recommended. The NEO-FFI has 60 items and measures the Big Five personality domains, namely Neuroticism, Extraversion, Openness, Agreeableness, and Conscientiousness. Participants score items on a five-point Likert scale, ranging from 1 = entirely disagree to 5 = entirely agree. In a Dutch sample of 356 nonclinical adults, Cronbach's alphas ranged between 0.69

and 0.82 for various subscales. In a subgroup of 135 adults the test–retest reliability after 6 months was 0.82, 0.87, 0.81, 0.75, and 0.80, respectively (Hoekstra, Ormel, & De Fruyt, 1996). In 2004, McCrae and Costa introduced a new version of the NEO-FFI, the NEO-FFI-R with 14 new items, especially for populations where literacy is likely to be a problem. However, the improvements of the psychometric properties over the original NEO-FFI appeared to be modest (McCrae, Costa Jr., & Martin, 2005). According to these authors, for most purposes, the original version of the instrument, with its established norms, will continue to suffice. Jones et al. (2011) found indications that the domains Neuroticism, Agreeableness, and Conscientiousness were related to antisocial and aggressive behavior. More specifically the research of Barlett and Anderson (2012) suggested that Agreeableness was indirectly negatively related to aggressive behavior via both aggressive emotions and aggressive attitudes. Neuroticism was indirectly related to aggressive behavior through aggressive emotions. Openness was indirectly related to aggressive behavior through aggressive attitudes. For violent behavior, Agreeableness and Openness were indirectly related to violent behavior through aggressive attitudes. Openness, Agreeableness, and Neuroticism all predicted physical aggression. No direct relations were found between the Big 5 and violent behavior. The NEO-FFI has been translated into Dutch (Hoekstra et al., 1996), French (Rolland, Parker, & Stumpf, 1998), German (Schmitz, Hartkamp, Baldini, Rollnik, & Tress, 2001), and Icelandic (Bjornsdottir et al., 2014).

The *Barratt Impulsiveness Scale-11* (BIS-11; Patton, Stanford, & Barratt, 1995) is a 30-item self-report questionnaire designed to assess the personality/behavioral construct of impulsiveness (Stanford et al., 2009). Items are scored on a four-point Likert scale, ranging from 1 ("Rarely/Never") to 4 ("Almost Always/Always"). The tenth version of the original BIS (Barratt, 1959), the BIS-10 (Barratt, 1985), was redesigned to measure the subtraits of Cognitive Impulsiveness (making quick decisions), Motor Impulsiveness (acting without thinking), and Non-Planning Impulsiveness (lack of "futuring" or forethought). A factor analysis of the BIS-11, completed by 412 university students, yielded six first-order factors, namely attention, motor, self-control, cognitive complexity, perseverance, and cognitive instability. An oblique rotation of the first-order factors showed the expected second-order factors Motor Impulsiveness and Non-planning Impulsiveness, but the third factor became labeled Attentional Impulsiveness and was defined as the inability to focus attention or concentrate. According to Stanford et al., the BIS-11 is sensitive to differences in levels of aggression. For instance, violent offenders appeared to score higher on the BIS-11 than nonviolent offenders and nonclinical volunteers (Smith, Waterman, & Ward, 2006). Dolan and Fullam (2004) found in a sample of 40 personality-disordered, violent offenders that impulsivity was significantly correlated with reactive aggression rather than with instrumental aggression. The BIS-11 has been translated into Chinese (Yao, Yang, Zhu, Auerbach, Abela, Pulleyblank, et al., 2007), Dialectal Arabic (Ellouze, Ghaffari, Zouari, Zouari, & M'rad, 2013), Dutch (Lijffijt & Barratt, 2005), German (Hartmann, Rief, & Hilbert, 2011), Italian (Fossati, Di Ceglie, Acquarini, & Barratt, 2001), Norwegian (Lindstrøm, Wyller, Halvorsen, Hartberg, & Lundqvist, 2017), Japanese (Someya et al., 2001), and Portuguese (Pechorro, Maroco, Ray, & Gonçalves, 2015).

The *State-Trait Anger Expression Inventory-2* (STAXI-2; Spielberger, 1999) is a self-report questionnaire designed to measure trait and state anger. It was derived from the original STAXI (Spielberger, 1988), which was designed to (a) understand the multidimensional components of anger that are distinct from the constructs of hostility and aggression, (b) specifically differentiate between state and trait anger, and (c) distinguish the experience of anger from the expression of anger (Eckhardt, Norlander, & Deffenbacher, 2004). The 44 items of the original STAXI are divided into six scales and two subscales measuring the experience and expression of anger. Experiences of anger are divided into State Anger and Trait Anger, the latter further divided into Angry Temperament and Angry Reaction. Anger expression is divided into Anger-Out, Anger-In, and Anger Control. The psychometric properties of the original STAXI have been evaluated among different populations (Mela et al., 2008) and different countries such as Norway (Haseth, 1996), Russia (Kassinove, Sukhodolsky, Eckhardt, & Tsytsarev, 1997), and Singapore (Bishop & Quah, 1998). In 1999, Spielberger released the STAXI-2, consisting of 42 of the 44 items from the original STAXI plus 15 additional items. The 57 items are divided into six scales, namely State Anger (15 items), Trait Anger (10 items), Anger Expression-Out (8 items), Anger Expression-In (8 items), Anger Control-Out (8 items), and Anger Control-In (8 items). Items consist of four-point scales that assess the intensity of anger at a particular moment and the frequency of anger experience, expression, and control. Factor analytic studies mostly support this new structure, although there is some degree of item overlap across the feeling angry and expressing anger verbally factors. An investigation by Etzler, Rohrmann, and Brandt (2014) with a German version of the STAXI-2 in 57 male inmates revealed that internal consistencies had high reliability and that subscale intercorrelations are close to those of the standardization sample. They also found that Anger Expression-Out and Anger Expression-In were related to the length of sentence and that Trait Anger was associated with the age of the first offense. The STAXI-2 has been translated into Chinese (Maxwell, Sukhodolsky, & Sit, 2009), Dutch (Hovens, Lievaart, & Rodenburg, 2014), Farsi (Khodayarifard, Spielberger, Lavasani, and Zardkhaneh (2013), French (Borteyroua, Bruchon-Schweitzer, & Spielberger, 2008), Spanish (Culhane & Morera, 2010), and Swedish (Lindqvist, Dåderman, & Hellström, 2003).

4.4.3 Recently Developed Self-Report Questionnaires

For several dynamic criminogenic factors, new self-report questionnaires have been developed, but it should be noted that these questionnaires are still at an experimental stage. It concerns questionnaires for the measurement of hostility, moral maturity, and attitudes toward women[2]. These three instruments have been developed in Dutch offender and nonclinical populations.

---

[2] Items, scoring, factors, and norms can be found in: Hornsveld, R. H. J. (2018), *Meetinstrumenten voor de forensische psychiatrie*. Rijswijk, NL: Challenger Press. Available at: https://www.agressiehanteringstherapie.nl/nl/menu/boeken.

The *Adapted Version* of Rosenzweig's (1978) *Picture-Frustration Study* (PFS-AV; Hornsveld, Nijman, Hollin, & Kraaimaat, 2007a) has been developed to measure hostility. The test asks participants to write down their reactions to 12 cartoon-like pictures. Respondents are instructed to examine the situation as shown in the pictures (e.g., to a shopkeeper: "This is the third time that this watch has stopped.") and to write the first appropriate reply in the blank text box that enters their mind. Answers are scored by an experienced and independent research assistant (psychologist) on a seven-point scale, ranging from 1 = not at all hostile to 7 = extremely hostile. In a sample of 231 Dutch violent forensic psychiatric patients, the internal consistency ($\alpha = 0.76$), test–retest reliability ($r = 0.67$), and interrater reliability ($r = 0.77$) of the PFS-AV were moderate to good. Furthermore, evidence was found for the convergent validity of the test as scores correlated with indices of agreeableness and aggressive behavior (Hornsveld et al., 2007).

The *Attitudes toward Women Inventory* (AWI; Hornsveld, Timonen, Kraaimaat, Zwets, & Kanters, 2014) comprises 12 items. Items are formulated as propositions, and respondents have to indicate their opinion on a five-point Likert scale, running from 1 = Completely disagree to 5 = Completely agree. Then, respondents have to clarify their opinion by completing a sentence, which starts with "I think this because ...." Starting from the score on the disagree/agree scale, the respondents' clarification in terms of masculine attitudes is scored using a seven-point Likert scale with the following scoring possibilities: 1 = Not at all, 2 = Minimal, 3 = Somewhat, 4 = Moderate, 5 = Strong, 6 = Very strong, and 7 = Extreme. In scoring the items, the assessor has some examples of each possibility at their disposal. The answers to questions regarding the (dis)agreement of a proposition are not further used. These questions are designed to stimulate respondents to think about their opinion before writing it down. In a sample of 78 Dutch forensic psychiatric inpatients and 36 amateur soccer players, the AWI showed an internal consistency of 0.82, a mean item-total correlation of 0.49, a mean inter-item correlation of 0.30, interrater reliability of 0.94, and a test–retest reliability of 0.85 (Hornsveld et al., 2014). A factor analysis yielded three provisional factors: (1) sexist behavior of men, (2) inappropriate behavior of women, and (3) duties of women. The validity of the AWI was supported in the patient group by negative correlations with the personality domains of agreeableness and conscientiousness and by positive correlations with hostility and verbal aggression. An alternative for the AWI is the *Hostility toward Women Scale* (Check, 2014) with 30 items. The scale appeared to be reliable and was found to consistently predict a number of self-report measures of rape-related attitudes, motivations, and behavior. Although the scale did not correlate exclusively with aggression against women, it predicted both the self-report and the behavioral criterion variables better than a measure of general hostility (Spielberger Trait Anger Scale).

The *Adapted Version of the Sociomoral Reflection Measure* (SRM-AV; Hornsveld, Kraaimaat, & Zwets, 2012) is intended for measuring moral maturity. The instrument comprises 20 items in the form of statements, divided over four subscales, namely: expecting decent behavior from others (for example: "How important do you think that others treat you with respect?"), addressing others for their misbehavior (for example: "Imagine: you see that a friend of yours is dealing with hard drugs, how important is it that this is forbidden?"), exhibiting decent behavior toward others (for example: "How important is it that people, in general, are honest?"), and helping needy people (for example: "Imagine: someone with a disability does not dare to cross the street, how important is it to help that person with crossing the road?"). Respondents are first asked how important they find the statement put in an item, followed by the question to write down the arguments for their opinion. For the scoring of the answers to the importance of a statement, a five-point scale is used, ranging from 1 = very unimportant to 5 = very important. The answers to the question about their reasons are scored using a seven-point scale. The points on this scale have been described by the four phases and three transition phases of Gibbs, Basinger, and Fuller (1992). Hornsveld et al. (2012) found in a sample of 80 Dutch forensic psychiatric inpatients that the interrater reliability was 0.84 and internal consistency (Cronbach's α) 0.94. In a subgroup of 71 patients, test–retest reliability appeared to be 0.77. The validity of the SRM-AV was supported by significant correlations with age and psychopathy, agreeableness, and verbal aggression.

4.4.4 Neuropsychological Tests

The *Cued Go No-Go Task* (Fillmore, 2003) is a reaction time task for measuring attention and impulsivity. It measures impulse control by the ability to inhibit instigated, "prepotent" responses. The task is presented on a screen and participants have to indicate their choice by pressing a computer key. Response prepotency is manipulated by presenting a preliminary go or no-go cue before the actual go or no-go target is displayed. The cues provide information concerning the probability that a go or no-go target will be presented. The cue-target relationship is manipulated so that the cues have a high probability of correctly signaling a go or no-go target (valid cues), and a low probability of incorrectly signaling a target (invalid cues). Valid cues tend to facilitate response inhibition and speed response execution, whereas invalid cue cues tend to impair response inhibition and slow response execution (Fillmore & Weafer, 2013). In case of an invalid go cue trial, following a fixation, the go cue is presented so that the subject prepares to respond to the expected go target. When the no-go target appears, the subject often fails to inhibit the response, and incorrectly responds to the no-go target. This is the critical trial condition that is used to assess the subject's inhibitory control over a prepotent response. Poor inhibitory control is evident in more failures to inhibit responses in this condition. The test comprises 250 trials and requires 15 min to complete. Some evidence for the validity of the cued go no-go task comes from its use in assessing clinical populations of children and young adults with ADHD which are also characterized by impulsivity. Studies using the cued go no-go task found that subjects with ADHD typically display more commission errors and slower response inhibition compared with controls (Derefinko et al., 2008; Roberts, Milich, & Fillmore, 2012; Weafer, Fillmore, & Milich, 2009).

4.4.5 Observation Checklists

Observation checklists can be divided into scales that ask staff members to record the behavior of a person over a past period and scales that staff members can use to register incidents. Examples of the first are the *Observation Scale for Aggressive Behavior* (OSAB; Hornsveld, Nijman, Hollin, & Kraaimaat, 2007b) and the *Forensic Inpatient Observation Scale* (FIOS; Timmerman, Vastenburg, & Emmelkamp, 2001), and of the second are the *Staff Observation Aggression Scale-Revised* (SOAS-R; Nijman et al., 1999) and the *Social Dysfunction and Aggression Scale* (SDAS; Wistedt et al., 1990).

The *Observation Scale for Aggressive Behavior* (OSAB; Hornsveld et al., 2007b) measures behavior on the ward. The scale comprises 40 items[3] spread over the subscales Irritation/Anger (e.g., "Hostility"), Anxiety/Gloominess (e.g., "Tense"), Aggressive Behavior (e.g., "Threats toward staff"), Social Behavior (e.g., "Gives his opinion adequately"), Antecedent (e.g., "Restraining measure"), and Sanction (e.g., "Must apologize"). The staff scores the behavior of inpatients in the preceding week on a four-point scale with 1 = no, 2 = seldom, 3 = occasionally, and 4 = frequently. The psychometric qualities of the OSAB were studied in a sample of 220 Dutch violent forensic psychiatric inpatients. Results showed that the internal consistency of the subscales varied from 0.63 to 0.93, interrater reliability correlations were between 0.49 and 0.81, whereas test–retest reliability ranged between 0.48 and 0.79.

The *Forensic Inpatient Observation Scale* (FIOS; Timmerman et al., 2001) has 35 items divided into six factors, namely Self-care, Social Behavior, Oppositional Behavior, Insight Offense/Problems, Verbal Skills, and Distress. A study of 78 Dutch forensic psychiatric inpatients found that the internal consistency of the scales ranged from 0.73 to 0.91 and that the scales appear to be measuring independent constructs. The interrater reliability of the scale was rather poor and ranged from 0.50 to 0.69. To examine the concurrent validity with the OSAB, Hornsveld et al. (2007b) correlated the OSAB with the FIOS subscales. Significant correlations were found between the OSAB Irritation/Anger and Aggressive Behavior subscales on the one hand and the FIOS Oppositional Behavior subscale on the other hand and between the OSAB Anxiety/Gloominess subscale and the FIOS Distress subscale. Moreover, the OSAB Social Behavior subscale showed a relatively high positive correlation with the FIOS Social Behavior subscale. Also, a significant negative relationship was found between the OSAB Aggressive Behavior subscale and the FIOS Social Behavior subscale. No significant correlations were found for either the OSAB or FIOS between the Aggressive and Oppositional Behavior subscales and the Social Behavior subscale successively.

The *Staff Observation Aggression Scale-Revised* (SOAS-R; Nijman et al., 1999) consists of five areas in which aggressive outbursts have to be recorded: (a) the

[3] Items and scoring can be found at https://www.agressiehanteringstherapie.nl/nl/menu/meetinstrumenten.

apparent provocation, which led to the aggressive event, (b) the means used by the patient during the aggressive event, (c) the target of aggression, (d) the consequence(s) for the victim(s) of the aggression, and (e) the measures taken to stop the aggression. Initially, good interrater reliability, intraclass correlation of .96 on SOAS scores was found in the study of Palmstierna and Wistedt (1987). However, in the studies by Nijman, Merkelbach, Allertz, and à (1997), and Steinert, Wölfle, and Gebhardt (1999, 2000), interobserver reliability was rather low and ranged from 0.61 to 0.74. Apart from that, significant correlations varied from 0.38 to 0.81 with other aggression measurement methods such as the use of a second observation scale and severity ratings of the staff (Nijman, Palmstierna, Almvik, & Stolker, 2005).

The *Social Dysfunction and Aggression Scale* (SDAS; Wistedt et al., 1990) was developed as an 11-item scale. The SDAS measures the presence of aggressive behavior over a range from mild to moderate to severe. The total SDAS scores have a range from 0 to 44 (scores can range from 0 = not present to 4 = extremely severe). A two-factor solution has been found of two items covering inward aggression (suicidal behavior and self-injurious behavior) and nine items covering outward aggression (nondirected verbal aggressiveness, directed verbal aggressiveness, irritability, negativism, dysphoric mood, socially disturbed behavior, physical violence to personnel, physical violence to others, and physical violence to things). The reliability of the SDAS has been found to be good, with a Cronbach's alpha of 0.79 and an intraclass correlation of 0.97 (Kobes, Nijman, & Bulten, 2012).

4.4.6 Conclusions and Recommendations

In our opinion, the instruments that are described in this chapter should be the first choice for the assessment of offenders or forensic psychiatric patients and for the evaluation of treatment programs for these populations. New self-report questionnaires have been described for some dynamic factors, but users should realize that these instruments are still at a developmental stage. For the observation checklists, preference is given to instruments that are developed explicitly for offenders or forensic psychiatric patients such as OSAB or FIOS. The SOAS-R and the SDAS are primarily intended for aggressive psychiatric patients in a hospital admittance ward, although recent research has supported their use among offenders or forensic psychiatric patients.

Although it is understandable that some authors want to continue working on the improvement of reliability and validity after the first publication of their instrument, often data are lacking comparisons between original and revised versions. For example, the HCR-20 already has a third version, some items of the NEO-FFI have been changed to improve readability, and new items have been added to the original version of the NAS-PI and AQ. If a particular country has carried out a relatively large amount of research into the psychometric properties of an original version of an instrument, then it seems in our opinion advisable to continue using that version when assessing offenders or patients and evaluating treatment programs.

4.5 Instruments for Sexual Interest

Meta-analytic evidence consistently shows that deviant sexual interest is a primary risk factor for sex offenses (Hanson & Bussière, 1998; Hanson & Morton-Bourgon, 2005). Consequently, a range of measurement instruments has been developed to measure sexual interest with the aim to differentiate between sex offenders and nonclinical populations, between sex offenders and nonsex offenders, and between subtypes of sex offenders.

4.5.1 Self-Report Questionnaire

A widely used self-report questionnaire for the measurement of sexual behavior is the *Multiphasic Sex Inventory* (MSI; Nichols & Molinder, 1984). This self-report questionnaire consists of statements about sexual activities, problems, and experiences. The *Multiphasic Sex Inventory-II* (MSI-II; Nichols & Molinder, 2000) is a revised version, which also includes other sexual matters such as erectile dysfunction, premature ejaculation, sado-masochism, and sexual addictions. The MSI-II asks explicit questions about sexual thoughts and behavior but is not time-bound, and questions are asked in varied tenses, which makes it difficult to assess change over time. The MSI-II includes among others scales of social sexual desirability, sexual knowledge, sexual obsessions, sexual orientation, and a lie scale. Schlank (1995) found that the MSI distinguishes clinically different subgroups of sex offenders (e.g., subgroup 4 that was more likely to include incest perpetrators against female children and subgroup 5 that was more likely to include rapists of adult females) and Kalichman, Henderson, Shealy, and Dwyer (1992) concluded that the MSI had moderate to good internal validity, but that some subscales may be assessing multiple dimensions. They also mentioned the possibility of respondents denying or faking their true level of sexual deviance. In a study by Stinson and Becker (2008), the MSI-II Rape scale had the strongest correlation with rape behavior, but they also noticed that the construction of the scales, the details of the samples used, and the sensitivity of the samples had not been published. With no published manual that includes information on development, reliability and validity, population characteristics, and normative data the MSI-II does not meet the published standards for use as a test, but may still provide insight into a person's sexual interest and how it relates to his or her sexual behavior (Akerman & Beech, 2012).

4.5.2 Psychophysiological Measure

The *Penile Plethysmograph* (PPG) is used extensively in Anglo-Saxon countries to assess sexual interest in males (Kalmus & Beech, 2005). The PPG measures change in genital tumescence by penile circumference or penile volume while viewing images or listening to audio stimuli. However, the opinions about the use of PPG for research purposes and for clinical assessment are divided. For example, Harris and Rice (1996) regarded PPG as the best available measure of men's sexual preferences, especially for researchers. In their opinion, there is also enough evidence of acceptable psychometric properties to warrant careful use in clinical assessment. PPG data would also correlate with paraphilic sexual preference and previous sexual offenses (Konopasky & Konopasky, 2000), and according to Hanson and Bussière (1998) PPG can be useful in predicting recidivism. Also, a meta-analytic review of McPhail et al. (2019) showed that phallometric tests for pedophilic and hebephilic interests predict sexual re-offending of child sexual abusers. Renaud et al. (2010), however, stated that the PPG has a weak test–retest reliability, does not discriminate between sexual interests, and is easily faked. Stinson and Becker (2008) reported that while the PPG provides an objective measure and is able to differentiate pedophiles from adult offenders, it cannot identify rapists preferring coerced sexual interactions. Also, 30% of the men in their sample did not show any clinically significant sexual arousal, which showed a further problem with the PPG, and there are indications that erection seems neither an adequate nor sufficient criterion for sexual arousal in men (Janssen, McBride, Yarber, Hill, & Butler, 2008). Renaud et al. (2009) reported that up to 80% of subjects who were asked to control their erectile response voluntarily succeeded through distraction techniques such as not concentrating on the stimulus, or thinking of non-arousing images. Research has also shown that prior use of drugs or alcohol can affect sexual functioning, which in turn could affect response in the PPG (Peugh & Belenko, 2001). Finally, Marshall (2014) concluded from the literature that the specificity and sensitivity of phallometry are satisfactory with child sexual abusers, although this may not be true for all subtypes of child sexual abusers. However, there are disagreements concerning the meaning of rapists' responses and no test has yet reliably identified deviance among exhibitionists. In his opinion, problems, therefore, remain with phallometric assessments and clinicians should be cautious in interpreting the meaning of the responses.

In summary, there are a number of problems with the PPG: (1) lack of standardization of stimulus materials and procedures; (2) low test–retest reliability; (3) low response rates; (4) poor specificity or discriminate validity; and (5) it being easy to fake (Kalmus & Beech, 2005). Moreover, in several countries such as the Netherlands, the PPG is not used for the assessment of sexual interest in sex offenders because of ethical objections.

4.5.3 Neurobiological Measures

In Chaps. 1 and 2, we already considered the role of testosterone and serotonin in deviant sexual interest. This relation is not linear since several studies have shown that sex offenders do not necessarily have a higher level of testosterone or a lowered level of serotonin than nonclinical males. Contextual factors are also important. However, SSRIs and antiandrogenic treatments are used frequently in sex offenders.

Briken, Hill, and Berner (2014) stated that a pharmacological treatment has to start with a thorough diagnostic and prognostic process. After such an indicative process, an algorithm for the pharmacological treatment of paraphilias and sex offenders should be used that recommends SSRI treatment as the first line for mild and less dangerous offenders. If there is an insufficient improvement and a moderate- to high-risk offense, CPA (cyproterone acetate) or MPA (medroxyprogesterone) could be considered. According to the clinical experience of Briken et al. (2014), there are moderate- to high-risk patients that do profit from antiandrogenic therapy, especially those patients who are preoccupied with uncontrollable sexual fantasies and urges in an addictive-like manner so that it is hard to work with them exclusively psychotherapeutically.

4.6 New Developments

4.6.1 Violent Offenders

Over the past decade, several new instruments have been developed, which generally succeed in distinguishing between subgroups of (sexual) offenders, but which cannot yet be used for the assessment of individual offenders. There is a chance that in the future these instruments can only be used for research purposes.

Several studies have investigated whether implicit antisocial attitudes are related to aggressive behavior. Implicit attitudes can be defined as automatic and unintentionally activated evaluative associations with a psychological object (Gawronski & Bodenhausen, 2006). These attitudes can be measured with implicit measures (Greenwald, Poehlman, Uhlmann, & Banji, 2009) such as the Implicit Association Test (IAT, Greenwald, McGhee, & Schwartz, 1998), a reaction-based categorization task that measures the strength of implicit associations in memory. Several studies have found support for the validity of the IAT in the assessment of offenders who show violent or other aggressive behavior. This could indicate that more positive implicit attitudes toward violence are usually associated with more violent behavior. A study by, for example, Eckhardt, Samper, Suhr, and Holtzwort-Munroe (2012) showed that a sample of domestic violent men had more positive implicit associations toward violence than a sample of nonviolent men, while no difference was found between the two samples in explicit attitudes toward violence. Therefore, aggressogenic attitudes may be able to influence aggressive behavior automatically and without conscious awareness (Eckhardt et al., 2012). Zwets et al. (2015a) used two IATs in their research among Dutch forensic psychiatric inpatients: a neutral IAT as a control condition and a violence-pleasant IAT. The results showed that implicit attitudes toward violence were not related to self-reporting measures of aggression, but there was a relatively low but positive relationship with the Antisocial facet of psychopathy. The researchers emphasized that the findings of this correlational research cannot be used for individual diagnostics.

Another development is the use of the Startle Probe Reflex (SPR) as a measure of the strength of emotions (Grillon & Baas, 2003). The eye blink startle reflex occurs when intensive auditory, visual, or tactile stimuli are suddenly administered. For example, psychopaths would be expected to show a different shock reflex from typical college students to negative images, but a usual shock reflex in positive images (Fowles & Dindo, 2006). The deviation in the fright reflex could be explained as being mainly related to the affective-interpersonal component and less to the impulsive-antisocial component of psychopathy (Vanman, Mejia, Dawson, Schell, & Raine, 2003). Grillon and Baas (2003), however, thought that the startle reflex as a diagnostic tool is limited.

Virtual Reality (VR) is a recently developed technique, with which people can experience certain artificial situations created by a computer as realistic by means of special stereoscopic glasses. For example, Virtual Reality Exposure Therapy (VRET) is already regularly used in the treatment of anxiety disorders, and a meta-analysis by Powers and Emmelkamp (2008) showed that VRET is as effective as practicing in vivo. In the treatment of social anxiety, VRET proved even more effective than in vivo exposure (Kampmann et al., 2016). It has been proposed that Virtual Reality could be used to assess potential behavior, and if so, it could be used in situations that can only occur in practice if a hospitalized forensic psychiatric patient or a detainee can take leave. However, no measuring instrument has been developed to date to explore the utility of virtual situations.

4.6.2 Sexually Violent Offenders

To gain more insight into the cognitive aspects of sexual offending, researchers have looked for alternative methods to measure sexual interest (Thornton & Laws, 2009). This has led to the development of a number of standardized cognitive tasks for measuring sexual interest, which could possibly replace the PPG (Banse, Schmidt, & Clarbour, 2010; Ciardha & Gormley, 2009).

One of those alternatives is measuring viewing time (VT). Harris, Rice, Quinsey, and Chaplin (1996) investigated VT as a measure of sexual interest in child abusers and typical heterosexual men. To this end, images of naked men and women of various ages were offered to both groups while the time being spent on looking at the relevant picture was measured. Furthermore, the participants had to indicate to what extent they found the individuals in the images sexually attractive. For a few participants, phallometric research was also done, using the same pictures. The VT data were found to discriminate between the two groups, but the differences were less than with the phallometric measurements. Two instruments that use VT are the Abel Assessment of Sexual Interest (AASI, Abel et al., 2004) and the Affinity Measure of Sexual Interest (Glasgow, 2009). However, the validity of both instruments has not yet been sufficiently demonstrated (Fisher & Smith, 1999). A study of Schmidt, Babchishin, and Lehmann (2017) comprised two meta-analyses of VT measures to determine their discrimination between child sexual abusers and non-child sexual as well as convergent validity (associations with other measures of sexual interest in children). On average, VT measures showed moderate discrimination between criterion groups and significant convergent validity with self-reports, penile plethysmography, Implicit Association Tests, and offense behavioral measures. However, they provided better discrimination for adults than adolescent samples. The authors concluded that at present, VT measures could be considered the best validated indirect latency-based measure of sexual interest in children and, thus, have to be preferred over corresponding IATs.

The Implicit Association Test (IAT) in sexual offenders focuses on the association between child/sex versus adult/sex constructs. The assumption is that when the child/sex association is stronger than the adult/sex association, this is indicative of a sexual preference for children. Kanters et al. (2014) investigated 123 violent forensic psychiatric inpatients, consisting of 28 child abusers, 36 rapists, and 59 nonsexually violent patients, using three IATs, namely a standard IAT, a submissive-sexy IAT, and a child-sex IAT. The results suggested that child sex offenders have a stronger sexual preference for submission than rapists and nonsexually violent patients. Moreover, submissive-sexy associations proved to distinguish the child abusers from the other patients better than the child-sex associations. Child abusers with stronger child-sex associations reported more social anxiety and hostility. Despite positive findings at a group level, the IAT cannot yet be used for individual offenders because the outcomes are open to multiple interpretations. Studies in which implicit associations of offenders were correlated with recidivism risk (Babchishin, Nunes, & Hermann, 2013) yielded correlations from −0.02 to 0.43. A study by Nunes, Firestone, and Baldwin (2007) showed a very inconsistent picture, as a result of which the predictive validity of this instrument could not be confirmed.

Hecker, King, and Scoular (2009) advocated using the Startle Probe Reflex for research into the sexual interest of sexual offenders. When people are surprised, they show a delayed fright when they look at images that they find sexually interesting compared to neutral or aversive images. Gress and Laws (2009) concluded that startle probe reflexes differentiate between sexual interest in adult women and sexual interest in adult men, but also that further research is needed to see if the startle probe reflex makes a distinction in arousal increase as a result of sexual or aversive stimuli.

Renaud et al. (2014) performed a study to determine how virtual reality (VR) modality compares to the standard auditory (SA) modality in their capacity to generate sexual arousal profiles and deviance differentials indicative of sexual interests. The PPG responses of 22 child sexual offenders and 42 non-deviant adult males were recorded. While both stimulus modalities generated significantly different genital arousal profiles for child sex abusers and non-deviant males, deviance differentials calculated from the VR modality allowed for significantly higher classification accuracy. Overall, results suggest that the VR modality allows significantly better group classification accuracy and discriminant validity than audio stimuli.

4.6.3 *Conclusions and Recommendations*

Unfortunately, an instrument that reliably and validly measures sexual interest is lacking, irrespective of the extent to which sexual interest is related to the tendency to commit sexual offenses. The PPG has the major disadvantage that this instrument may not be used in all countries for the assessment of sexually violent offenders because of ethical objections. New developments such as the IAT or VT indicate that these instruments can distinguish between, for example, a sample of sex offenders and a sample of nonsex offenders. However, these instruments do not seem suitable for making statements about individual sex offenders. For the time being, a combination of the usual with the new instruments seems most appropriate (Akerman & Beech, 2012).

4.7 Case Formulation

The data from measuring instruments must be related to each other so that a treatment plan can be drawn up with specific treatment objectives. Then, it can be established for which objectives a (group) treatment is offered and for which an individual or partner relationship therapy is indicated. In formulating the treatment goals, the psychometric properties of the measurement instruments used must be considered: the outcome of instruments with good psychometric properties must outweigh those with less good psychometric properties. For offenders, treatment plans should not only be determined in consultation with the individual offender but also with the person responsible for the treatment and who represents the institution or prison and indirect society.

Cognitive behavioral case formulation can be defined as an idiographic theory of the person and his or her life situation, which includes problems as well as triggering and maintaining variables, including cognitions (thoughts and beliefs), that have relevance for treatment planning (Mumma, 2011). Several studies have shown that case formulation helps to guide effective treatment decision-making (Dudley, Ingham, Sowerby, & Freeston, 2015). Also, these studies demonstrated that both reliability and quality of case formulation were associated with levels of clinical experience and accreditation status (Kuyken, Fothergill, Musa, & Chadwick, 2005; Kuyken, Padesky, & Dudley, 2008). As a consequence, a case formulation for an individual client or patient should be conducted by an experienced cognitive-behaviorally trained therapist or by a cognitive-behavioral therapist in training, supervised by a more experienced colleague.

Case formulation in the form of a heuristic model for the development and maintenance of individual problems should be based on information of the static and dynamic factors. Information on these factors may come from files, interviews, and specific assessment instruments such as risk assessment instruments, observation scales, and self-report questionnaires. Hart, Gresswell, and Braham (2011) used for

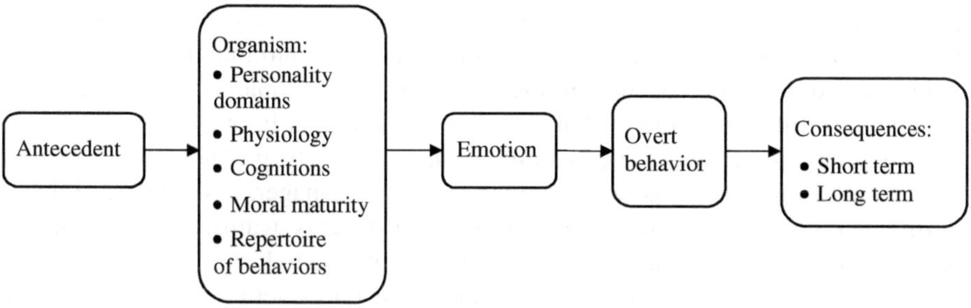

Fig. 4.1 A heuristic model for individual problem behaviors

their functional analyses the A-B-C format in which the A refers to Antecedents or stimuli thought to have triggered or elicited the behavior in question, B to the Behavior itself, to be described in terms of overt or covert behaviors, and C to the Consequences that follow the behavior. In this book, the A-B-C format is expanded with an O factor and consequences are divided into consequences in the short term and on the long run (Fig. 4.1).

The O factor refers to the psychological makeup of the individual regarding his or her personality domains, physiological characteristics, (distorted) cognitions, moral maturity, and repertoire of social and coping skills (Hornsveld, Kraaimaat, Zwets, & Kanters, 2017). Examples of a heuristic model for nonsexually violent and sexually violent offenders have been described in Chap. 2.

4.7.1 *Dynamic Factors*

Empirical research provides a good understanding of the factors that are related to violent behavior. Andrews and Bonta (2010) formulated eight factors, the Central Eight that are associated with general recidivism, namely history of antisocial behavior, antisocial personality pattern, antisocial cognition, antisocial associates, family/marital circumstances, school/work, leisure/recreation, and substance abuse. A meta-analysis by Hanson and Morton-Bourgon (2005) demonstrated that deviant sexual interests and antisocial orientation / lifestyle instability are the primary risk factors associated with sexual recidivism. Other empirically supported risk factors for sexual recidivism are poor problem-solving skills and offense-supportive cognitions (Hanson & Harris, 2000, Hanson & Harris, 2001; Mann et al., 2010), whereas several variables commonly addressed in sex offender treatment (e.g., the motivation for treatment, denial of sexual offense(s), psychological distress, victim empathy) have little or no relationship with sexual recidivism (Hanson & Morton-Bourgon, 2005; Mann et al., 2010).

From the empirical studies mentioned, dynamic criminogenic factors vary from individual characteristics (e.g., impulsivity) to broad domains or areas of interest (e.g., education/work). To design an individual treatment plan, it is important that these characteristics and domains are further translated into individual personality domains and situation-specific problem behaviors. A problem behavior may be exhibited in different domains, but it is also possible that in one domain there are several problem behaviors. For example, an impulsivity problem may manifest itself in inadequate responses to commands from a manager, in domestic violence during a conflict with a partner, or in too strong protests against the decision of a referee during a soccer game. Or an offender is not able to keep his job because he cannot manage the critical remarks of his boss, he dares not to communicate with his colleagues during lunchtime, or he cannot stand up for his rights when there are problems in the workplace.

For the treatment of violent offenders, therapists have various treatment programs at their disposal nowadays (see Chap. 5). Such programs have the advantage that they offer the therapist structure and concrete guidelines. However, most programs focus on the common dynamic criminogenic factors of offenders and do not take the specific problems of an individual offender into account. Information on all problem behaviors should feed into a personal heuristic model (case formulation) before an offender is assigned to a treatment program. Once a heuristic model has been formulated, functional analyses of the various specific problem behaviors can be made, and an individual treatment plan with particular treatment objectives can be established (Hart, Sturmey, Logan, & McMurran, 2011). With the aim to promote treatment motivation, an instrument for the measurement of protective factors should be used, such as the Structured Assessment of PROtective Factors for Violence Risk (SAPROF; De Vries Robbé, De Vogel, Koster, & Bogaerts, 2015).

4.7.2 Case Formulation for Violent Offenders

An example of a functional analysis is described in vignette 1, Anthony (nonsexually violent offender).

Vignette 1: Background and Core Problems of Anthony

Anthony (18 years old) was raised in a family with two children. The biological father left the family when Anthony was 8 years old. Shortly afterwards, the mother got acquainted with another man with whom she remarried 2 years later. It did not go well between Anthony and his stepfather, and in quarrels the latter often used violence. When Anthony was 16 years old, he had become so strong that he could take on his stepfather and consequently beat him up during a fight. After this, the abuse by his stepfather stopped. In the meantime, Anthony performed poorly at school, partly because of a conduct disorder. He was absent frequently and failed to obtain a diploma. However, he had met a group of peers who were hanging out on the street. They argued a lot. With a number of these peers, Anthony committed several robberies at petrol stations or shops. Anthony was convicted and sentenced

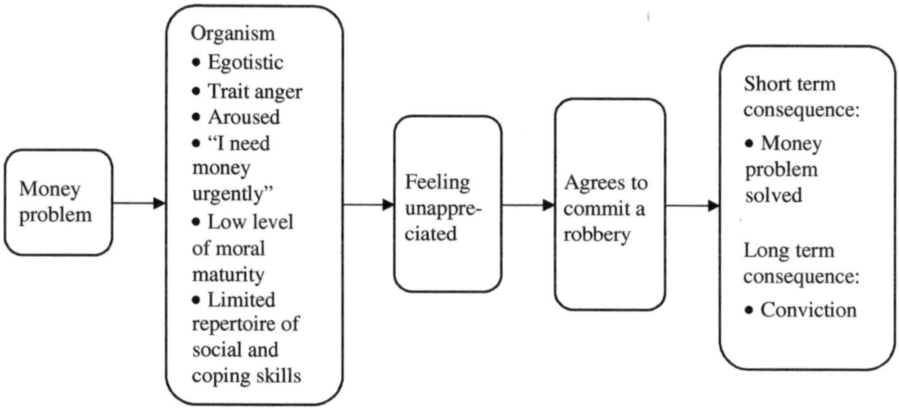

Fig. 4.2 Functional analysis of one of Anthony's problem behaviors

to a 1-year prison term, followed by treatment at a forensic psychiatric outpatient clinic. Figure 4.2 suggests that Anthony must learn to earn money legally and for that objective has to follow among others a moral reasoning and social skills training.

4.7.3 Case Formulation for Sexually Violent Offenders

Examples of functional analyses are described in two vignettes, Juan (rapist) in vignette 2 and Eric (child sex abuser) in vignette 3.

Vignette 2: Background and Core Problems

Juan (38 years old) was born in a large family from the Caribbean. Both parents had several children from previous relationships. When Juan was 12 years old, he was placed in a boarding school because of persistent behavioral problems. At the boarding school, Juan came in contact with soft and hard drugs, and he displayed inappropriate sexual behavior toward his female classmates. As an adult, Juan had employment problems and he regularly ended up in jail because of burglaries, assaults, or robberies. He also conceived five children with three different women. Under the influence of drugs, he threatened a random stranger with a knife and forced her to go with him to a quiet place in a park where he raped her. Juan was sentenced to detention under hospital order for threat and rape. Figure 4.3 suggests that Juan must learn how to deal with anger as a result of rejection, in combination with learning to convert sexist cognitions into prosocial cognitions.

Vignette 3: Background and Core Problems of Eric

Eric (55 years old) had his first sexual experience when he was 8 years old and an older classmate showed him how to masturbate. At the age of 12, Eric began peeking at adult women. Eric married at the age of 30. There was sexual contact during the

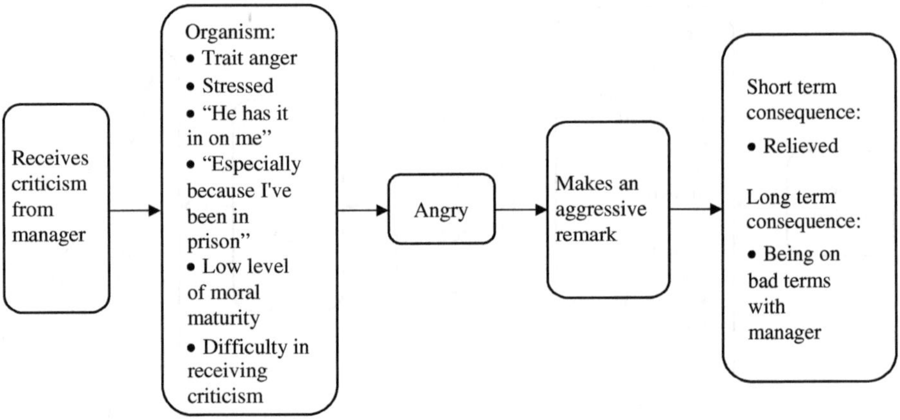

Fig. 4.3 Functional analysis of one of Juan's problem behaviors

marriage and the couple conceived a daughter. Initially, Eric only downloaded pornography, but soon he started to exhibit and masturbate in front of adult women. After Eric was arrested and sentenced to outpatient treatment, he was abandoned by his wife. Eric, however, continued to exhibit and his sexual interest slowly shifted toward children. Eventually, Eric raped several underage girls who were friends of his daughter. He was arrested again and sentenced to detention under hospital order.

The analysis in Fig. 4.4 might indicate a treatment with cognitive restructuring (the replacement of cognitive distortions by prosocial cognitions), in combination with medical intervention.

4.7.4 Functional Analyses During Treatment

Conducting functional analyses is not only desirable in the assessment phase but is also required in the course of treatment, for example, if an offender or patient has a new problem or if unexpected problems occur during treatment. A therapist/trainer should, therefore, be an experienced and well-trained clinician or be supervised by such a colleague. For example, Eric practiced how to start a conversation with an adult woman. During that role-play, it emerged that Eric suffers from many more behavioral shortcomings than thought initially (Fig. 4.5).

The analysis shows that after starting the conversation with the woman, Eric immediately decided to invite her for a coffee at his home. He showed no insight into the circumstances in which it is appropriate to invite a woman to drink coffee with a man she hardly knew and no insight into the several phases of intimacy during getting acquainted. This meant that it must be explained to Eric that making acquaintance with somebody can only be followed by an invitation when it has gone through increasing phases of intimacy and that each phase requires different skills. Therefore, Eric had to first exercise a situation in which he had a short conversation on the weather and nothing else.

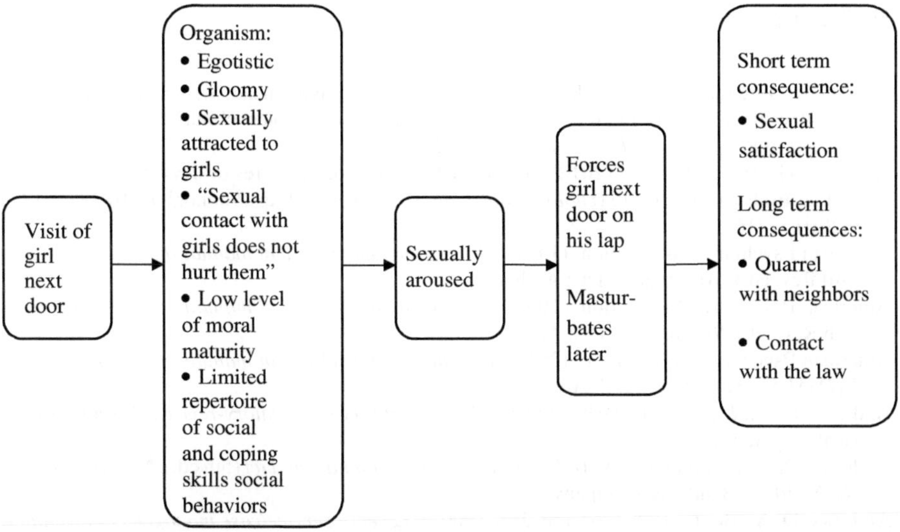

Fig. 4.4 Functional analysis of one of Eric's problem behaviors

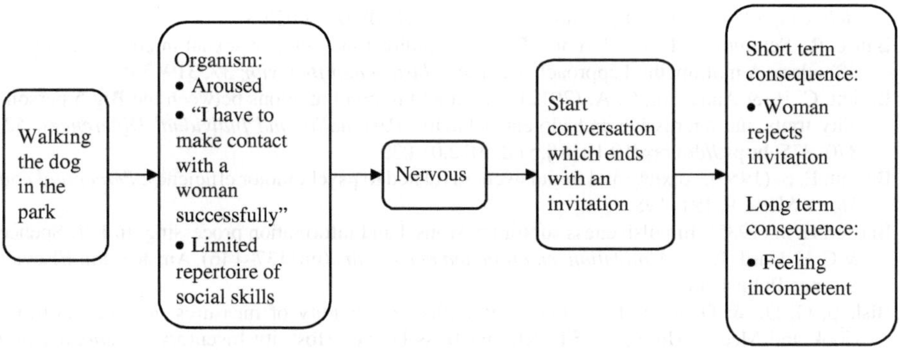

Fig. 4.5 Functional analysis of Eric's situation in making contact with adult women

4.8 Conclusions and Recommendations

Before assigning offenders to a treatment program, a treatment plan for each offender should be formulated. Such a treatment plan has to be based on the dynamic criminogenic needs that the offender has in common with other offenders and on specific additional individual problem behaviors (case formulation). For an inventory of all relevant problem behaviors, a thorough assessment of each offender is necessary. For such an assessment, reliable and valid instruments should be used which have been tested in several populations in various nations. The latter will facilitate the international exchange of data. The literature has shown that experienced and well-educated clinicians should perform the formulation of individual treatment plans (Kuyken et al., 2005).

References

Abel, G. G., Jordan, A., Rouleau, J. L., Emerick, R., Barboza-Whitehead, S., & Osborn, C. (2004). Use of visual reaction time to assess male adolescents who molest children. *Sexual Abuse: A Journal of Research and Treatment, 16*, 255–265.

Akerman, G., & Beech, A. R. (2012). A systematic review of measures of deviant sexual interest and arousal. *Psychiatry, Psychology and Law, 19*, 118–143. https://doi.org/10.1080/13218719.2010.547161

American Psychiatric Association. (1987). *Diagnostic and statistical manual of mental disorders* (3rd Rev. ed.). Washington, DC: Author.

American Psychiatric Association. (1994). *Diagnostic and statistical manual of mental disorders* (4th Rev. ed.). Washington, DC: Author.

American Psychiatric Association. (2013). *Diagnostic and statistical manual of mental disorders 5 (DSM-5)*. Washington, DC: Author.

Andrews, D. A., & Bonta, J. (1995). *LSI-R: The level of service inventory-revised*. Toronto: Multi-Health Systems.

Andrews, D. A., & Bonta, J. (2010). *The psychology of criminal conduct* (5th ed.). New Providence, NJ: Matthew Bender & Company.

Andrews, D. A., Bonta, J., & Wormith, J. S. (2004). *Level of service/case management inventory: An offender assessment system*. North Tonawanda, NY: Multi-Health Systems.

Babchishin, K. M., Nunes, K. L., & Hermann, C. A. (2013). The validity of implicit association test (IAT) measures of sexual attraction to children: A meta-analysis. *Archives of Sexual Behavior, 42*, 487–499. https://doi.org/10.1007/s10508-012-0022-8

Banse, R., Schmidt, A. F., & Clarbour, J. (2010). Indirect measures of sexual interest in child sex offenders: A multimethod approach. *Criminal Justice and Behavior, 37*, 319–335.

Barlett, C. P., & Anderson, C. A. (2012). Direct and indirect relations between the Big 5 personality traits and aggressive and violent behavior. *Personality and Individual Differences, 52*, 870–875. https://doi.org/10.1016/j.paid.2012.01.029

Barratt, E. S. (1959). Anxiety and impulsiveness related to psychomotor efficiency. *Perceptual and Motor Skills, 9*, 191–198.

Barratt, E. S. (1985). Impulsiveness subtraits: Arousal and information processing. In J. T. Spence & C. E. Izard (Eds.), *Motivation, emotion and personality* (pp. 137–146). Amsterdam: Elsevier Science Publishers.

Bishop, G. D., & Quah, S. H. (1998). Reliability and validity of measures of anger/hostility: Cook and Medley Ho Scale, STAXI, and Buss-Durkee Hostility Inventory. *Personality and Individual Differences, 24*, 867–878.

Bjornsdottir, G., Jonsson, F. H., Hansdotti, I., Almarsdottir, A. B., Heimisdottir, M., Tyrfingsson, T., et al. (2014). Psychometric properties of the Icelandic NEO-FFI in a general population sample compared to a sample recruited for a study on the genetics of addiction. *Personality and Individual Differences, 58*, 71–75. https://doi.org/10.1016/j.paid.2013.10.010

Boer, D. P., Wilson, R. J., Gauthier, C. M., & Hart, S. D. (1997). Assessing risk for sexual violence: Guidelines for clinical practice. In C. D. Webster & M. A. Jackson (Eds.), *Impulsivity: Theory, assessment, and treatment* (pp. 326–342). New York: Guilford.

Bonta, J., & Andrews, D. A. (2007). *Risk-need responsivity model for offender assessment and rehabilitation*. Ottawa: Public Safety Canada.

Borteyroua, X., Bruchon-Schweitzer, M., & Spielberger, C. D. (2008). The French adaptation of the STAXI-2, C. D. Spielberger's State-Trait Anger Expression Inventory. *L'Encéphale, 34*, 249–255. https://doi.org/10.1016/j.encep.2007.06.001

Briken, P., Hill, A., & Berner, W. (2014). Pharmacotherapy of sexual offenders and men who are at risk of sexual offending. In D. P. Boer, R. Eher, L. A. Craig, M. H. Miner, & F. Pfäfflin (Eds.), *International perspectives on the assessment and treatment of sexual offenders* (pp. 437–449). Chichester: Wiley-Blackwell.

Bryant, F. B., & Smith, B. D. (2001). Refining the architecture of aggression: A measurement model for the Buss-Perry Aggression Questionnaire. *Journal of Research in Personality, 35*, 138–167.

Buss, A. H., & Perry, M. (1992). The aggression questionnaire. *Journal of Personality and Social Psychology, 63*, 452–459.

Buss, A. H., & Warren, W. L. (2000). *The Aggression Questionnaire (AQ) manual*. Los Angeles, CA: Western Psychological Services.

Check, J. V. P. (2014). *The hostility toward women scale*. Thesis, University of Manitoba, Manitoba. http://hdl.handle.net/1993/23279

Ciardha, C. Ó., & Gormley, M. (2009). Comparing two implicit cognitive measures of sexual interest: A pictorial modified Stroop task and the Implicit Association Test. In D. Thornton & D. R. Laws (Eds.), *Cognitive approaches to the assessment of sexual interest in sexual offenders* (pp. 85–99). Chichester: Wiley.

Costa Jr., P. T., & McCrae, R. R. (1992). *Revised NEO Personality Inventory (NEO-PI-R) and NEO Five-Factor Inventory (NEO-FFI): Professional manual*. Odessa, FL: Psychological Assessment Resources.

Craig, L. A., Beech, A. R., & Cortoni, F. (2013). What works in assessing risk in sexual and violent offenders. In L. A. Craig, L. Dixon, & T. A. Gannon (Eds.), *What works in offender rehabilitation: An evidence-based approach to assessment and treatment* (pp. 94–114). Chichester: Wiley.

Culhane, S. E., & Morera, O. F. (2010). Reliability and validity of the Novaco Anger Scale and Provocation Inventory (NAS-PI) and State-Trait Anger Expression Inventory-2 (STAXI-2) in Hispanic and Non-Hispanic white student samples. *Hispanic Journal of Behavioral Sciences, 32*, 586–606. https://doi.org/10.1177/0739986310381458

De Vries Robbé, M., de Vogel, V., Koster, K., & Bogaerts, S. (2015). Assessing protective factors for sexually violent offending with the SAPROF. *Sexual Abuse: A Journal of Research and Treatment, 27*, 51–70. https://doi.org/10.1177/1079063214550168

Derefinko, K. J., Adams, Z. W., Milich, R., Fillmore, M. T., Lorch, E. P., & Lynam, D. R. (2008). Response style differences in inattentive and combined subtypes of Attention-Deficit/Hyperactivity Disorder. *Journal of Abnormal Child Psychology, 36*, 745–758. https://doi.org/10.1007/s10802-007-9207-3

Dolan, M., & Fullam, R. (2004). Behavioural and psychometric measures of impulsivity in a personality disordered population. *Journal of Forensic Psychiatry & Psychology, 15*, 426–450.

Douglas, K. S., Hart, S. D., Webster, C. D., Belfrage, H., & Guy, L. S. (2014). Historical-Clinical-Risk Management-20, Version 3 (HCR-20^{V3}): Development and overview. *International Journal of Forensic Mental Health, 13*, 93–108. https://doi.org/10.1080/14999013.2014.906519

Drenth, P. J. D., & Sijtsma, K. (2006). *Testtheorie. Inleiding in de theorie van de psychologische test en zijn toepassingen [Testtheory. Introduction to the theory of the psychological test and its applications]*. Houten, NL: Bohn Stafleu van Loghum.

Dudley, R., Ingham, B., Sowerby, K., & Freeston, M. (2015). The utility of case formulation in treatment decision making; the effect of experience and expertise. *Journal of Behavior Therapy and Experimental Psychiatry, 48*, 66–74. https://doi.org/10.1016/j.jbtep.2015.01.009

Eckhardt, C., Norlander, B., & Deffenbacher, J. (2004). The assessment of anger and hostility: A critical review. *Aggression and Violent Behavior, 9*, 17–43. https://doi.org/10.1016/S1359-1789(02)001167

Eckhardt, C. I., Samper, R., Suhr, L., & Holtzwort-Munroe, A. (2012). Implicit attitudes toward violence among male perpetrators of intimate partner violence: A preliminary investigation. *Journal of Interpersonal Violence, 27*, 471–491. https://doi.org/10.1177/0886260511421677

Eher, R., Matthes, A., Schilling, F., Haubner-MacLean, T., & Rettenberger, M. (2012). Dynamic risk assessment in sexual offenders using STABLE-2000 and STABLE-2007: An investigation of predictive and incremental validity. *Sexual Abuse: A Journal of Research and Treatment, 24*, 5–28. https://doi.org/10.1177/1079063211403164

Ellouze, F., Ghaffari, O., Zouari, O., Zouari, B., & M'rad, M. F. (2013). Validation of the dialectal Arabic version of Barratt's impulsivity scale, the BIS-11. *L'Encéphale, 39*, 13–18. https://doi.org/10.1016/j.encep.2012.06.034

Etzler, S. L., Rohrmann, S., & Brandt, H. (2014). Validation of the STAXI-2: A study with prison inmates. *Psychological Test and Assessment Modeling, 56*, 178–194.

Fernandez, Y., Harris, A. J. R., Hanson, R. K., & Sparks, J. (2012). *Stable-2007 coding manual: Revised 2012*. Ottawa: Public Safety Canada.

Fillmore, M. T. (2003). Drug abuse as a problem of impaired control: Current approaches and findings. *Behavioral & Cognitive Neuroscience Reviews, 2*, 179–197. https://doi.org/10.1177/1534582303257007

Fillmore, M. T., & Weafer, J. (2013). Behavioral inhibition and addiction. In J. MacKillop & H. de Wit (Eds.), *The Wiley-Blackwell handbook of addiction psychopharmacology* (pp. 135–164). Chichester: Wiley-Blackwell.

First, M. B., Spitzer, R. L., Williams, J. B. W., & Benjamin, L. S. (2015). *Structured clinical interview for DSM-5 personality disorders (SCID-5-PD)*. Arlington, VA: American Psychiatric Association.

First, M. B., Williams, J. B. W., Karg, R. S., & Spitzer, R. L. (2015). *Structured clinical interview for DSM-5 disorders, clinician version (SCID-5-CV)*. Arlington, VA: American Psychiatric Association.

Fisher, L., & Smith, G. (1999). Statistical adequacy of the Abel Assessment for Interest in Paraphilias. *Sexual Abuse: A Journal of Research and Treatment, 11*, 195–205.

Fossati, A., Di Ceglie, A., Acquarini, E., & Barratt, E. S. (2001). Psychometric properties of an Italian version of the Barratt Impulsiveness Scale-11 (BIS-11) in nonclinical subjects. *Journal of Clinical Psychology, 57*, 815–828.

Fossati, A., Maffei, C., Acquarini, E., & Di Ceglie, A. (2003). Multigroup confirmatory component and factor analyses of the Italian version of the Aggression Questionnaire. *European Journal of Psychological Assessment, 19*, 54–65.

Fowles, D. C., & Dindo, L. (2006). A dual-deficit model of psychopathy. In C. J. Patrick (Ed.), *Handbook of psychopathy* (pp. 14–34). New York: Guilford.

Freedman, R., Lewis, D. A., Michels, R., Pine, D. S., Schultz, S. K., Tamminga, C. A., et al. (2013). The initial field trials of DSM-5: New blooms and old thorns. *American Journal of Psychiatry, 170*, 1–5. https://doi.org/10.1176/appi.ajp.2012.12091189

Gawronski, B., & Bodenhausen, G. V. (2006). Associative and propositional processes in evaluation: An integrative review of implicit and explicit attitude change. *Psychological Bulletin, 132*, 692–731. https://doi.org/10.1037/0033-2909.132.5.692

Genoud, P. A., & Zimmermann, G. (2009). *French version of the 12-item Aggression Questionnaire: Preliminary psychometric properties*. 11th Congress of the Swiss Psychological Society, Neuchâtel.

Gibbs, J. C., Basinger, K. S., & Fuller, D. (1992). *Moral maturity: Measuring the development of sociomoral reflection*. Hillsdale, NJ: Erlbaum. https://doi.org/10.1037/031668.

Glasgow, D. V. (2009). The development of a self-report assessment of paedophile sexual interest incorporating a Viewing Time validity measure, Chapter 3. In D. Thornton & D. R. Laws (Eds.), *Cognitive approaches to the assessment of sexual interest in sexual offenders*. Chichester: Wiley.

Greenwald, A. G., McGhee, D. E., & Schwartz, J. L. K. (1998). Measuring individual differences in implicit cognition: The implicit association test. *Journal of Personality and Social Psychology, 85*, 1464–1480. https://doi.org/10.1037/0022-3514.74.6.1464

Greenwald, A. G., Poehlman, T. A., Uhlmann, E. L., & Banji, M. R. (2009). Understanding and using the Implicit Association Test: III. Meta-analysis of predictive validity. *Journal of Personality and Social Psychology, 97*, 17–41. https://doi.org/10.1037/a0015575

Gress, C. L. Z., & Laws, R. D. (2009). Measuring sexual deviance: Attention-based measures. In A. R. Beech, L. A. Craig, & K. D. Browne (Eds.), *Assessment and treatment of sex offenders: A handbook* (pp. 109–128). Chichester: Wiley-Blackwell.

Grillon, C., & Baas, J. (2003). A review of the modulation of the startle reflex by affective states and its application in psychiatry. *Clinical Neurophysiology, 114*, 1557–1579. https://doi.org/10.1016/S1388-2457(03)00202-5

Grove, W. M. (2005). Clinical versus statistical prediction: The contribution of Paul E. Meehl. *Journal of Clinical Psychology, 61*, 1233–1243. https://doi.org/10.1002/jclp.20179

Hanson, R. K. (2000). *Risk assessment*. Beaverton, OR: ATSA: Association for the Treatment of Sexual Abusers. Informational package, ATSA.

Hanson, R. K., & Bussière, M. T. (1998). Predicting relapse: A meta-analysis of sexual offender recidivism studies. *Journal of Consulting and Clinical Psychology, 66*, 348–362. https://doi.org/10.1037/0022-006X.66.2.348

Hanson, R. K., & Harris, A. J. R. (2000). Where should we intervene? Dynamic predictors of sexual offense recidivism. *Criminal Justice and Behavior, 27*, 6–35. https://doi.org/10.1177/0093854800027001002

Hanson, R. K., & Harris, A. J. R. (2001). A structured approach to evaluating change among Sexual offenders. *Sexual Abuse: A Journal of Research and Treatment, 13*, 105–122. https://doi.org/10.1177/107906320101300204

Hanson, R. K., & Harris, A. J. R. (2012). *Acute-2007 coding manual*. Ottawa: Public Safety Canada.

Hanson, R. K., & Morton-Bourgon, K. E. (2005). The characteristics of persistent sexual offenders: A meta-analysis of recidivism studies. *Journal of Consulting and Clinical Psychology, 73*, 1153–1163. https://doi.org/10.1037/0022-006X.73.6.1154

Hanson, R. K., & Morton-Bourgon, K. E. (2009). The accuracy of recidivism risk assessments for sexual offenders: a meta-analysis of 118 prediction studies. *Psychological Assessment, 21*, 1–21. https://doi.org/10.1037/a0014421

Hare, R. D. (1991). *The hare psychopathy checklist-revised*. Toronto: Multi-Health Systems.

Hare, R. D. (2003). *Hare psychopathy checklist-revised (PCL-R)* (2nd ed.). Toronto: Multi-Health Systems.

Harris, A. J. R., Phenix, A., Hanson, R. K., & Thornton, D. (2003). *STATIC-99 coding rules revised-2003*. Ottawa: Solicitor General Canada.

Harris, G. T., & Rice, M. E. (1996). The science in phallometric measurement of male sexual interest. *Current Directions in Psychological Science, 5*, 156–160.

Harris, G. T., Rice, M. E., Quinsey, V. L., & Chaplin, T. C. (1996). Viewing Time as a measure of sexual interest among child molesters and normal heterosexual men. *Behaviour Research and Therapy, 34*, 389–394.

Hart, A. J. P., Gresswell, D. M., & Braham, L. G. (2011). Formulation of serious violent offending using multiple sequential functional analysis. In P. Sturmey & M. McMurran (Eds.), *Forensic case formulation* (pp. 129–152). Chichester: Wiley.

Hart, S., Sturmey, P., Logan, C., & McMurran, M. (2011). Forensic case formulation. *International Journal of Forensic Mental Health, 10*, 118–126. https://doi.org/10.1080/14999013.2011.577137

Hart, S. D., Webster, C. D., Belfrage, H., Guy, L. S., & Wilson, C. M. (2014). Historical-Clinical-Risk Management-20, Version 3 (HCR-20^{V3}): Development and overview. *International Journal of Forensic Mental Health, 13*, 93–108. https://doi.org/10.1080/14999013.2014.906519

Hartmann, A. S., Rief, W., & Hilbert, A. (2011). Psychometric properties of the German version of the Barratt Impulsiveness Scale-11 (BIS-11) for adolescents. *Perceptual and Motor Skills, 112*, 353–368. https://doi.org/10.2466/08.09.10.PMS.112.2.353-368

Haseth, K. J. (1996). The Norwegian adaptation of the State-Trait Anger Expression Inventory. In C. Spielberger & I. Sarason (Eds.), *Stress and emotion: Anxiety, anger, and curiosity* (Vol. 16, pp. 83–106). Washington, DC: Taylor & Francis.

Hecker, J. E., King, M. W., & Scoular, R. J. (2009). The Startle Probe Reflex: An alternative approach to the measurement of sexual interest. In D. Thornton & D. R. Laws (Eds.), *Cognitive approaches to the assessment of sexual interest in sexual offenders* (pp. 203–224). Chichester: Wiley-Blackwell.

Hoekstra, H. A., Ormel, J., & De Fruyt, F. (1996). *Handleiding NEO Persoonlijkheidsvragenlijsten [Manual NEO personality questionnaires]*. Lisse: Swets Test Services.

Hornsveld, R. H. J. (2018). Meetinstrumenten voor de forensische psychiatrie *[Measuring instruments for forensic psychiatry]*. Rijswijk, NL: Challenger Press. Available at: https://www.agressiehanteringstherapie.nl/nl/menu/boeken

Hornsveld, R. H. J., Kraaimaat, F. W., Bouwmeester, S., Polak, M. A., & Zwets, A. J. (2014). Behavior on the ward of personality disordered inpatients and chronically psychotic inpatients during a three-year stay in a Dutch forensic psychiatric hospital. *The Journal of Forensic Psychiatry and Psychology, 25*, 684–704. https://doi.org/10.1080/14789949.2014.947308

Hornsveld, R. H. J., Kraaimaat, F. W., & Zwets, A. J. (2012). The Adapted Version of the Sociomoral Reflection Measure (SRM-AV) in Dutch forensic psychiatric patients. *International Journal of Forensic Mental Health, 11*, 1–9. https://doi.org/10.1080/14999013.2012.723667

Hornsveld, R. H. J., Kraaimaat, F. W., Zwets, A. J., & Kanters, T. (2017). Beyond Aggression Replacement Training: Cognitive-behavioral programs for Dutch (sexually) violent forensic psychiatric inpatients, Chapter 82. In P. Sturmey (Ed.), *Handbook of violence and aggression*. Chichester: Wiley-Blackwell.

Hornsveld, R. H. J., Muris, P., Kraaimaat, F. W., & Meesters, C. (2009). The Aggression Questionnaire in Dutch violent forensic psychiatric patients and secondary vocational students. *Assessment, 16*, 181–192.

Hornsveld, R. H. J., Muris, P. E. H. M., & Kraaimaat, F. W. (2011). The Novaco Anger Scale-Provocation Inventory (1994 version) in Dutch forensic psychiatric patients. *Psychological Assessment, 23*, 937–944. https://doi.org/10.1037/a0024018

Hornsveld, R. H. J., Nijman, H. L. I., Hollin, C. R., & Kraaimaat, F. W. (2007a). An adapted version of the Rosenzweig Picture-Frustration Study (PFS-AV) for the measurement of hostility in violent forensic psychiatric patients. *Criminal Behaviour and Mental Health, 17*, 45–56.

Hornsveld, R. H. J., Nijman, H. L. I., Hollin, C. R., & Kraaimaat, F. W. (2007b). Development of the Observation Scale for Aggressive Behavior (OSAB) for Dutch forensic psychiatric inpatients with an antisocial personality disorder. *International Journal of Law and Psychiatry, 30*, 480–491. https://doi.org/10.1016/j.ijlp.2007.09.009

Hornsveld, R. H. J., Timonen, B., Kraaimaat, F. W., Zwets, A. J., & Kanters, T. (2014). The Attitudes toward Women Inventory (AWI) in Dutch violent forensic psychiatric inpatients. *Journal of Forensic Psychology Practice, 14*, 383–397. https://doi.org/10.1080/15228932.2014.964105

Hovens, J. E., Lievaart, M., & Rodenburg, J. (2014). *STAXI-2: Vragenlijst over boosheid: [Manual of the Dutch version of the State Trait Anger Expression Inventory (STAXI-2)]*. Amsterdam: Hogrefe.

Iftikhar, R., & Malik, F. (2014). Translation and validation of Aggression Questionnaire in a Pakistani children cohort. *Pakistan Journal of Social and Clinical Psychology, 12*, 39–45.

Janssen, E., McBride, K., Yarber, W., Hill, B. J., & Butler, S. (2008). Factors that influence sexual arousal in men: A focus group study. *Archives of Sexual Behavior, 37*, 252–265.

Jones, S. E., Miller, J. D., & Lynam, D. R. (2011). Personality, antisocial behavior, and aggression: A meta-analytic review. *Journal of Criminal Justice, 39*, 329–337.

Kalichman, S. C., Henderson, M. C., Shealy, L. S., & Dwyer, M. (1992). Psychometric properties of the Multiphasic Sex Inventory in assessing sex offenders. *Criminal Justice and Behavior, 19*, 384–396.

Kalmus, E., & Beech, A. R. (2005). Forensic assessment of sexual interest: A review. *Aggression and Violent Behavior, 10*, 193–218. https://doi.org/10.1016/j.avb.2003.12.002

Kampmann, I. L., Emmelkamp, P. M. G., Hartanto, D., Brinkman, W. P., Zijlstra, B. J. H., & Morina, N. (2016). Exposure to virtual social interactions in the treatment of social anxiety disorder: A randomized controlled trial. *Behaviour Research and Therapy, 77*, 147–156. https://doi.org/10.1016/j.brat.2015.12.016

Kanters, T., Hornsveld, R. H. J., Nunes, K. L., Huijding, J., Zwets, A. J., Snowden, R. J., Muris, P., & Van Marle, H. J. C. (2014). Are child abusers attracted to submissiveness? Assessment of sex-related cognition with the Implicit Association Test. *Sexual Abuse: A Journal of Research and Treatment, 28*, 448–468. https://doi.org/10.1177/1079063214544330

Kanters, T., Hornsveld, R. H. J., Nunes, K. L., Zwets, A. J., Muris, P., & Van Marle, H. J. C. (2017). The Sexual Violence Risk-20: Factor structure and psychometric properties. *The Journal of Forensic Psychiatry & Psychology, 28*, 368–387. https://doi.org/10.1080/14789949.2017.1284887

Kassinove, H., Sukhodolsky, D. G., Eckhardt, C. I., & Tsytsarev, S. V. (1997). Development of a Russian state-trait anger expression inventory. *Journal of Clinical Psychology, 53*, 543–557.

Kay, S. R., Fiszbein, A., & Opler, L. A. (1987). The Positive and Negative Syndrome Scale (PANSS) for schizophrenia. *Schizophrenia Bulletin, 13*, 261–276.

Kay, S. R., Opler, L. A., & Lindenmayer, J. (1988). Reliability and validity of the Positive and Negative Syndrome Scale for Schizophrenics. *Psychiatry Research, 23*, 99–110.

Khan, A., Yavorsky, C., Liechti, S., Opler, M., Rothman, B., DiClemente, G., et al. (2013). A rasch model to test the cross-cultural validity in the positive and negative syndrome scale (PANSS) across six geo-cultural groups. *BMC Psychology, 1*(5), 1–18.

Khodayarifard, M., Spielberger, C. D., Lavasani, M. G., & Zardkhaneh, S. A. (2013). Psychometric properties of Farsi Version State-Trait Anger Expression Inventory-2 (FSTAXI-2). *Procedia—Social and Behavioral Sciences, 82*, 325–329. https://doi.org/10.1016/j.sbspro.2013.06.269

Klepfisz, G., Daffern, M., & Day, A. (2016). Understanding dynamic risk factors for violence. *Psychology, Crime & Law, 22*, 124–137. https://doi.org/10.1080/1068316X.2015.1109091

Kobes, M. H. B. M., Nijman, H. L. I., & Bulten, E. B. H. (2012). Assessing aggressive behavior in forensic psychiatric patients: Validity and clinical utility of combining two instruments. *Archives of Psychiatric Nursing, 26*, 487–494.

Konopasky, R. J., & Konopasky, A. W. B. (2000). Remaking penile plethysmography. In D. R. Laws, S. M. Hudson, & T. Ward (Eds.), *Remaking relapse prevention with sex offenders: A source book* (pp. 257–284). Thousand Oaks, CA: Sage.

Kuyken, W., Fothergill, C. D., Musa, M., & Chadwick, P. (2005). The reliability and quality of cognitive case formulation. *Behaviour Research and Therapy, 43*, 1187–1201. https://doi.org/10.1016/j.brat.2004.08.007

Kuyken, W., Padesky, C. A., & Dudley, R. (2008). The science and practice of case conceptualization. *Behavioural and Cognitive Psychotherapy, 2008*(36), 757–768. https://doi.org/10.1017/S1352465808004815

Lammers, S., Keulen-de Vos, M. E., De Groot, A., & Uzieblo, K, (2015). Diagnostiek van psychopathie.[Diagnosing psychopathy]. In W. Canton, D. van Beek, L. Gijs, E. Klein-Haneveld, I. Jeandarme, & L. Claes Eds.), *Handboek Antisociale Persoonlijkheidsstoornis en Psychopathie [Handbook on Antisocial Personality Disorder and Psychopathy]* pp.159-180. Utrecht, NL: De Tijdstroom.

Lijffijt, M., & Barratt, E. S. (2005). Dutch version of the Barratt Impulsiveness Scale-11 (BIS-11). http://www.impulsivity.org/measurement/bis11_Dutch

Lindqvist, J. K., Dåderman, A. M., & Hellström, A. (2003). Swedish adaptations of the Novaco Anger Scale-1998, the Provocation Inventory, and the State-Trait Anger Expression Inventory-2. *Social Behavior and Personality, 31*, 773–788.

Lindqvist, J. K., Dåderman, A. M., & Hellström, A. (2005). Internal reliability and construct validity of the Novaco Anger Scale-1998-S in a sample of violent prison inmates in Sweden. *Psychology, Crime & Law, 11*, 223–237.

Lindstrøm, J. C., Wyller, N. G., Halvorsen, M. M., Hartberg, S., & Lundqvist, C. (2017). Psychometric properties of the Norwegian version of the Barratt Impulsiveness Scale-11 (BIS-11). *Brain and Behavior, 7*, e00605. https://doi.org/10.1002/brb3.605

McPhail, I. V., Hermann, C. A., Fernane, S., Fernandez, Y. M., Nunes, K. L., & Cantor, J. M. (2019). Validity in phallometric testing for sexual interests in children: A meta-analytic review. *Assessment, 26*, 535–551. https://doi.org/10.1177/1073191117706139

Mann, R. E., Hanson, R. K., & Thornton, D. (2010). Assessing risk sexual recidivism: Some proposals on the nature of psychologically meaningful risk factors. *Sexual Abuse: A Journal of Research and Treatment, 22*, 191–217. https://doi.org/10.1177/1079063210366039

Marshall, W. L. (2014). Phallometric assessments of sexual interests: An update. *Current Psychiatry Reports, 16*, 428.

Mattick, R. P., & Clarke, J. C. (1998). Development and validation of measures of social phobia scrutiny fear and social interaction anxiety. *Behaviour Research and Therapy, 36*, 455–470.

Maxwell, J. P., Sukhodolsky, D. G., & Sit, C. H. P. (2009). Preliminary validation of a Chinese version of the State-Trait Anger Expression Inventory-2. *Asian Journal of Social Psychology, 12*, 1–11. https://doi.org/10.1111/j.1467-839X.2008.01264.x

McCrae, R. R., & Costa Jr., P. T. (2004). A contemplated revision of the NEO Five-Factor Inventory. *Personality and Individual Differences, 36*, 587–596. https://doi.org/10.1016/S0191-8869(03)00118-1

McCrae, R. R., Costa Jr., P. T., & Martin, T. A. (2005). The NEO-PI-3: A more readable Revised NEO Personality Inventory. *Journal of Personality Assessment, 84*, 261–270. https://doi.org/10.1207/s15327752jpa8403_05

Mela, M., Balbuena, L., Duncan, C. R., Wong, S., Gu, D., Polvi, N., et al. (2008). The STAXI as a measure of inmate anger and a predictor of institutional offending. *The Journal of Forensic Psychiatry & Psychology, 19*, 396–406. https://doi.org/10.1080/14789940802164090

Morgan, R. D., Kroner, D. G., & Mills, J. F. (2012). *Re-entry: Dynamic risk assessment*. Rockville, MD: National Institute of Justice/NCJRS. https://www.ncjrs.gov/pdffiles1/nij/grants/238075.pdf

Mumma, G. H. (2011). Validity issues in cognitive-behavioral case formulation. *European Journal of Psychological Assessment, 27*, 29–49. https://doi.org/10.1027/1015-5759/a000054

Nagi, C., Ostapiuk, E. B., Craig, L. A., Hacker, D., & Beech, A. R. (2009). Using the revised Problem Identification Checklist to predict inpatient and community violence: A pilot study. *British Journal of Forensic Practice, 11*, 4–13.

Nakano, K. (2001). Psychometric evaluation of the Japanese adaptation of the Aggression Questionnaire. *Behaviour Research and Therapy, 39*, 853–858.

Narrow, W. E., Clarke, D. E., Kuramoto, S. J., Kupfer, D. J., Greiner, L., & Regier, D. A. (2013). DSM-5 field trials in the United States and Canada, part III: Development and reliability testing of a cross-cutting symptom assessment for DSM-5. *American Journal of Psychiatry, 170*, 71–82. https://doi.org/10.1176/appi.ajp.2012.12071000

Nichols, H. R., & Molinder, I. (2000). Multiphasic sexual inventory II. Unpublished manuscript.

Nichols, H. R., & Molinder, L. (1984). The multiphasic sex inventory manual. Unpublished manuscript.

Nijman, H. L. I., Merkelbach, H. L. G. J., Allertz, W. W. F., & à Campo, J. M. L. G. (1997). Prevention of aggressive incidents on a closed psychiatric ward. *Psychiatric Services, 48*, 694–698.

Nijman, H. L. I., Muris, P., Merckelbach, H. L. G. J., Palmstierna, T., Wistedt, B., Vos, A. M., et al. (1999). The Staff Observation Aggression Scale-Revised (SOAS-R). *Aggressive Behavior, 25*, 197–209. https://doi.org/10.1002/(SICI)1098-2337(1999)25:3<197::AID-AB4>3.0.CO;2-C

Nijman, H. L. I., Palmstierna, T., Almvik, R., & Stolker, J. J. (2005). Fifteen years of research with the Staff Observation Aggression Scale: A review. *Acta Psychiatrica Scandinavica, 111*, 12–21. https://doi.org/10.1111/j.1600-0447.2004.00417.x

Novaco, R. W. (1994). Anger as a risk factor for violence among the mentally disordered. In J. Monahan & H. J. Steadman (Eds.), *Violence and mental disorder* (pp. 21–59). Chicago, IL: University of Chicago Press.

Novaco, R. W. (2003). *The Novaco Anger Scale and Provocation Inventory: Manual*. Los Angeles, CA: Western Psychological Services.

Nunes, K. L., Firestone, P., & Baldwin, M. W. (2007). Indirect assessment of cognitions of Child sexual abusers with the implicit association test. *Criminal Justice and Behavior, 34*, 454–475. https://doi.org/10.1177/0093854806291703

Olivares, J., García-López, L. J., & Hidalgo, M. D. (2001). The Social Phobia Scale and the Social Interaction Anxiety Scale: Factor structure and reliability in a Spanish-speaking population. *Journal of Psychoeducational Assessment, 19*, 69–80.

Ostapiuk, E., Stringer, I., & Craig, L. A. (2000). *Some modifications and revisions to the Problem Identification Checklist.* Unpublished manuscript, Forensic Psychology Practice Ltd., Sutton and Coldfield.

Palmstierna, T., & Wistedt, B. (1987). Staff observation aggression scale, SOAS: Presentation and evaluation. *Acta Psychiatrica Scandinavica, 76*, 657–663. https://doi.org/10.1111/j.1600-0447.1987.tb02936.x

Patton, J. H., Stanford, M. S., & Barratt, E. S. (1995). Factor structure of the Barratt impulsiveness scale. *Journal of Clinical Psychology, 6*, 768–774.

Pechorro, P., Maroco, J., Ray, J. V., & Gonçalves, A. (2015). Psychometric properties of the Barratt Impulsiveness Scale version 11 among a Portuguese sample of incarcerated juvenile offenders. *Psychology, Crime & Law, 21*, 1–17. https://doi.org/10.1080/1068316X.2015.1054386

Peters, L. (2000). Discriminant validity of the Social Phobia and Anxiety Inventory (SPAI), the Social Phobia Scale (SPS) and the Social Interaction Anxiety Scale (SIAS). *Behaviour Research and Therapy, 38*, 943–950.

Peugh, J., & Belenko, S. (2001). Alcohol, drugs and sexual function: A review. *Journal of Psychoactive Drugs, 33*(3), 223–232. https://doi.org/10.1177/0306624X17691242

Philipse, M. W. G., Koeter, M. W. J., Van der Staak, C. P. F., & Van den Brink, W. (2006). Reliability and discriminant validity of dynamic reoffending risk indicators in forensic clinical practice. *Criminal Justice and Behavior, 32*, 643–664.

Powers, M. B., & Emmelkamp, P. M. G. (2008). Virtual reality exposure therapy for anxiety disorders: A meta-analysis. *Journal of Anxiety Disorders, 22*, 561–569. https://doi.org/10.1016/j.janxdis.2007.04.006

Prentky, R. A., Barbaree, H. E., & Janus, E. S. (2015). *Sexual predators. Society, risk, and the law.* New York: Routledge.

Quinsey, V. L., Coleman, G., Jones, B. G., & Altrows, I. (1997). Proximal antecedents of eloping and reoffending among mentally disordered offenders. *Journal of Interpersonal Violence, 12*, 794–813.

Quinsey, V. L., Harris, G. T., Rice, M. E., & Cormier, C. (2005). *Violent offenders: Appraising and managing risk* (2nd ed.). Washington, DC: American Psychological Association.

Quinsey, V. L., Jones, G. B., Book, A. S., & Barr, K. N. (2006). The dynamic prediction of antisocial behavior among forensic psychiatric patients. A prospective field study. *Journal of Interpersonal Violence, 21*, 1539–1565. https://doi.org/10.1177/0886260506294238

Renaud, P., Chartier, S., Rouleau, J., Proulx, J., Décarie, J., Trottier, D., et al. (2009). Gaze behavior nonlinear dynamics assessed in virtual immersion as a diagnostic index of sexual deviancy: Preliminary results. *Journal of Virtual Reality and Broadcasting, 6*, 3.

Renaud, P., Goyette, M., Chartier, S., Zhornitski, S., Trottier, D., Rouleau, J., et al. (2010). Sexual affordances, perceptual-motor invariance extraction, and intentional nonlinear dynamics: Sexually deviant and non-deviant patterns in male subjects. *Nonlinear Dynamics, Psychology, and Life Sciences, 14*, 463–489.

Renaud, P., Trottier, D., Rouleau, J., Goyette, M., Saumur, C., Boukhalfi, T., et al. (2014). Using immersive virtual reality and anatomically correct computer-generated characters in the forensic assessment of deviant sexual preferences. *Virtual Reality, 18*, 37–47. https://doi.org/10.1007/s10055-013-0235-8

Rettenberger, M., Boer, D. P., & Eher, R. (2011). The predictive accuracy of risk factors in the Sexual Violence Risk-20 (SVR-20). *Criminal Justice and Behavior, 38*, 1009–1027. https://doi.org/10.1177/0093854811416908

Rettenberger, M., Matthes, A., Boer, D. P., & Eher, R. (2010). Prospective actuarial risk assessment: A comparison of five risk assessment instruments in different sexual offender subtypes. *International Journal of Offender Therapy and Comparative Criminology, 54*, 169–186. https://doi.org/10.1177/0306624X08328755

Reyna, C., Ivacevich, M. G. L., Sanchez, A., & Brussino, S. (2011). The Buss-Perry Aggression Questionnaire: Construct validity and gender invariance among Argentinean adolescents. *International Journal of Psychological Research, 4*, 30–37.

Rice, M. E., Harris, G. T., Quinsey, V. L., & Cyr, M. (1990). Planning treatment programs in secure psychiatric facilities. In D. Weisstub (Ed.), *Law and mental health: International perspectives* (Vol. 5, pp. 162–230). New York: Pergamon.

Roberts, W., Milich, R., & Fillmore, M. T. (2012). Constraints on information processing capacity in adults with ADHD. *Neuropsychology, 26*, 695–703. https://doi.org/10.1037/a0030296

Rolland, J. P., Parker, W. D., & Stumpf, H. (1998). A psychometric examination of the French translations of NEO-PI-R and NEO-FFI. *Journal of Personality Assessment, 71*, 269–291. https://doi.org/10.1207/s15327752jpa7102_13

Rosenzweig, S. (1978). *Aggressive Behavior and the Rosenzweig Picture-Frustration Study*. New York: Praeger.

Santisteban, C., Alvarado, J. M., & Recio, P. (2007). Evaluation of a Spanish version of the Buss and Perry Aggression Questionnaire: Some personal and situational factors related to the aggression scores of young subjects. *Personality and Individual Differences, 42*, 1453–1465. https://doi.org/10.1016/j.paid.2006.10.019

Schlank, A. M. (1995). The utility of the MMPI and the MSI for identifying a sexual offender typology. *Sexual Abuse: A Journal of Research and Treatment, 2*, 185–194.

Schmidt, A. F., Babchishin, K. M., & Lehmann, R. J. B. (2017). A meta-analysis of viewing time measures of sexual interest in children. *Archives of Sexual Behavior, 46*, 287–300.

Schmitz, N., Hartkamp, N., Baldini, C., Rollnik, J., & Tress, W. (2001). Psychometric properties of the German version of the NEO-FFI in psychosomatic outpatients. *Personality and Individual Differences, 31*, 713–722.

Smith, P., Waterman, M., & Ward, N. (2006). Driving aggression in forensic and non-forensic populations: Relationships to self-reported levels of aggression, anger, and impulsivity. *British Journal of Psychology, 97*, 387–403.

Someya, T., Sakado, K., Seki, T., Kojima, M., Reist, C., Tang, S. W., et al. (2001). The Japanese version of the Barratt Impulsiveness Scale, 11th version (BIS-11): Its reliability and validity. *Psychiatry and Clinical Neurosciences, 55*, 111–114. https://doi.org/10.1046/j.1440-1819.2001.00796.x

Spielberger, C. D. (1988). *State-Trait-Anger-Expression-Inventory*. Palo Alto, CA: Consulting Psychologist Press.

Spielberger, C. D. (1999). *State-Trait Anger Expression Inventory-2 (STAXI-2). Professional manual*. Tampa, FL: Psychological Assessment Resources.

Stanford, M. S., Mathias, C. W., Dougherty, D. M., Lake, S. L., Anderson, N. E., & Patton, J. H. (2009). Fifty years of the Barratt Impulsiveness Scale: An update and review. *Personality and Individual Differences, 47*, 385–395. https://doi.org/10.1016/j.paid.2009.04.008

Steinert, T., Wölfle, M., & Gebhardt, R. P. (1999). No correlation of serum cholesterol levels with measures of violence in patients with schizophrenia and non-psychotic disorders. *European Psychiatry, 14*, 346–348. https://doi.org/10.1016/S0924-9338(99)00157-1

Steinert, T., Wölfle, M., & Gebhardt, R. P. (2000). Measurement of violence during in-patient treatment and association with psychopathology. *Acta Psychiatrica Scandinavica, 102*, 107–112. https://doi.org/10.1034/j.1600-0447.2000.102002107.x

Stinson, J. D., & Becker, J. V. (2008). Assessing sexual deviance: A comparison of physiological, historical, and self-report measures. *Journal of Psychiatric Practice, 14*, 379–388.

Tharp, A. T., DeGue, S., Valle, L. A., Brookmeyer, K. A., Massetti, G. M., & Matjasko, J. L. (2012). A systematic qualitative review of risk and protective factors for sexual violence perpetration. *Trauma, Violence, & Abuse, 14*, 133–167. https://doi.org/10.1177/1524838012470031

Thornton, D., Kelley, S. M., & Nelligan, K. E. (2017). Protective factors and mental illness in men with a history of sexual offending. *Aggression and Violent Behavior, 32*, 29–36. https://doi.org/10.1016/j.avb.2016.12.003

Thornton, D., & Laws, D. R. (2009). Introduction. In D. Thornton & D. R. Laws (Eds.), *Cognitive approaches to the assessment of sexual interest in sexual offenders* (pp. 1–5). Chichester: Wiley.

Timmerman, I. G. H., Vastenburg, N. C., & Emmelkamp, P. M. G. (2001). The Forensic Inpatient Observation Scale (FIOS): Development and validity. *Criminal Behavior and Mental Health, 11*, 144–162.

Turner, S. M., Beidel, D. C., Dancu, C. V., & Stanley, M. A. (1989). An empirically derived inventory to measure social fears and anxiety: The Social Phobia and Anxiety Inventory. *Psychological Assessment, 1*, 35–40.

Van Dam-Baggen, R., & Kraaimaat, F. (1999). Assessing social anxiety: The Inventory of Interpersonal Situations (IIS). *European Journal of Psychological Assessment, 15*, 25–38.

Van der Gaag, M., Cuijpers, A., Hoffman, T., Remijsen, M., Hijman, R., De Haan, L., et al. (2006a). The five-factor model of the Positive and Negative Syndrome Scale I: Confirmatory factor analysis fails to confirm 25 published five-factor solutions. *Schizophrenia Research, 85*, 273–279. https://doi.org/10.1016/j.schres.2006.04.001

Van der Gaag, M., Cuijpers, A., Hoffman, T., Remijsen, M., Hijman, R., De Haan, L., et al. (2006b). The five-factor model of the Positive and Negative Syndrome Scale II: A ten-fold cross-validation of a revised model. *Schizophrenia Research, 85*, 280–287. https://doi.org/10.1016/j.schres.2006.03.021

Vanman, E. J., Mejia, V. Y., Dawson, M. E., Schell, A. M., & Raine, A. (2003). Modification of the startle reflex in a community sample: Do one or two dimensions of psychopathy underlie emotional processing? *Personality and Individual Differences, 35*, 2007–2021. https://doi.org/10.1016/S0191-8869(03)00052-7

Von Collani, G., & Werner, R. (2005). Self-related and motivational constructs as determinants of aggression. An analysis and validation of a German version of the Buss-Perry Aggression Questionnaire. *Personality and Individual Differences, 38*, 1631–1643. https://doi.org/10.1016/j.paid.2004.09.027

Weafer, J., Fillmore, M. T., & Milich, R. (2009). Increased sensitivity to the disinhibiting effects of alcohol in adults with ADHD. *Experimental and Clinical Psychopharmacology, 17*, 113–121. https://doi.org/10.1037/a0015418

Wistedt, B., Rasmussen, A., Pedersen, L., Malm, U., Träskman-Bendz, L., Wakelin, J., et al. (1990). The development of an observer-scale for Measuring Social Dysfunction and Aggression. *Pharmacopsychiatry, 23*, 249–252. https://doi.org/10.1055/s-2007-1014514

Wu, B., Lan, T., Hu, T., Lee, S., & Liou, J. (2015). Validation of a five-factor model of a Chinese Mandarin version of the Positive and Negative Syndrome Scale (CMV-PANSS) in a sample of 813 schizophrenia patients. *Schizophrenia Research, 169*, 489–490. https://doi.org/10.1016/j.schres.2015.09.011

Yao, S., Yang, H., Zhu, X., Auerbach, R. P., Abela, J. R., Pulleyblank, R. W., et al. (2007). An examination of the psychometric properties of the Chinese version of the Barratt Impulsiveness Scale, 11th version in a sample of Chinese adolescents. *Perceptual and Motor Skills, 104*, 1169–1182. https://doi.org/10.2466/pms.104.4.1169-1182

Zwets, A. J., Hornsveld, R. H. J., Muris, P., Huijding, J., Kanters, T., Snowden, R. J., & Van Marle, H. (2015a). Implicit attitudes toward violence and their relation to psychopathy, aggression, and socially adaptive behaviors in forensic psychiatric forensic inpatient sample. *International Journal of Law and Psychiatry, 39*, 13–22. https://doi.org/10.1016/j.ijlp.2015.01.016

Zwets, A. J., Hornsveld, R. H. J., Neumann, C., Muris, P., & Van Marle, H. J. C. (2015b). The four-factor model of the Psychopathy Checklist-Revised: Validation in a Dutch forensic inpatient sample. *International Journal of Law and Psychiatry, 39*, 13–22. https://doi.org/10.1016/j.ijlp.2015.01.016

Chapter 5
Cognitive-Behavioral Treatment (CBT) Programs for Violent Offenders and Sexually Violent Offenders: What Substantive Conditions Must Be Met?

Ruud H. J. Hornsveld, Floris W. Kraaimaat, Luk A. C. L. Gijs, and Emma J. Palmer

5.1 Introduction

Forty years ago, Martinson (1976, 1979) concluded that the search for programs that might reduce recidivism in offenders was useless because nothing works. Nowadays there is increasing evidence that this critique was wrong because there is a growing body of evidence that supports the conclusion that many programs and practices can reduce recidivism (Weisburd, Farrington, & Gill, 2017). However, there is also evidence of less effective practices and, importantly, of practices that may even cause harm. Therefore, this chapter attempts to determine the substantive conditions of effective treatment programs for violent and sexually violent offenders.

The original version of this chapter was revised. The correction to this chapter is available at https://doi.org/10.1007/978-3-030-27840-3_12

R. H. J. Hornsveld (✉)
Erasmus University Medical Center, Rotterdam, The Netherlands
e-mail: ruud.hornsveld@ziggo.nl

F. W. Kraaimaat
Radboud University Nijmegen, Nijmegen, The Netherlands

L. A. C. L. Gijs
KU Leuven, Leuven, Belgium

E. J. Palmer
University of Leicester, Leicester, UK

R. H. J. Hornsveld et al. (eds.), *Assessment and Obligatory Treatment of Violent and Sexually Violent Offenders*, Advances in Preventing and Treating Violence and Aggression, https://doi.org/10.1007/978-3-030-27840-3_5

5.2 Programs for Offenders

The first cognitive-behavioral programs for offenders were developed during the 1970s, mainly in the Anglo-Saxon countries, followed by several Western European countries, sometimes almost a decade later. Most of these programs had or have a cognitive-behavioral approach that is based on social learning principles. Studies on the effect of these programs were conducted by comparing the rate of recidivism of a sample of treated offenders with that of a matched sample of untreated offenders. For example, the Reasoning and Rehabilitation program (R&R) designed by Ross, Fabiano, and Ewles (1988) was delivered in Canada and the United States in the early 1990s. This program is based on the proposal that offenders cannot realize their goals because they lack the necessary cognitive and behavioral skills. In 36 two-hour sessions, 6–12 participants extend or modify their cognitions and skills in such a way that the individual recidivism risk factors decrease. Robinson and Porporino (2001) reviewed several studies on the effects of R&R, including a study in more than 4000 Canadian offenders who completed the R&R program between 1989 and 1994 (Robinson, 1995). The recidivism rate in this study turned out to be 19.7% for R&R participants and 24.8% for the control group a year after discharge, which indicates a reduction of 20.5% in the treatment group.

A modified version of R&R was implemented in the United Kingdom from 1993 onwards, namely the Enhanced Thinking Skills (ETS) program with 20 sessions. Friendship, Blud, Erikson, Travers, and Thornton (2003a) compared a group of 667 offenders who followed R&R or ETS with a control group of 1801 offenders. Treatment turned out to produce a robust reduction in the probability of reconviction when other relevant variables were controlled for. For treated offenders, the percentage point reduction in reconviction was 14% in medium-low risk offenders and 11% in medium-high risk offenders. For the low- and high-risk offenders there was a trend in the expected direction, although the difference was not statistically significant.

Lipsey, Chapman, and Landenberger (2001) studied cognitive-behavioral programs focused on teaching new cognitive skills. The participants in these studies were defined as general criminal offenders, juveniles or adults, who are treated while on probation, incarcerated, or in aftercare/parole. Participants were at random or matched assigned to a cognitive-behavioral program or treatment-as-usual. A meta-analysis of fourteen studies from 1985 that met this condition showed that cognitive-behavioral programs were indeed effective interventions. Treated offenders on average recidivated at a rate of about two-thirds that of offenders in the treatment-as-usual control groups. Moreover, the most effective programs reduced recidivism rates to about one-third of the rate for untreated controls. However, most of the substantial recidivism reductions were produced by the programs that were designed by researchers, and no other comparisons were made for instance between the effects of programs in correctional institutions and those for offenders on probation or parole.

Landenberger and Lipsey (2005) performed a meta-analysis of 58 studies on the effects of cognitive-behavioral treatment programs on the recidivism of adult and juvenile offenders to find out which factors contributed to the positive effects of these programs.

Participants in these studies were criminal offenders, either juveniles or adults, treated while on probation, incarcerated/institutionalized, or during aftercare/parole, and were drawn from a general offender population. Offender samples that were selected for, or restricted to, persons committing specific types of offenses were not included. They found that the factors independently related to the effect sizes were (a) the risk level of the offenders, (b) the quality of the program implementation, and (c) the content of the program. The inclusion of anger management and interpersonal problem-solving in the program were associated with more substantial effects, while victim impact and behavior modification were associated with smaller effects. None of the major CBT brand-name programs, for instance, R&R (Ross et al., 1988) or Aggression Replacement Training (ART; Goldstein, Glick, & Gibbs, 1998), produced larger effects on recidivism than the other programs. According to these researchers, high-quality implementation, close monitoring of the performance of the programs, and adequate training for the providers seem to most strongly characterize effective CBT (Lipsey, Landenberger, & Wilson, 2007).

Pearson, Lipton, Cleland, and Yee (2002) conducted a meta-analysis of 69 research studies, published between 1968 and 1996, on the effectiveness of behavioral and cognitive-behavioral treatment in reducing recidivism for offenders. They defined behavior modification/behavior therapy as arranging contingencies of positive reinforcement to develop and maintain appropriate patterns of behavior, such as contingency contracting and token economies. Cognitive-behavioral treatments were described as treatments that include attention to cognitive and emotional processes that function between the stimuli received and the overt behaviors enacted, for example, problem-solving skills training and anger management training. They found that reduced recidivism was mainly reported in cognitive-behavioral interventions, rather than programs with standard behavior modification approaches. However, no information was provided whether or not the cognitive-behavioral programs were individually or group oriented.

5.2.1 Group Programs for Offenders

A meta-analysis of 20 studies of group-oriented cognitive behavioral programs for offenders was performed by Wilson, Allen, and MacKenzie (2000; cited in Lipsey et al., 2001). These programs were found to reduce recidivism by 20–30% compared to untreated control groups. However, some studies concerned general samples of offenders, others specialized types of offenders, for example, sex offenders, drug offenders, driving under the influence cases, or batterers. Therefore, much of the variability in effects found across studies may have been due to differences between types of offenders. In a later study, Wilson, Bouffard, and MacKenzie (2005) investigated the effectiveness of cognitive-behavioral group programs for offenders in 20 studies. They found that all higher quality studies reported positive effects favoring the cognitive-behavioral treatment programs. Specifically, actual reductions in recidivism were observed for Moral Reconation Therapy (Little & Robinson, 1986), R&R (Ross et al., 1988), and various cognitive-restructuring programs. More specifically, there was evidence for the effectiveness of programs that focus on cognitive skills and cognitive restructuring as well as programs that emphasize moral teachings and reasoning.

5.3 Programs for Violent Offenders

Turning specifically to programs for violent offenders, the effectiveness of cognitive behavioral group programs has been examined in some ways, including meta-analyses, systematic or narrative reviews, or studies examining the evaluation of individual programs. For instance, Dowden and Andrews (2000) conducted a meta-analysis of 35 studies to examine the effectiveness of correctional treatment in reducing violent recidivism. As expected, cognitive-behavioral and social learning strategies were associated with substantially larger treatment effects than those produced by non-behavioral approaches. Also, programs that predominantly targeted criminogenic needs produced greater treatment effects than programs that predominantly targeted non-criminogenic needs.

Polaschek and Collie (2004) reviewed nine studies on treatment programs with a cognitive-behavioral approach, and had an appropriate methodological rigor: two cognitive programs, three anger management programs, and four programs that used multiple intervention targets and strategies. Although most programs had small to large positive effects on violent and nonviolent recidivism, little could be concluded about the most promising theoretical framework for future program development.

A systematic review of 11 high-quality research reports was conducted by Joliffe and Farrington (2007) to assess the evidence on the effectiveness of interventions with adult male violent offenders and to identify potential mediators and moderators. Analysis of the reports suggested that interventions with violent offenders were effective both at reducing general and violent recidivism. Violent offenders with extensive criminal histories were more likely to recidivate than general offenders and tended to be more challenging to engage in treatment. Also, there was some evidence to suggest that those interventions of greater overall duration were more effective and that the greater duration per session was associated with greater effect for both general and violent recidivism. However, what could not be assessed in this review is what the optimal dosage of intervention might be. The evidence also suggested that interventions which addressed cognitive skills, anger control, used role play and relapse prevention and had offenders to complete homework were more effective than those interventions that did not.

5.3.1 Group Programs for Violent Offenders

Cortoni, Nunes, and Latendresse (2006) evaluated the Canadian Violence Prevention Program (VPP) for incarcerated violent offenders, who have committed at least two violent offenses and who are at high risk to commit future violent crimes. The goal of the VPP is to reduce the likelihood of violent recidivism among the male offender population. The intervention phase of the VPP consists of the following modules: Making Change (6 sessions), Violence Awareness (12 sessions), Anger Control (12 sessions), Solving Problems (10 sessions), Social Attitudes (10 sessions), Positive Relationships (8 sessions), Conflict Resolution (8 sessions), Positive Lifestyles (8 sessions), Self-Control (8 sessions), and Violence Prevention (12 sessions). Although VPP is not explicitly called a cognitive behavioral program, the modules indicate a cognitive-behavioral approach because they are, according to the researchers, based on social learning and information-processing theories. Five-hundred treated offenders were compared to a matched, non-treated comparison group of 466 offenders. Results showed that offenders who had completed the program had significantly lower rates of recidivism than the non-treated offenders.

Finally, Polaschek, Yesberg, Bell, Casey, and Dickson (2016) compared 121 violent offenders who had completed treatment in a New Zealand high-risk special treatment unit with 154 violent offenders who were eligible to attend the treatment program but had not done so. The treatment comprised a structured, closed-group cognitive-behavioral intervention combined with a "hierarchical democratic therapeutic community approach." The group intervention included sessions on areas such as offense-supportive thinking, mood management, problem-solving skills, and relapse prevention planning. In addition to the treatment program, offenders took part in several activities within the unit community and developed a reintegration plan for release from prison. The program was delivered to closed groups of 10 offenders for approximately 250 h over 25 weeks and remained in the treatment unit for 10–12 months. Completers of the treatment program were found significantly less likely to breach parole, to be reconvicted for any offense, to be reconvicted for violence, and to be imprisoned for a new offense within 12 months after release.

5.3.2 Aggression Replacement Training (ART)

ART is a North American multimodal intervention developed by Goldstein et al. (1998) to improve prosocial behavior in children and adolescents who perform aggressive and violent behaviors. However, as this intervention was the starting point for the development of the treatment programs as described in Chap. 6, it will also be considered here. Goldstein et al. (1998) regarded aggressive behavior as a result of inadequate emotional control, a limited repertoire of social skills, and a lack of moral standards and values. Consequently, ART has three main components, namely anger management, social skills, and moral reasoning. In the original version, ART takes 10 weeks with three sessions per week, one for each component. The groups usually include 6–8 participants. Homework assignments are given during all modules of ART in order to achieve generalization of the learned skills to new situations. In 1999, the state of Washington (USA) decided to investigate ART together with Functional Family Therapy (FFT; Alexander & Parsons, 1982) and Multisystemic Therapy (MST; Henggeler, 1999). In a study by the Washington State Institute for Public Policy (WISP) an experimental group of 704 juvenile offenders with a medium to high recidivism risk was compared with a control group of 525 juvenile offenders. ART resulted in 24% lower recidivism than a control group throughout 18 months in the experimental group (Barnoski, 2004).

More recent research has yielded mixed results. Gunderson and Svartdal (2010) found that the behavior of 77 Norwegian children (girls and boys) who followed ART improved according to trainers, parents, and teachers but in the control sample of 63 children positive changes were also observed. Similar findings were yielded in a study by Koposov, Gunderson, and Svartdal (2014) who investigated ART in a sample of 145 Russian children (girls and boys). They found a significant improvement of social skills among children who had followed ART but in the control sample of 90 children an improvement in social skills and a reduction of problem behaviors were also found. A study by Langeveld, Gunderson, and Svartdal (2012) in 112 Norwegian children and adolescents (girls and boys) showed that after ART social competence was significantly improved and behavioral problems significantly decreased. During awaiting period before the start of the training program, no changes in social competence and behavioral problems were found. Finally, Hornsveld, Kraaimaat, Muris, Zwets, and Kanters (2015) explored the effects of ART in a group of 62 Dutch violent young men aged 16–21 years, who were required to follow a treatment program in a forensic psychiatric outpatient clinic. During the waiting period, the patients did not change on most measures, although they displayed a significant increase in anger. The training produced significant decreases in physical aggression and social anxiety and showed trends toward a decline in self-reported hostility, general aggression, and anger. After the training, the patients scored comparably with a reference group on measures of hostility and aggressive behavior. However, Brännström, Kaunitz, Andershed, South, and Smedslund (2016) concluded from 16 studies that there is insufficient support for the effectiveness of ART. They also noted that almost half of the studies were conducted by researchers who had an interest in the research.

ART has been applied not only to juvenile but also to adult offenders. Hatcher et al. (2010) studied ART in a group of British violent adult offenders serving community sentences in the Probation Service. An experimental group of 53 violent offenders who were required to follow ART was compared with a matched control group of 53 violent offenders who were not obliged to follow the training. Twenty offenders in the experimental group were reconvicted, compared with 27 offenders in the comparison control group. Because of these findings, Hatcher et al. (2010) concluded that “the ART programme may be effective with adult males in community settings” (p. 529). Hornsveld, Nijman, and Kraaimaat (2008) found some support for the effectiveness of an ART-based program in a sample of 89 Dutch violent forensic psychiatric inpatients, while an exploratory study by Zwets et al. (2016) in Dutch violent forensic psychiatric inpatients demonstrated that ART in combination with psychomotor therapy (PMT) resulted in clinically significant improvements of observed social behavior, observed aggressive behavior, and self-reported anger, but there were no differences in treatment effects between the experimental sample of 22 inpatients group and the control sample of 15 inpatients on primary outcome measures. However, on secondary outcome measures, the experimental sample displayed somewhat more improvement than the control sample.

5.3.3 Conclusions and Recommendations

The above studies show that programs that follow a cognitive-behavioral approach are the most successful in reducing recidivism among offenders in general and in violent offenders in particular. There are also strong indications that programs that focus on criminogenic risk factors yield better results than programs that do not. These studies also suggest that interventions that aim to teach prosocial cognitive skills and to learn to control anger, using role play, relapse prevention, and homework assignments, are more effective than interventions that do not. A limitation, however, is that the meta-analyses do not provide information about the treatment integrity of the programs studied. Manuals turn out not to be public and hardly any mention is made of the knowledge and experience of those who led the programs.

5.4 Programs for Sexually Violent Offenders

Group treatment with sex offenders is utilized far more frequently than individual treatment. A 2013 survey of North American sex offender programs showed that 90% of the programs were group based, although there are hardly studies which explored whether one modality is more effective than another (Serran, Marshall, Marshall, & O'Brien, 2013).

5.4.1 Recidivism of Treated and Untreated Sex Offenders

Studies on the effect of the first cognitive-behavioral programs for sexual offenders were conducted by comparing the rate of recidivism of a sample of treated sex offenders with that of a matched sample of untreated sex offenders. The programs focused not only on the modification of deviant sexual orientations but also on improvement of relational skills and a more mature sexual orientation (Barlow, 1973). Due to the introduction of the relapse prevention model in the early 1980s (Pithers, Marques, Gibat, & Marlatt, 1983), modules were added to promote empathy, social skills, relational skills, anger management, and self-esteem (Marshall & Hollin, 2014; Marshall & Laws, 2003). Pithers, Kashima, Cumming, Beal, and Buell (1988) defined relapse as a process of successive steps which result in sexually violent behavior, namely negative mood, fantasies about deviant sexual behavior, distorted cognitions, making plans for committing sexual offenses, deviant masturbation fantasies, and finally committing the offense. Therefore, the relapse prevention-based programs aimed to provide sex offenders insight into the situations that trigger an offense and into the various associated thoughts, feelings, and behaviors involved. Also, sex offenders learned coping skills for dealing with future problems or risk situations, and they had to draw up a plan that would minimize the risk of unexpected risk situations (Marshall & Anderson, 2000).

The most influential study on the effect of a program for sexual offenders that included a relapse prevention component was the Sex Offender Treatment and Evaluation Project in California (SOTEP; Marques, Day, Nelson, & West, 1994). In their controlled study, Marques, Wiederanders, Day, Nelson, and Van Ommeren (2005) compared an experimental group of 259 sex offenders with a matched group of 225 sex offenders who did not follow the program but participated in the investigation, and a control group of 220 sex offenders who did not follow the program and did not want to participate in the study. The treatment program at the Atascadero State Hospital lasted 2 years and included three sessions of 90 min a week. After discharge, participants in the clinical program followed a 1-year aftercare program (SOAP). Noteworthy, the researchers found no difference between the three conditions for sexual or violent recidivism throughout 8 years, but the sex offenders who "met the program's treatment goals had lower re-offense rates than those who did not" (p. 79). However, in the study of Marques et al. (2005) the base rate of recidivism for the untreated offenders was low (13–14%) compared to 10.8% in the experimental group.

More or less parallel to developments in the United States, the Sex Offender Treatment Program (SOTP) was implemented in Britain in 1992 (Grubin & Thornton, 1994). This program included a Core and a Better Lives Booster program for all offenders, as well as an Extended program that provides a more prolonged and more intensive program for high-risk and high-need sex offenders with specific modules on assessment grounds. The Core program consisted of challenging distorted cognitions, promoting empathy, and drawing up an offense scenario to develop relapse prevention strategies. For example, the modules of the Extended program focused on a lack of social skills or insufficient anger management. Finally, the Booster program consisted of integrated skills training, which reconsidered the relapse prevention strategies from the Core program and the Extended Program skills. Individual group meetings could also be added to the group meetings of the three programs. The Core and Booster programs lasted 140–160 h (Grubin & Thornton, 1994). However, an evaluation of the SOTP by Friendship, Mann, and Beech (2003b), comparing a group of 647 treated sex offenders to a group of 1910 matched untreated sex offenders, yielded disappointing results. After 2 years, the percentage of sexual recidivism in the treated group was not significantly lower than in the untreated group, but significant differences were found between the two groups in the recidivism rate when sexual offenses were combined with violent offenses. Friendship and colleagues (2003b) attributed the results primarily to the low base rate of sex offenses, but also to insufficient treatment integrity (Hollin, 1995). Other debilitating factors were that the program changed in between (Mann & Thornton, 2000), the training level of the therapists/trainers (psychologists, recruitment staff, and prison guards) varied greatly, and supervision appeared to be insufficient. A recent large-scale evaluation (Mews, Di Bella, & Purver, 2017) concluded that the Core SOTP was not producing reductions in reconviction (and perhaps in some cases, increased reconvictions) and so the SOTP suite of program was withdrawn by the English and Welsh Prison Service.

However, an evaluation of international studies in the period 1970–1998 by Grossman, Martis, and Fichtner (1999) indicated that both hormonal interventions and cognitive-behavioral therapy programs lead to a 30% reduction in recidivism. Outpatient treatments were more effective than clinical treatments, possibly because the outpatients had a lower recidivism risk than the participants in the clinical programs. An early meta-analysis conducted by Hanson et al. (2002) reviewed 43 studies conducted before 2000. Averaged across all studies, the sexual offense recidivism rate was lower for the treatment groups (12.3%) than the comparison groups (16.8%). Currently, mainly cognitive-behavioral treatments are associated with reductions in both sexual recidivism (from 17.4% to 9.9%) and general recidivism (from 51% to 32%). Older forms of treatment (operating before 1980) appeared to have little effect.

A meta-analysis of 69 studies including 22,181 sex offenders by Lösel and Schmucker (2005) also showed that programs with a relapse prevention component produce positive results, while approaches such as castration, hormone treatment, and some psychotherapeutic approaches show no impact at all. Similar findings were found by De Ruiter, Veen, and Greeven (2008) in a meta-analysis of five studies with a total of 578 rapists, which demonstrated that cognitive behavioral therapy aimed at relapse prevention resulted in a decrease in sexual and general recidivism. The authors concluded that the positive treatment effects found were mainly observed after intensive and relatively long-term intramural treatment, which in some cases was followed by an outpatient care program.

As an alternative to the principles of relapse prevention, Ward and Hudson (2000) developed a Self-Regulation Model with a focus on the various ways in which individuals realize key goals. The model has nine stages for sex offenders: event, desire for forbidden sex, determination of goals, determination of approach, being in a high-risk situation, relapse, sexual offense, evaluation after the offense, and attitude toward future offenses. The authors distinguished four pathways that result in a sexual offense, namely (a) *avoidant/passive:* the offender loses self-control, (b) *avoidant/active:* the offender firstly shows avoidance behavior but loses self-control, (c) *approach/automatic:* the offender commits the sexual offense without thinking, and (d) *approach/explicit:* the offender commits the sexual offense consciously and feels sexually satisfied (Ward & Hudson, 2000). Following the pathways of this model, Bickley and Beech (2002) could classify 87 child sexual abusers to one of these four paths. Approach sex offenders reported more cognitive distortions, among others, on the consequences of the abuse for the victims than avoiding sex offenders with boys or boys and girls as victims. Avoidant sex offenders often had a long-term relationship with an adult partner during the offense and had mostly abused girls. Compared to *active* sex abusers, *passive* sex abusers more often blamed the circumstances and were more often convicted of sexual offenses. Yates and Kingston (2006) also supported the Self-Regulation Model and investigated 80 intra-familial child sexual abusers, extra-familial child sexual abusers, and rapists. On intra-familial child sexual abusers, *avoidant/passive* path was found to be applicable, and to rapists both the *approach/automatic* and the *approach/explicit* path. The validity and usability of the Self-Regulation Model in a treatment context were later evaluated by Kingston, Yates, and Olver (2014) in a group of 275 male sex offenders following one of Canada's Correctional Service (Yates et al., 2000) treatment programs. Results indicated that participation in treatment resulted in moderate to large sized improvements from pretreatment to posttreatment on a dynamic risk assessment measure and several self-reported treatment targets. These changes were, in some cases, differentially associated with self-regulation pathways, suggesting that offense pathway is a clinically relevant variable when evaluating treatment change. Concerning outcome, individuals following the *approach* pathways, particularly the *approach-automatic* pathway, demonstrated higher failure rates than individuals following *avoidant* pathways. However, many of these differences were less pronounced when taking risk of recidivism into account. Because no control group was used in this study, the empirical support for the Self-Regulation Model is for the time being limited.

A population study by Hanson and Harris (2000) of the dynamic risk factors in 208 recidivated and 201 matched non-recidivated Canadian sex offenders revealed that the first group was characterized by limited social support, positive attitudes toward sexual violence, antisocial lifestyles, limited self-control strategies, and problems with supervision. Also, the recidivists appeared to have experienced more subjective tension and anger before the new offense. The different types of sex offenders appeared to provide similar risk factors, although fewer factors were significant among the girl's sexual abusers than among the boy's sexual abusers, or the rapists. These findings may be on the conservative side because the recidivists had followed significantly fewer treatment programs than the non-recidivists.

In a critical discussion of the relapse prevention model, Hanson (2000) suggested that treatment programs should focus more on risk factors that initiate criminal behavior (for example, deviant sexual interests) and risk factors that prevent relapse (for example, self-regulation strategies) than on risk factors that can result in a sexual offense. Hanson's (2000) critique is in line with the Risk-Need-Responsivity principles advocated by Andrews and Bonta (2010) who showed that recidivism risk of violent offenders is related to antisocial history, antisocial personality, antisocial cognitions, antisocial network, family and/or relationship problems, limited education and/or no work, insufficient leisure activities, and substance abuse. Hanson, Bourgon, Helmus, and Hodgson (2009) found that these factors also apply to sex offenders. A meta-analysis of 23 high-quality studies revealed that the recidivism risk of treated sex offenders (10.9%) was significantly lower than for untreated sex offenders (19.2%). Programs based on the Risk-Need-Responsivity principles gave the greatest decrease in sexual and general recidivism. Smid, Kamphuis, Wever, and Van Beek (2014) conducted a survey in which a sample of 106 Dutch treated sex offenders was compared to a group of 188 untreated sexual offenders, using the Static-99R. The treatment lasted an average of 8 years and 4 months and consisted of individual or group psychotherapy, a relapse prevention program, practical training and/or education, and any medication. The researchers found a treatment effect in the high-risk offenders, but not in the average- or low-risk offenders, comparing the pre-measurement with the post-measurement.

Some studies into the effectiveness of treatment programs concerned only child sexual abusers. Långström et al. (2013) found evidence of a reduction in recidivism risk as a result of pharmacological, psychological, or psychoeducational interventions based on eight methodologically sound studies in child sexual abusers. Grønnerød, Grønnerød, and Grøndahl (2015) supported this finding in their meta-analysis of 14 studies with a robust research design on psychotherapeutic interventions, which showed that the effect sizes of such interventions in this population are very small. Out of ten studies conducted by Walton and Chou (2015), which investigated the impact of psychological interventions on child abusers, there were only three who could demonstrate a lower recidivism risk. These three well-controlled studies involved cognitive-behavioral treatment programs.

In 2004, Ward and Marshall suggested that treatment of negative offense-related behavior in sex offenders (for example, cognitive distortions) should be complemented by promoting positive behavior (for example, intimate relationships skills), thus giving them the chance to reduce future offenses. Ward and colleagues introduced the Good Lives Model, which focuses on the potential of sex offenders to improve the quality of their lives. According to this model, ten main aspects of existence have to be addressed in the preparation of a treatment plan: healthy life, knowledge, play and work, independence, inner peace, relationships, community spirit, spirituality, happiness, and creativity (Wills, Yates, Gannon, & Ward, 2013). However, Marshall and Marshall (2014) noted that, to date, hardly any controlled research has been conducted on the effectiveness of Good Lives Model-based treatment programs. Therefore, they advocated a balanced approach, addressing both negative and positive behaviors (Marshall et al., 2005). Their treatment program (Marshall, Marshall, Serran, & Fernandez, 2006) focuses on both negative factors and sexual abuse in childhood, inability to attachment and intimacy, deviant sexual interests or sexual compulsion as well as strengthening positive (protective) factors such as learning coping skills, emotion regulation, and building a more or less satisfying existence. Marshall, Marshall, Serran, and O'Brien (2013) concluded that effective programs meet four criteria: (1) they focus on dynamic criminological factors, (2) are offered in a user-friendly manner, (3) apply procedures that allow criminogenic needs to be changed, and (4) place treatment in a positive framework according to the principles of the Good Lives Model. In a study by Olver, Marshall, Marshall, and Nicholaichuk (2018), the early version of Rockwood's prison-based sex offender program that has elements of a strength-based approach was compared with sex offender treatment programs of the Correctional Service of Canada and with no-treatment sex offenders. Both treatment groups displayed significantly lower rates of both sexual and violent reoffending when compared with the no-treatment sex offenders, but the Rockwood program generated the lowest recidivism rates.

5.4.2 Recidivism and Other Treatment Outcomes

The promising results of cognitive-behavioral treatment programs for sexually violent offenders at the beginning of the twenty-first century were followed by studies in which the differences between a pretest at the beginning and a posttest at the end of a program were related to recidivism risk, and no longer was a comparison made between treated and untreated groups.

Williams, Wakeling, and Webster (2007) found that 211 British sex offenders who had followed the Adapted Sex Offender Treatment Program (ASOTP) for lower intellectually functioning sex offenders scored afterwards significantly better on the dynamic items of risk assessment instruments. The program included sexual education, accountability for the offense, victimization, and the learning of coping skills. For evaluating purposes, self-report questionnaires that measured cognitive distortions, attitudes about victims, victim empathy, coping skills, self-esteem, and loneliness were used. Recidivism risk at the beginning of the treatment did not influence changes in problem behaviors, nor did the type of crime. In a follow-up study of 3773 British sex offenders who had completed treatment, Wakeling, Beech, and Freemantle (2013) calculated significant changes of the four domains in the Structured Assessment of Risk and Need (Thornton, 2002): (1) sexual interests; (2) pro-offending attitudes; (3) socio-affective problems; and (4) self-regulation problems. Analyses indicated that those whose scores were in the average range before and after treatment were reconvicted at a significantly lower rate than those whose scores were not in the average range after treatment on selected psychometric scales. Additionally, participants who were deemed to have changed overall on three of the four risk domains were reconvicted at a lower rate than those who were deemed not to have changed on these domains. An overall treatment change status was also computed, but this did not add significantly to the predictive validity of a modified version of an actuarial risk assessment tool (RM2000, Thornton et al., 2003).

Olver, Kingston, Nicholaichuk, and Wong (2014) also found among 392 detained sex offenders that change in self-report questionnaires for cognitive distortions, aggression/hostility, empathy, loneliness, intimacy, and taking responsibility correlated with recidivism risk when controlling for pre-measurements. Noteworthy in this study, however, was that the investigated offenders at the pre-measurement did not score "in a particularly pathological manner on the battery of psychometric measures" (p. 549).

Due to the sensitivity of self-report questionnaires for socially desirable responding, in a number of studies treatment results have been measured using risk assessment instruments. In addition to self-report questionnaires for cognitive distortions, intimacy, and loneliness, in their study of 313 Canadian sex offenders Nunes, Babchishin, and Cortoni (2011) used three risk assessment instruments, including the Stable 2000 (Hanson, Harris, Scott, & Helmus, 2007) for the measurement of psychological risk factors. The treatment consisted of a short version (40–48 h) or an extended version (200–224 h) of the National Sex Offender

Program (NaSOP), including self-regulation, cognitive distortions, deviant sexual arousal and fantasy, social skills, anger- and emotion regulation, empathy, and victim-empathy. The short program was given to both community and detained sex offenders, the long program was intended exclusively for detained sex offenders. Nunes et al. (2011) found that investigated sex offenders improved on both self-report questionnaires and risk assessment instruments, but those who followed the short program showed a greater improvement than those who completed the long program. However, the participants in the short program had a lower recidivism risk, measured with the Static-99 (Hanson & Thornton, 1999), than the participants in the long program. Olver, Wong, Nicholaichuk, and Gordon (2007) showed in their study of 321 Canadian sex offenders that positive changes in the psychological items of the Violence Risk Scale-Sexual Offender Version (VRS-SO, Wong, Olver, Nicholaichuk, & Gordon, 2003) were related to a decline in recidivism risk. All psychological risk factors together also contributed to improved predictions of sexual recidivism. In a combined study by Olver, Beggs Christofferson, Grace, and Wong (2014), these findings were confirmed in a larger group of Canadian and New Zealand sex offenders. However, Beggs and Grace (2011) believed that there is stronger evidence of the relationship between treatment outcome and recidivism risk when using different behavioral measurement instruments. Therefore, in their study of 218 sex offenders, they used three different instruments for determining treatment outcome, namely self-report questionnaires, the psychological items of the VRS-SO, and a modified version of the Standard Goal Attainment Scaling (SGAS; Hogue, 1994). The combined score on the three measurements for treatment results correlated significantly positive with recidivism risk. Consequently, the authors concluded that positive treatment results contributed to a decrease in recidivism risk.

5.4.3 Conclusions and Recommendations

Studies comparing a treated and an untreated sample of sex offenders as well as studies where the differences between a pre- and post-measurement were related to recidivism after discharge, resulted in a significant but modest reduction of recidivism. However, these studies have several methodological shortcomings. Firstly, most effect studies do not distinguish any subgroups (e.g., intrafamilial child sexual abusers versus extrafamilial child sexual abusers) with their specific risk factors. Thus, it remains unclear on which of these factors a treatment program should be focused and for which subgroup this should be meant. Another problem is that, just as with programs for violent offenders, the manuals for the programs studied are usually not public, although the interventions used are sometimes briefly described (Olver & Wong, 2013). As a result, it is difficult to determine what exactly the content of the programs was, and which interventions were effective and which were not. Which behavioral change must be achieved in order to decide on discharge or subsequent treatment in a community program remains unnoticed. Besides, it is unclear how the problems of individual participants were analyzed and then addressed in conjunction with the group program. No outcome study, except Friendship et al. (2003), reported on treatment integrity (Hollin, 1995), namely that treatment was conducted by well-trained and supervised therapists who followed the treatment manual (Mann, 2009).

Consequently, Brooks-Gordon, Bilby, and Wells (2006) concluded by an analysis of nine studies that "the uncertainty on the effectiveness of psychological interventions remains" (p. 460). A Cochrane review of ten studies in which included 944 sex offenders also concluded that psychological treatments, both behavioral and psychodynamic, do not automatically result in a decline in recidivism risk (Dennis et al., 2012). In their opinion, the state of affairs is characterized as follows: "Currently available evidence does not support the belief that once the individual has been treated, their risk of offending is reduced" (p. 2). Several studies have found that high-risk sex offenders benefit more from treatment programs than those with average or low recidivism (Beggs & Grace, 2011; Olver et al., 2007; Olver, Nicholaichuk, Kingston, & Wong, 2014; Smid et al., 2014; Wakeling et al., 2013). Beggs and Grace (2011) noted, however, that "higher pretreatment scores leave more room to show genuine improvement" (p. 185).

5.5 General Conclusions

Treatment programs for offenders are effective when they focus on the dynamic factors that are related to criminal behavior (Andrews & Bonta, 2010). These factors are antisocial personality pattern, antisocial cognition, antisocial associates, family/marital circumstances, school/work, leisure/recreation, and substance abuse. The factor "antisocial personality pattern" refers in most offenders to an antisocial personality disorder (Raine, 1993). An antisocial personality disorder may hardly be cured, but it is an important factor that refers to the ability and the motivation to change behavior. Further, the factors "antisocial associates," "family/marital circumstances, school/work," and "leisure/recreation" are broad domains which require several functional analyses for the determination of the various problem behaviors that are playing an important role in such a domain (Chap. 4). Substance abuse is a problem behavior for which we refer to Leukefeld, Gullotta, and Gregrich (2011) or Weekes, Moser, Wheatley, and Matheson (2013).

For the time being, the advice of Mann, Hanson, and Thornton (2010) should be followed regarding the content of cognitive-behavioral programs for sexually violent offenders. In the first place, these programs have to focus on empirically supported risk factors such as deviant sexual interest, offense-supportive attitudes, emotional congruence with children, lack of intimate relationships with adults, impulsiveness, poor problem solving, resistance to control, rancor, and antisocial associates. In the second place, programs should be devoted to promising risk factors such as hostility toward women, antisocial personality pattern, lack of concern for others (callousness), and inadequate coping skills. Finally, programs should not pay attention to factors such as depression, general social skills deficits, poor victim empathy, and lack of motivation.

Several publications stress other non-substantive factors that are related to the effectiveness of treatment programs for offenders, such as the education and experience of the providers and in closed institutions of the staff on the ward, facilities for research on the effectiveness of the program, and finally the support of the management during the implementation and the performance of the program. These conditions are part of treatment integrity (Cooke & Philip, 2001), which are discussed in Chap. 8.

References

Alexander, J. F., & Parsons, B. V. (1982). *Functional family therapy: Principles and procedures*. Carmel, CA: Brooks/Cole.

Andrews, D. A., & Bonta, J. (2010). *The psychology of criminal conduct* (5th ed.). New Providence, NJ: Matthew Bender & Company.

Barlow, D. H. (1973). Increasing heterosexual responsiveness in the treatment of sexual deviation. *Behavior Therapy, 4*, 655–671.

Barnoski, R. (2004). *Outcome evaluation of Washington State's research-based programs for juvenile offenders*. Olympia, WA: Washington State Institute for Public Policy. Retrieved October 3, 2016, from http://wsipp.wa.gov/pub.asp?docid=04-01-1201

Beggs, S. M., & Grace, R. C. (2011). Treatment gain for sexual offenders against children predicts reduced recidivism: A comparative validity study. *Journal of Consulting and Clinical Psychology, 79*, 182–192. https://doi.org/10.1037/a0022900

Bickley, J. A., & Beech, A. R. (2002). An investigation of the Ward and Hudson pathways of the sexual offense process with child abusers. *Journal of Interpersonal Violence, 17*, 371–393. https://doi.org/10.1177/0886260502017004002

Brännström, L., Kaunitz, C., Andershed, A., South, S., & Smedslund, G. (2016). Aggression Replacement Training (ART) for reducing antisocial behavior in adolescents and adults: A systematic review. *Aggression and Violent Behavior, 27*, 30–41. https://doi.org/10.1016/j.avb.2016.02.006

Brooks-Gordon, B., Bilby, C., & Wells, H. (2006). A systematic review of psychological interventions for sexual offenders I: Randomised control trials. *The Journal of Forensic Psychiatry & Psychology, 17*, 442–466. https://doi.org/10.1080/14789940600819341

Cooke, D. J., & Philip, L. (2001). To treat or not to treat? An empirical perspective. In C. R. Hollin (Ed.), *Handbook of offender assessment and treatment* (pp. 17–34). Chichester: Wiley.

Cortoni, F., Nunes, K., & Latendresse, M. (2006). *An examination of the effectiveness of the Violence Prevention Program*. Research Report R-178. Ottawa: Correctional Service Canada.

De Ruiter, C., Veen, V., & Greeven, P. (2008). De effectiviteit van psychologische behandeling bij volwassen verkrachters: bevindingen van een meta-analyse [The effectiveness of psychological treatment in adult rapists: Findings from a meta-analysis]. *Tijdschrift voor Seksuologie [Dutch Journal of Sexology], 32*, 28–41.

Dennis, J. A., Khan, O., Ferriter, M., Huband, N., Powney, M. J., & Duggan, C. (2012). Psychological interventions for adults who have sexually offended or are at risk of offending (Review). *The Cochrane Library, 12*. Chichester: Wiley.

Dowden, C., & Andrews, D. A. (2000). Effective correctional treatment and violent reoffending: A meta-analysis. *Canadian Journal of Criminology and Criminal Justice, 42*, 449–467.

Friendship, C., Blud, L., Erikson, M., Travers, R., & Thornton, D. (2003a). Cognitive-behavioural treatment for imprisoned offenders: An evaluation of HM Prison Service's cognitive skills programmes. *Legal and Criminological Psychology, 8*, 103–114.

Friendship, C., Mann, R. E., & Beech, A. R. (2003b). Evaluation of a national prison-based treatment program for sexual offenders in England and Wales. *Journal of Interpersonal Violence, 18*, 744–759.

Goldstein, A. P., Glick, B., & Gibbs, J. C. (1998). *Aggression Replacement Training: A comprehensive intervention for aggressive youth* (2nd ed.). Champaign, IL: Research Press.

Grønnerød, C., Grønnerød, J. S., & Grøndahl, P. (2015). Psychological treatment of sexual offenders against children: A meta-analytic review of treatment outcome studies. *Trauma, Violence, & Abuse, 16*, 280–290. https://doi.org/10.1177/1524838014526043

Grossman, L. S., Martis, B., & Fichtner, M. D. (1999). Are sex offenders treatable? A research overview. *Psychiatric Services, 50*, 349–361.

Grubin, D., & Thornton, D. (1994). A national program for the assessment and treatment of sex offenders in the English prison system. *Criminal Justice and Behavior, 21*, 55–71. https://doi.org/10.1177/0093854894021001005

Gunderson, K., & Svartdal, F. (2010). Diffusion of treatment interventions: Exploration of "secondary" treatment diffusion. *Psychology, Crime & Law, 16*, 233–249. https://doi.org/10.1080/10683160802612924

Hanson, R. K. (2000). Treatment outcome and evaluation problems (and solutions). In D. R. Laws, S. M. Hudson, & T. Ward (Eds.), *Remaking relapse prevention with sex offenders: A sourcebook* (pp. 485–499). Thousand Oaks, CA: Sage.

Hanson, R. K., Bourgon, G., Helmus, L., & Hodgson, S. (2009). The principles of effective correctional treatment also apply to sexual offenders: A meta-analysis. *Criminal Justice and Behavior, 36*, 865–891. https://doi.org/10.1177/0093854809338545

Hanson, R. K., & Harris, A. J. R. (2000). *Dynamic predictors of sexual recidivism based on comparing 208 recidivists and 201 non-recidivists on community supervision.* Unpublished raw data.

Hanson, R. K., Gordon, A., Harris, A. J. R., Marques, J. K., Murphy, W., Quinsey, V. L., et al. (2002). First report of the collaborative outcome data project on the effectiveness of psychological treatment for sex offenders. *Sexual Abuse: A Journal of Research and Treatment, 14*, 169–194.

Hanson, R. K., Harris, A. J. R., Scott, T., & Helmus, L. (2007). *Assessing the risk of sexual offenders on community supervision: The Dynamic Supervision Project.* Corrections Research User Report No. 2007-05. Ottawa: Public Safety Canada.

Hanson, R. K., & Thornton, D. (1999). *Static 99: Improving actuarial risk assessment for sex offenders*. User Report No. 99-02. Ottawa: Corrections Research, Department of the Solicitor General of Canada.

Hatcher, R. M., Palmer, E. J., McGuire, J., Hounsome, J. C., Bilby, C. A. L., & Hollin, C. R. (2010). Aggression Replacement Training with adult male offenders within community settings: A reconviction analysis. *The Journal of Forensic Psychiatry & Psychology, 19*, 517–532. https://doi.org/10.1080/14789940801936407

Henggeler, S. W. (1999). Multisystemic therapy: An overview of clinical procedures, outcomes, and policy implications. *Child Psychology & Psychiatry Review, 4*, 2–10. https://doi.org/10.1017/S1360641798001786

Hogue, T. E. (1994). Goal attainment scaling: A measure of clinical impact and risk assessment. *Issues in Criminological & Legal Psychology, 21*, 96–102.

Hollin, C. R. (1995). The meaning and implications of "treatment integrity". In J. McGuire (Ed.), *What works: Reducing reoffending-guidelines from research and practice* (pp. 195–208). Chichester: Wiley.

Hornsveld, R. H. J., Kraaimaat, F. W., Muris, P., Zwets, A. J., & Kanters, T. (2015). Aggression Replacement Training for violent young men in a forensic psychiatric outpatient clinic. *Journal of Interpersonal Violence, 30*, 3174–3191. https://doi.org/10.1177/0886260514555007

Hornsveld, R. H. J., Nijman, H. L. I., & Kraaimaat, F. W. (2008). Aggression Control Therapy for violent forensic psychiatric patients: First results. *Psychology, Crime & Law, 14*, 1–18. https://doi.org/10.1080/10683160701340569

Joliffe, D., & Farrington, D. P. (2007). *A systematic review of the national and international evidence on the effectiveness of interventions with violent offenders*. London: Ministry of Justice.

Kingston, D. A., Yates, P. M., & Olver, M. E. (2014). The self-regulation model of sexual offending: Intermediate outcomes and posttreatment recidivism. *Sexual Abuse: A Journal of Research and Treatment, 26*, 429–449. https://doi.org/10.1177/10790632134958964

Koposov, R., Gunderson, K., & Svartdal, F. (2014). Efficacy of Aggression Replacement Training among children from north-west Russia. *International Journal of Emotional Education, 6*, 14–24.

Landenberger, N. A., & Lipsey, M. W. (2005). The positive effects of cognitive-behavioral programs for offenders: A meta-analysis of factors associated with effective treatment. *Journal of Experimental Criminology, 1*, 451–476.

Langeveld, J. H., Gunderson, K. K., & Svartdal, F. (2012). Social competence as a mediating factor in reduction of behavioral problems. *Scandinavian Journal of Educational Research, 56*, 381–399. https://doi.org/10.1080/00313831.2011.594614

Långström, N., Enebrink, P., Laurén, E., Lindblom, J., Werkö, S., & Hanson, R. K. (2013). Preventing sexual abusers of children from reoffending: Systematic review of medical and psychological interventions. *British Medical Journal, 347*, f4630. https://doi.org/10.1136/bmj.f4630

Leukefeld, C., Gullotta, T. P., & Gregrich, J. (2011). *Handbook of evidence-based substance abuse treatment in criminal justice settings*. New York: Springer.

Lipsey, M. W., Chapman, G. L., & Landenberger, N. A. (2001). Cognitive-behavioral programs for offenders. *Annals of the American Academy of Political and Social Science, 578*, 144–157.

Lipsey, M. W., Landenberger, N. A., & Wilson, S. J. (2007). Effects of cognitive-behavioral programs for criminal offenders. *Campbell Systematic Reviews, 6*, 1–27.

Little, G. L., & Robinson, K. D. (1986). *How to escape your prison*. Memphis, TN: Eagle Wing Books.

Lösel, F., & Schmucker, M. (2005). The effectiveness of treatment for sexual offenders: A comprehensive meta-analysis. *Journal of Experimental Criminology, 1*, 117–146.

Mann, R. E. (2009). Sex offender treatment: The case for manualization. *Journal of Sexual Aggression, 15*, 121–131. https://doi.org/10.1080/13552600902907288

Mann, R. E., Hanson, R. K., & Thornton, D. (2010). Assessing risk sexual recidivism: Some proposals on the nature of psychologically meaningful risk factors. *Sexual Abuse: A Journal of Research and Treatment, 22*, 191–217. https://doi.org/10.1177/1079063210366039

Mann, R. E., & Thornton, D. (2000). An evidence-based relapse prevention program. In D. R. Laws, S. M. Hudson, & T. Ward (Eds.), *Remaking relapse prevention with sex offenders: A sourcebook* (pp. 341–350). Thousand Oaks, CA: Sage.

Marques, J. K., Day, D. M., Nelson, C., & West, M. A. (1994). Effects of cognitive-behavioral treatment on sex offender recidivism: Preliminary results of a longitudinal study. *Criminal Justice and Behavior, 21*, 28–54.

Marques, J. K., Wiederanders, M., Day, D. M., Nelson, C., & Van Ommeren, A. (2005). Effects of a relapse prevention program on sexual recidivism: Final results from California's Sex Offenders Treatment and Evaluation Project (SOTEP). *Sexual Abuse: A Journal of Research and Treatment, 17*, 79–107. https://doi.org/10.1007/s11194-005-1212-x

Marshall, W. L., & Anderson, D. (2000). Do relapse prevention components enhance treatment effectiveness. In D. R. Laws, S. M. Hudson, & T. Ward (Eds.), *Remaking relapse prevention with sex offenders: A sourcebook* (pp. 39–55). Thousand Oaks, CA: Sage.

Marshall, W. L., & Hollin, C. (2014). Historical developments in sex offender treatment. *Journal of Sexual Aggression, 21*, 1–11. https://doi.org/10.1080/13552600.2014.980339

Marshall, W. L., & Laws, D. R. (2003). A brief history of behavioral and cognitive behavioral approaches to sexual offenders: Part 2. The modern era. *Sexual Abuse: A Journal of Research and Treatment, 15*, 93–120.

Marshall, W. L., & Marshall, L. E. (2014). The future of sexual offender treatment programs. In D. P. Boer, R. Eher, L. A. Craig, M. H. Miner, & F. Pfäfflin (Eds.), *International perspectives on the assessment and treatment of sexual offenders* (pp. 707–740). Chichester: Wiley-Blackwell.

Marshall, W. L., Marshall, L. E., Serran, G. A., & Fernandez, Y. M. (2006). *Treating sexual offenders: An integrated approach*. New York: Routledge.

Marshall, W. L., Marshall, L. E., Serran, G. A., & O'Brien, M. D. (2013). What works in reducing sexual offending. In L. A. Craig, L. Dixon, & T. A. Gannon (Eds.), *What works in offender rehabilitation: An evidence-based approach to assessment and treatment* (pp. 173–191). Chichester: Wiley.

Marshall, W. L., Ward, T., Mann, R. E., Moulden, H., Fernandez, Y. M., Serran, G., et al. (2005). Working positively with sexual offenders: Maximizing the effectiveness of treatment. *Journal of Interpersonal Violence, 20*, 1096–1114. https://doi.org/10.1177/0886260505278514

Martinson, R. (1976). California research at the crossroads. *Crime & Delinquency, 22*, 180–191.

Martinson, R. (1979). New findings, new views: A note of caution regarding sentencing reform. *Hofstra Law Review, 7*, 243–258.

Mews, A., Di Bella, L., & Purver, M. (2017). *Impact evaluation of the prison-based Core Sex Offender Treatment Programme*. London: Ministry of Justice.

Nunes, K. L., Babchishin, K., & Cortoni, F. (2011). Measuring treatment change in sex offenders: Clinical and statistical significance. *Criminal Justice and Behavior, 38*, 157–173. https://doi.org/10.1177/0093854810391054

Olver, M. E., Beggs Christofferson, S. M., Grace, R. C., & Wong, S. C. P. (2014). Incorporating change information into sexual offender risk assessment using the Violence Risk Scale-Sexual Offender Version. *Sexual Abuse: A Journal of Research and Treatment, 26*, 472–499. https://doi.org/10.1177/1079063213502679

Olver, M. E., Kingston, D. A., Nicholaichuk, T. P., & Wong, S. C. P. (2014). A psychometric examination of treatment change in a multisite sample of treated Canadian federal sexual offenders. *Law and Human Behavior, 38*, 544–559. https://doi.org/10.1037/lhb0000086

Olver, M. E., Marshall, L. E., Marshall, W. L., & Nicholaichuk, T. P. (2018). A long-term outcome assessment of the effects on subsequent reoffense rates of a prison-based CBT/RNR sex offender treatment program with strength-based elements. *Sexual Abuse*. https://doi.org/10.1177/1079063218807486

Olver, M. E., Nicholaichuk, T. P., Kingston, D. A., & Wong, S. C. P. (2014). A multisite examination of sexual violence risk and therapeutic change. *Journal of Consulting and Clinical Psychology, 82*, 312–324. https://doi.org/10.1037/a0035340

Olver, M. E., & Wong, S. C. P. (2013). A description and research review of the Clearwater Sex Offender Treatment Programme. *Psychology, Crime & Law, 19*, 477–492. https://doi.org/10.1080/1068316X.2013.758983

Olver, M. E., Wong, S. C. P., Nicholaichuk, T., & Gordon, A. (2007). The validity and reliability of the Violence Risk Scale-Sexual Offender version: Assessing sex offender risk and evaluating therapeutic change. *Psychological Assessment, 19*, 318–329. https://doi.org/10.1037/1040-3590.19.3.318

Pearson, F. S., Lipton, D. S., Cleland, C. M., & Yee, D. S. (2002). The effects of behavioral/cognitive-behavioral programs on recidivism. *Crime & Delinquency, 48*, 476–496.

Pithers, W. D., Kashima, K. M., Cumming, G. F., Beal, L. S., & Buell, M. M. (1988). Relapse prevention of sexual aggression. *Annals of the New York Academy of Sciences, 528*, 244–260. https://doi.org/10.1111/j.1749-6632.1988.tb50868.x

Pithers, W. D., Marques, J. K., Gibat, C. C., & Marlatt, G. A. (1983). Relapse prevention with sexual aggressiveness: A self-control model of treatment and maintenance of change. In J. G. Greer & I. R. Stuart (Eds.), *The sexual aggressor: Current perspectives on treatment* (pp. 214–239). New York: Van Nostrand Reinhold.

Polaschek, D. L. L., & Collie, R. M. (2004). Rehabilitating serious violent adult offenders: An empirical and theoretical stocktake. *Psychology, Crime & Law, 10*, 321–334. https://doi.org/10.1080/10683160410001662807

Polaschek, D. L. L., Yesberg, J. A., Bell, R. K., Casey, A. R., & Dickson, S. R. (2016). Intensive psychological treatment of high-risk violent offenders: Outcomes and pre-release mechanisms. *Psychology, Crime & Law, 22*, 344–365. https://doi.org/10.1080/1068316X.2015.1109088

Raine, A. (1993). *The psychopathology of crime: Criminal behavior as a clinical disorder* (p. 1993). San Diego, CA: Academic Press.

Robinson, D. (1995). *The impact of cognitive skills training on post-release recidivism among Canadian federal offenders*. No. R-41. Research Branch. Ottawa: Correctional Sevice Canada.
Robinson, D., & Porporino, F. J. (2001). Programming in cognitive skills: The reasoning and rehabilitation programme. In C. R. Hollin (Ed.), *Handbook of offender assessment and treatment* (pp. 179–194). Chichester: Wiley.
Ross, R. R., Fabiano, E. A., & Ewles, C. D. (1988). Reasoning and rehabilitation. *International Journal of Offender Therapy and Comparative Criminology, 32*, 29–35.
Serran, G. A., Marshall, W. L., Marshall, L. E., & O'Brien, M. D. (2013). Group or individual therapy in the treatment of sexual offenders. In L. A. Craig, L. Dixon, & T. A. Gannon (Eds.), *What works in offender rehabilitation: An evidence-based approach to assessment and treatment* (pp. 452–467). Chichester: Wiley-Blackwell.
Smid, W. J., Kamphuis, J. H., Wever, E. C., & Van Beek, D. J. (2014). Treatment referral for sex offenders based on clinical judgment vs. actuarial risk assessment: Match and analysis of mismatch. *Journal of Interpersonal Violence, 28*, 2273–2289. https://doi.org/10.1177/0886260512475313
Thornton, D. (2002). Constructing and testing a framework for dynamic risk assessment. *Sexual Abuse: A Journal of Research and Treatment, 14*, 139–153.
Thornton, D., Mann, R., Webster, S., Blud, L., Travers, R., Friendship, C., & Erikson, M. (2003). Distinguishing between and combining risks for sexual and violent recidivism. In R. A. Prentky, E. S. Janus, & M. C. Seton (Eds.), *Understanding and managing sexually coercive behavior. Annals of the New York Academy of Sciences, 989*, 223–235.
Wakeling, H., Beech, A. R., & Freemantle, N. (2013). Investigating treatment change and its relationship in a sample of 3773 sex offenders in the UK. *Psychology, Crime & Law, 19*, 233–252. https://doi.org/10.1080/1068316X.2011.626413
Walton, J. S, & Chou, S. (2015). The effectiveness of psychological treatment for reducing recidivism in child molesters: a systematic review of randomized and nonrandomized studies. *Trauma, Violence, & Abuse, 16*, 401–417. https://doi.org/10.1177/15248380145379
Ward, T., & Hudson, S. M. (2000). A self-regulation model of relapse prevention. In D. R. Laws, S. M. Hudson, & T. Ward (Eds.), *Remaking relapse prevention with sex offenders: A sourcebook* (pp. 79–101). Thousand Oaks, CA: Sage.
Ward, T., & Marshall, W. L. (2004). Good lives, aetiology and the rehabilitation of sex offenders: A bridging theory. Journal of Sexual Aggression: Special Issue: *Treatment & Treatability, 10*, 153–169.
Weekes, J. R., Moser, A. E., Wheatley, M., & Matheson, F. I. (2013). What works in reducing substance-related offending. In L. A. Craig, L. Dixon, & T. A. Gannon (Eds.), *What works in offender rehabilitation: An evidence-based approach to assessment and treatment* (pp. 237–254). Chichester: Wiley.
Weisburd, D., Farrington, D., & Gill, C. (2017). What works in crime prevention and rehabilitation. An assessment of systematic reviews. *Criminology & Public Policy, 16*, 415–449. https://doi.org/10.1111/1745-9133
Williams, F., Wakeling, H., & Webster, S. (2007). A psychometric study of six self-report measures for use with sexual offenders with cognitive and social functioning deficits. *Psychology, Crime & Law, 13*, 505–522. https://doi.org/10.1080/10683160601060739
Wills, G., Yates, P., Gannon, T., & Ward, T. (2013). How to integrate the good lives model into treatment programs for sexual offending: An introduction and overview. *Sexual Abuse: A Journal of Research and Treatment, 25*, 123–142.
Wilson, D., Allen, L., & MacKenzie, D. (2000). *Quantitative review of cognitive behavioral programs*. College Park, MD: University of Maryland.
Wilson, D. B., Bouffard, L. A., & Mackenzie, D. L. (2005). A quantitative review of structured, group-oriented, cognitive-behavioral programs for offenders. *Criminal Justice and Behavior, 32*, 172–204. https://doi.org/10.1177/0093854804272889
Wong, S., Olver, M. E., Nicholaichuk, T. P., & Gordon, A. (2003). *The Violence Risk Scale-Sexual Offender version (VRS-SO)*. Saskatoon: Regional Psychiatric Centre and University of Saskatchewan.

Yates, P. M., Goguen, B. C., Nicholaichuk, T. P., Williams, S. M., Long, C. A., Jeglic, E., et al. (2000). *National sex offender programs (Moderate, low, and maintenance intensity levels)*. Ottawa: Correctional Service of Canada.

Yates, P. M., & Kingston, D. A. (2006). The self-regulation model of sexual offending: The relationship between offense pathways and static and dynamic sexual offense risk. *Sexual Abuse: Journal of Research and Treatment, 18*, 259–227. https://doi.org/10.1177/107906320601800304

Zwets, A. J., Hornsveld, R. H. J., Muris, P., Kanters, T., Langstraat, E., & Van Marle, H. J. C. (2016). Psychomotor therapy as an additive intervention for violent forensic psychiatric inpatients: A pilot study. *International Journal of Forensic Mental Health, 15*, 222–234. https://doi.org/10.1080/14999013.2016.1152613

Part II
Practice

Chapter 6
Treatment Programs for Violent Offenders and Sexually Violent Offenders

Ruud H. J. Hornsveld and Floris W. Kraaimaat

6.1 Introduction

Although there is until now no evidence for the effectiveness of group treatment above individual treatment, group treatment is almost universally regarded as the preferred treatment option for violent offenders (Jennings & Sawyer, 2003; Russell, 2002; Serran, Marshall, Marshall, & O'Brien, 2013). The benefits of group treatment relate to cost-effectiveness, an environment of participants with similar problems, a wide range of antisocial cognitions, and less pressure on the participants (Stinson & Becker, 2013).

In our opinion, practicing prosocial skills preferably takes place in groups using role-playing. Treatment programs for offenders have become considerably more cognitive and less behavioral over time. However, Fernandez, Shingler, and Marshall (2006) stated that a better balance between cognitive and behavioral change techniques would facilitate the achievement of treatment goals and provide trainers with strategies for managing group interactions. Designing interventions that are likely to maximize generalization of treatment gains is essential to provide offenders with opportunities to exercise new skills in their everyday life, whether that is in prison, in a forensic psychiatric hospital, or in the community (Fernandez, Shingler, & Marshall, 2006).

R. H. J. Hornsveld (✉)
Erasmus University Medical Center, Rotterdam, The Netherlands
e-mail: ruud.hornsveld@ziggo.nl

F. W. Kraaimaat
Radboud University Nijmegen, Nijmegen, The Netherlands

R. H. J. Hornsveld et al. (eds.), *Assessment and Obligatory Treatment of Violent and Sexually Violent Offenders*, Advances in Preventing and Treating Violence and Aggression, https://doi.org/10.1007/978-3-030-27840-3_6

Russell (2002) stated that treatment groups for men provide a unique experience for most men who typically have not had the opportunities to openly and honestly explore their beliefs about intimate relationships. This kind of self-exploration and self-confrontation is still rare in traditional male culture. Men in groups frequently identify with experiences of other group members, learn from examples provided by others, and give advice to others. Furthermore, a group environment may encourage breaking male taboos, such as admitting weakness and challenging traditional beliefs associated with masculinity. According to Marshall, Anderson, and Fernandez (1999), group treatment for sex offenders is more effective than individual treatment because other participants are regarded as more credible than trainers, especially when addressing cognitive distortions.

Advantages of closed treatment groups in comparison with open treatment groups are that all participants receive the same treatment, the group process is not disturbed by the arrival of new participants, and trainers become better informed about the specific problems of all participants (Stinson & Becker, 2013). Whereas open groups should be considered when new participants are regularly admitted to shortening the waiting list period for treatment.

6.2 Treatment Program for Violent Offenders

The development of this treatment program for violent offenders was based on the heuristic model of violent offenders (Chap. 2) and the Aggression Replacement Training (ART) of Goldstein, Glick, and Gibbs (1998) was chosen as a starting point because this training is solidly based on cognitive-behavioral theory (Hollin, 2004; Polaschek, 2006). The *Basic program* for violent offenders (Table 6.1) contains three components, namely Anger Management (sessions 1–5), Social Skills (sessions 6–10), and Moral Reasoning (sessions 11–15).

Table 6.1 Flowchart of treatment modules for violent offenders

Group	Violent offenders	Sessions
Assessment		≥3
Basic program	• Anger Management	≥5
	• Prosocial Skills	≥5
	• Moral Reasoning	≥5
Extended program	• Prosocial Thinking	≥5
	• Consequences of Behavior	≥5
	• Prosocial Network	≥5
	• Contact with Women	≥5
	• Work and Leisure	≥5
Assessment		≥2
Evaluation	• Discussing participant's reports	≥2
Generalization and maintenance	• Self-Regulation Skills	

6.2.1 *Anger Management*

The aim of this module is that participants learn to reduce the frequency of their anger outbursts through self-regulation. Participants learn to observe the behavior of others, to distinguish observations from interpretations, and to recognize the emotional consequences of interpretations. Participants also learn to lower their arousal level, to distinguish different emotions, and to realize the consequences of behavior in the short and long term. During the Anger Management module, the behavioral chain is used as described in Chap. 4, namely the A-O-E-B-C format.

6.2.2 *Prosocial Skills*

The purpose of this module is to teach participants new social skills or to improve existing social skills so that they behave more assertively in social situations, that is, achieve their goals without harming the interests of others. This module is based on the method of Van Dam-Baggen and Kraaimaat (2014), which holds in this case that participants choose at least 5 from 12 social skills, such as responding on a refusal, criticizing, and complimenting someone. Then, a group ranking is composed of individual choices.

During the first session, each participant is asked to indicate on a five-point scale how much tension he/she experiences in five generally formulated situations. The participants exercise in the first meeting with the situation that gives them the least tension. In the subsequent sessions, those situations are exercised that the participants have come up with. Next, they mention five exercise situations from easy to difficult. Before practicing, the goals ("What do you want to achieve?") and criteria ("What do I pay attention to?") are listed, after which the participants get a handout of possible goals and criteria. Participants start practicing with easy situations, i.e., situations that give little tension. Finally, the hierarchy is further processed per participant per meeting.

6.2.3 *Moral Reasoning*

During the module Moral Reasoning of the program, participants discuss, based on problem situations, moral dilemmas to achieve a more mature moral stage. Also, participants are asked to report moral problems they have been faced with and how they have solved these problems.

The *Basic program* for violent offenders with 15 sessions was extended with five modules for dynamic criminogenic risk factors such as antisocial attitudes, antisocial network, relational problems, and work/leisure problems. The five modules of the *Extended program* are Prosocial Thinking (sessions 16–20), Consequences of Behavior (sessions 21–25), Prosocial Network (sessions 26–30), Contact with

Women (sessions 31–35), and Work and Leisure (sessions 26–40). During the sessions of the various modules, a theme is discussed firstly, followed by practicing related prosocial behaviors.

6.2.4 *Prosocial Thinking*

The Prosocial Thinking module addresses knowing how to convert cognitions that may lead to antisocial behavior into cognitions that may lead to prosocial behavior. During each session, participants have to answer questions on possible antisocial cognitions which may lead to a problem situation in which somebody exhibits aggressive behavior. Five antisocial cognitions are discussed and exercised during role-playing exercises, which address not putting yourself in somebody else's shoes, egocentricity, denial, suspiciousness, and blaming others.

6.2.5 *Consequences of Behavior*

The Consequences of Behavior module is about the short-term and long-term consequences of prosocial and antisocial behavior. Five themes are discussed and exercised, namely responsibility, subservience, respect, cooperation, and honesty. In each session, consequences of behavior on the short and the long term are discussed by asking participants to answer questions on a problem situation in which somebody has shown aggressive behavior. The discussions are followed by practicing new behavior utilizing role-playing.

6.2.6 *Prosocial Network*

The Prosocial Network module teaches how to engage in prosocial contact and to refrain from or end antisocial contact. During each session, a problem situation is exercised by presenting participants a problem situation in which a person has to figure out how to behave appropriately. Five problem situations are exercised, first through discussions, then by role-playing, namely making acquaintance, making an appointment, deepening a contact, informing others about your rehabilitation or treatment program, and responding to a rejection.

6.2.7 *Contact with Women*

In the Contact with Women module, participants learn how to behave appropriately toward women. Using a problem situation with accompanying questions, participants discuss how to act respectfully toward women. The five problem situations that are exercised are: showing your need for intimacy, responding to a rejection, responding to an approach, talking about sex, and deepening intimacy. Discussions are followed by practicing new behavior that is related to the discussed problem behaviors.

6.2.8 Work and Leisure

During this module, participants learn specific social skills for performing paid work or unpaid voluntary work and for recreation in the form of sports, hobby, or the like. It concerns five combinations of social skills, namely responding to a compliment and maintaining contact, standing up for yourself and responding to a refusal, refusing and giving your opinion, responding to criticism and asking for help, and criticizing and complimenting someone. The five combinations are exercised using role-playing.

6.3 Treatment Program for Sexually Violent Offenders

Based on the heuristic models of rapists and child sexual abusers (Chap. 2), different basic programs were developed for these two subgroups of sex offenders (Table 6.2). The *Basic program* for rapists is similar to the program for violent offenders because they often display also non-sexually aggressive behavior (Wilson, Mouilso, Gentile, Calhoun, & Zeichner, 2015). It comprises the modules Anger Management (sessions 1–5), Prosocial Skills (sessions 6–10), and Moral Reasoning (session 11–15).

The *Basic program* for child sexual abusers focusses on Emotion Management (sessions 1–5) that follows the module Anger Management for violent offenders but emphasizes also emotions other than anger, for example, fear or gloom, but the procedure is the same, by using the A-O-E-B-C behavioral chain. The method applied in module Prosocial Skills (sessions 6–10) is similar to the Prosocial Skills module for violent offenders, but the focus in both subgroups is mainly on interpersonal skills in intimate situations. The moral problems that are discussed during the module Moral Reasoning are devoted in rapists and child sexual abusers to situations with sexual content. Participants are asked to report moral problems regarding sexual behavior they have been faced with and how they have solved these problems.

After the *Basic program,* rapists and child sexual abusers participate together in a *Specific program* that comprises the modules Psychoeducation (sessions 26–35), Cognitive Distortions (sessions 36–50), and three modules that are equal to the modules for the violent offenders, namely Prosocial Network (sessions 51–55), Contact with Women (sessions 56–60), and Work and Leisure (sessions 61–65). The last module of the Specific program is called Management of Risk Situations (sessions 66–71).

Table 6.2 Flowchart of treatment modules for sexually violent offenders

Group	Sexually violent offenders			
Subgroups	Rapists	Sessions	Child sexual abusers	Sessions
Assessment		≥3		≥3
Basic program	• Anger Management	≥5	• Emotion management	≥5
	• Prosocial Skills	≥5	• Prosocial Skills	≥5
	• Moral Reasoning	≥5	• Moral Reasoning	≥5
Group	Rapists and child sexual abusers			
Specific program	• Psychoeducation			≥10
	• Cognitive Distortions			≥15
	• Prosocial Network			≥5
	• Contact with Women			≥5
	• Work and Leisure			≥5
	• Management of Risk Situations			≥5
Assessment				≥3
Generalization and Maintenance	Self-Regulation Skills			

6.3.1 Psychoeducation

During the module Psychoeducation, information is provided on several aspects of sexuality, such as the art of making love, problems when making love, sexual diversity, sexually transmitted diseases (STDs), contraception, pornography, and internet addiction. A brochure with information about the various aspects of sexuality is available on www.Agressiehanteringstherapie.nl/nl/menu/boeken/. After the provision of the information, a discussion takes place during which the participants are allowed to give their opinion on the subject, but they also get to hear what the consequences are of the information provided for their behavior, and what the norms and values are in their country regarding sexuality.

6.3.2 Cognitive Distortions

The purpose of the Cognitive Distortions module is that participants learn to replace cognitive distortions that are related to a sexual offense with prosocial cognitions. During the group sessions, participants have to answer questions about problem situations in which someone is sexually violent. The module consists of approximately 15 sessions and is dedicated to five cognitive distortions related to rapists and five related to child abusers. The cognitive distortions of rapists are: (1) women are unknowable, because in their view women mislead men and do not say what they want; (2) women are sex objects, because they think that women are always sexually receptive to the needs of men, though they are not still aware of this; (3) male sexual drive is uncontrollable, which means that in their view the sexual need in men can be so high that it becomes dangerous for women if they do not answer to that need; (4) entitlement, because they see it as their right to punish a woman and to force her, when she does not respond directly to the sexual needs of a man; and finally (5) dangerous world, which means that in their view the world is a hostile and threatening place and that people in general are dangerous. The cognitive distortions of child sexual abusers are: (1) children as sexual objects, which means that they see children as loving sex with adults and are continually looking for it; (2) nature of harm, because they think that sexual contact between adults and children is not harmful to the child unless violence is used; (3) uncontrollability, that stands for the opinion that some men have such a strong sexual need that their behavior is not always under control; (4) entitlement, because men are superior and have a right to have sex with inferior people such as children; and finally (5) dangerous world, which refers to the thought that the world is a threatening environment full of hostile people.

6.3.3 Management of Risk Situations

The Management of Risk Situations module focuses on coping with high-risk situations in which participants make a functional analysis of their most important problem behaviors with the aid of the trainers. Participants have to demonstrate through role-playing to what extent they can resolve various risky situations adequately. If needed, the number of sessions can be extended.

6.4 Evaluation and Reports

At the end of the program, a few sessions are dedicated to treatment evaluation. The same risk assessment instruments as at the beginning of the treatment program are administered to reevaluate the risk of (sexual) recidivism. An evaluation report for each participant is made from the risk assessment and clinical impressions of the trainers during the treatment. This report describes the participant's treatment goals, his or her motivation during the program, clinical impressions of the progress made by the participant, and the risk assessment at the end of the treatment program. If the participant has made insufficient progress, it is advised to offer him additional treatment. If the risk of recidivism remains consistently high even after several treatment attempts, care in a long-stay institution should be considered. The evaluation report is discussed with the participants before it is sent to the relevant officials, such as a primary treating physician.

6.5 Conditions

Trainers should have a *manual* at their disposal and participants a *workbook* in which they can make their homework assignments. These homework assignments are given for the generalization of learned skills to new situations. All training sessions last about 90 min. For the participants who need assistance in making their homework assignments, *homework sessions* of 90 min between the treatment sessions have to be organized. The group can be divided into two subgroups so that each participant can receive 45 min of guidance for making the homework assignments.

The training sessions are led by two *trainers,* preferably a man and a woman. The training sessions take place in a group room with armchairs, tables, and chairs. Also, present are a blackboard, a video camera, and playback equipment. *Role-playing* with the use of video equipment and an actress is an essential part of the program. The video allows a participant to review his behavior and an instructed actress enhances the realism of the training situations. After discussing the feedback, the role-play is rehearsed when necessary.

In the description of the two programs, *numbers of sessions* are mentioned. However, the number of sessions can be extended if the circumstances so require, for example, because a group consists of relatively slowly learning participants or because a subject is particularly relevant for the majority of the participants.

6.6 Clinical Experience

6.6.1 Violent Offenders

The *Anger Management* module usually does not cause too many problems for the trainers because the participants are informed about the behavior chain and the exercises they have to do during the sessions are not too difficult. More problems occur with the *Prosocial Skills* module. Participants have to introduce their problem situations, and then some participants state that they do not experience them or abandon further participation. The latter mainly applies to programs in a community center or a forensic psychiatric outpatient clinic. The *Moral Reasoning* module is entirely new for most participants. They have not learned to recognize moral problem situations and certainly not to manage them. For the entire Basic program, the trainers must ensure that participants do not get the feeling that they are back in school. However, on every step of the desired behavior must be responded as much positive as possible.

The Extended or Specific program is primarily meant for offenders staying in a closed setting. Then, the chance of dropping out is less probable. When practicing with role-playing, care must be taken to ensure that all participants are covered and that the focus is on desired behavior and less on undesirable behavior. This means that participants react positively to each other as much as possible. Participants who are intractable or who seek to disrupt the group process must be taken separately after the session and receive a warning unless the trainers feel that the behavior is not structural and/or is partly motivated by the individual problems of a participant.

6.6.2 *Case Vignette*

Examples of participant's behavior during the Basic program for violent offenders are described in vignette 1 (see for Anthony's case formulation subchapter 4.7.2).

6.6.2.1 Vignette 1: Anthony

In the forensic psychiatric outpatient clinic, Anthony did not fail to attend to the Basic program once. However, he manifested himself as the most dominant participant and, strangely, the other participants accepted his role. Anthony sometimes went so far as to behave as a sort of co-trainer who ensured that the other participants made their homework assignments. As a result, he was taken apart at the end of a few sessions to make it clear to him that he must participate in the program to learn how to change his behavior. Therefore, he became pointed out the short- and long-term consequences of his dominant behavior (module Consequences of Behavior, subchapter 10.6) so that he realized somewhat that these long-term consequences could be detrimental to him. At the same time, he was praised for his active contribution to the group, provided that he controls his tendency to dominate.

6.6.3 *Sexually Violent Offenders*

At the start of the module *Psychoeducation*, participants generally showed little knowledge of sexuality and intimate relationships. Most were raised in an environment in which women and gay persons are discriminated. Others said to know all about sex because they regularly see porn movies. Some participants believed that sexual violence is allowed in certain threatening situations. Various participants were sexually abused during childhood. Child sexual abusers tended to give socially desirable answers but sometimes stated that sexual contact with a minor should be allowed. Rapists often expressed sexist views on sexual diversity and interacting with women. Therefore, trainers had to emphasize regularly that sexual contact with children and violence against women and men are morally unacceptable and legally prohibited.

During the module *Cognitive Distortions*, trainers had to ensure that rapists did not continuously disqualify the child sex abusers and, in this way making their own sexually deviant behavior under-addressed. Noteworthy was that child sexual abusers often gave comprehensive answers to the homework assignments to emphasize that they are not sexually attracted to children. Group sessions turned out to be strenuous for the participants. When fatigue increased, and self-control decreased, participants were more likely to make sexist comments that reflected their cognitive distortions. Participants were confronted with their cognitive distortions constructively, to prevent that the atmosphere became unpleasant. Trainers need to proceed in such a way that an open and safe therapeutic environment is guaranteed. Too much stress among the participants impedes addressing cognitive distortions.

The module *Prosocial Skills* showed significant differences in skills between child sexual abusers and rapists. Rapists generally appeared to have a good repertoire of social skills, and they often learned quickly to replace inadequate and / or antisocial behavior with prosocial behavior. Noteworthy were their hostile attitudes against women, which were explicitly addressed during role-playing. Rapists appeared to give insufficient attention to the possible negative consequences of their behavior. The child sexual abusers generally behaved somewhat awkward, and they initially struggled to change their inappropriate social behavior. When, after several sessions, the child sexual abusers became more at ease, they were able to make better use of the given feedback, especially by reviewing the video recording of the role-play.

During the *Management of Risk Situations* module, most participants were further informed about the mandatory aftercare program in an outpatient treatment facility. Some child sexual abusers appeared to have learned remarkably little of the clinical program, and they hardly seemed to realize the difficulties that await them in the community. They seemed to persist in justifying sexual contact with minors that made an admission in a long-stay institution almost inevitable.

6.6.4 Case Vignettes

Examples of participant's behavior during the Basic program and Specific program are described in two vignettes, Juan (rapist) in vignette 2 and Eric (child sexual abuser) in vignette 3 (see for Juan's and Eric's case formulation subchapter 4.7.3).

6.6.4.1 Vignette 2: Juan

In the module *Prosocial Skills* (subchapter 10.3), Juan demonstrated he already possessed good social skills. His initial contact with women was adequate, but Juan got intrusive when relationships became more intimate. Therefore, Juan was thought to consider both the short- and long-term consequences of his behavior (subchapter 10.6). Juan also learned to interpret the signals of women more adequately, so he could better assess whether or not they are interested in him (subchapter 10.8). In the module *Psychoeducation* (subchapter 11.3), Juan regularly made sexist statements. He stated, for instance, that some women get sexually aroused by forced sexual contact. Juan learned that women are equal to men and that several of his behaviors towards women are unacceptable. Noteworthy was that Juan saw his former partner(s) solely as the mother of his children rather than as his wife or partner. During the module *Cognitive Distortions* (subchapter 11.4), Juan indicated that his misogynistic behavior could be explained by cognitions such as: "I am entitled to have sex," "Women like sex all the time," and "We live in a dangerous world." Juan's homework assignments consisted of describing alternative thoughts and behavior for past situations in which he acted condescending and/or aggressive towards women. In addition to the pharmacological treatment for his deviant sexual behavior, Juan also received treatment for his drug addiction.

6.6.4.2 Vignette 3: Eric

During the module *Psychoeducation* (subchapter 11.3), it was emphasized that pedophilia is not a socially accepted sexual interest and that sexual contact with minors is prohibited. In the module *Cognitive Distortions* (subchapter 11.4), Eric's cognitions that initiated and justified his deviant sexual behavior were addressed. That were "I am entitled to have sex," "My victims have suffered no physical pain," and "I did not ejaculate inside my victims." Eric received homework assignments in which he had to memorize situations where he had these thoughts. Then, Eric had to visualize (and write down) appropriate alternative behavior for that given situation. When discussing his homework assignments, we noticed Eric's tendency to minimize his deviant sexual behavior. During the modules *Prosocial Skills* (subchapter 10.3) and *Contact with Women* (subchapter 10.8), Eric had to role-play a casual meeting with an adult woman (played by an actress) and during the module Work and Leisure (subchapter 10.9) a job interview for voluntary work. In both cases, he demonstrated his limited social skills by mentioning unexpectedly that he was a convicted sex offender, but they should not be afraid of him. For his deviant sexual interests, Eric received pharmacological treatment.

6.7 Additional Interventions

Preferably, participants follow the modules of the program in the described order. Sometimes it may be necessary to conduct an individual interview with a participant, for example, because he threatens to drop out or because a further exploration of a particular problem behavior has become topical. Also, the heuristic model can show that another treatment is also indicated, for problems such as trauma, depression, or substance dependence. By participating in the program for violent or sexually violent offenders with an individual or group treatment for these problems, offenders can be offered a tailor-made program.

The program for sexually violent offenders does not include interventions that are pre-eminently aimed at reducing deviant sexual interest. In our opinion, this may be better achieved through psychopharmacological interventions, although there are indications that treatment focused on most problem behaviors and attitudes except deviant sexual interest, may result in a decrease in deviant sexual interest (Brown, 2011; Gee, Ward, & Eccleston, 2003; Marshall, 1997; Marshall, Marshall, Serran, & O'Brien, 2013).

6.8 Conclusions and Recommendations

In this chapter, two cognitive-behavioral programs have been presented: one for violent and one for sexually violent offenders (child sexual abusers and rapists). In our opinion, programs are not cookbooks that have to be strictly followed, but a methodology that requires improvisation if this is in the interest of the participants. This does require that the trainers are well trained and have experience in treating groups with limited-motivated participants (see also Chap. 8).

The main finding of our clinical experience and research is that a change in aggressive behaviors, including sexually aggressive behavior, is difficult to achieve in a closed setting for male offenders because of the structure and control. Therefore, we recommended attention to the strengthening of prosocial behavior instead of focusing solely on the reduction of negative behaviors (Hornsveld, Kraaimaat, Bouwmeester, Polak, & Zwets, 2014). For the exercise of new prosocial behavior, including prosocial sexual behavior, the use of Virtual Reality apparatus seems to be useful (Kampmann et al., 2016). Follow-up assessment of program effectiveness on several occasions after discharge is essential.

References

Brown, S. (2011). *Treating sex offenders. An introduction to sex offender treatment programmes*. London: Routledge.

Gee, D., Ward, T., & Eccleston, L. (2003). The function of sexual fantasies for sexual offenders: A preliminary model. *Behaviour Change, 20*, 44–60. https://doi.org/10.1375/bech.20.1.44.24846

Hollin, C. R. (2004). Aggression Replacement Training: The cognitive-behavioral context. In A. P. Goldstein, R. Nensén, B. Daleflod, & M. Kalt (Eds.), *New perspectives on aggression replacement training* (pp. 3–19). Chichester: Wiley.

Jennings, J. L., & Sawyer, S. (2003). Principles and techniques for maximizing the effectiveness of group therapy with sex offenders. *Sexual Abuse: A Journal of Research and Treatment, 15*, 251–267.

Kampmann, I. L., Emmelkamp, P. M. G., Hartanto, D., Brinkman, W. P., Zijlstra, B. J. H., & Morina, N. (2016). Exposure to virtual social interactions in the treatment of social anxiety disorder: A randomized controlled trial. *Behaviour Research and Therapy, 77*, 147–156. https://doi.org/10.1016/j.brat.2015.12.016

Marshall, W. L. (1997). The relationship between self-esteem and deviant sexual arousal in nonfamilial child molesters. *Behavior Modification, 21*, 86–96.

Marshall, W. L., Anderson, D., & Fernandez, Y. (1999). *Cognitive-behavioral treatment of sexual offenders*. Chichester: Wiley.

Polaschek, D. L. L. (2006). Violent offender programmes: Concept, theory, and practice. In C. R. Hollin & E. J. Palmer (Eds.), *Offending behaviour programmes. Development, application, and controversies* (pp. 113–154). Chichester: Wiley.

Russell, M. N. (2002). Changing beliefs of spouse abusers. In J. McGuire (Ed.), *Offender rehabilitation and treatment: Effective programmes and policies to reduce re-offending* (pp. 243–258). Chichester: Wiley.

Stinson, J. D., & Becker, J. V. (2013). *Treating sex offenders. An evidence-based manual.* New York: Guilford.

Van Dam-Baggen, R., & Kraaimaat, F. (2014). Cognitive-behavioral group therapy for social anxiety and social incompetence: A social skills perspective. Maarn/Nijmegen. Open Access book: http://www.floriskraaimaat.nl/pdfiles/sstjune2014.pdf

Chapter 7
Self-Management Skills for Generalization and Maintenance of Treatment Results

Ruud H. J. Hornsveld and Floris W. Kraaimaat

7.1 Introduction

Publications are scarce on how offenders can maintain or, when necessary, expand the improvements in their behavior after the end of a treatment program. This problem mainly occurs with offenders who have followed a rehabilitation or treatment program in a penitentiary or forensic psychiatric institution successively. In addition to the written transfer of an offender's file to a counseling or treatment team from a probation institution or a forensic psychiatric outpatient clinic, it is essential that offenders themselves have the necessary skills to make a more or less smooth transition from a closed setting to the community. This may be achieved by learning offender's self-management skills in order to familiarize themselves with new situations and acquire new behaviors. Generally, self-management procedures are of interest to advance an individual's self-control.

7.2 Self-Regulation Theories of Bandura and Zimmerman

Bandura (1977, 1991, 1997, 2001) is one of the leading theorists on observational learning and self-regulation theory (SRT). Observational or vicarious learning is learning from viewing others performing a complex behavior. An application of observational learning is the behavioral change method of modeling. Modeling and underlying conditions were extensively studied and found to be an effective method

R. H. J. Hornsveld (✉)
Erasmus University Medical Center, Rotterdam, The Netherlands
e-mail: ruud.hornsveld@ziggo.nl

F. W. Kraaimaat
Radboud University Nijmegen, Nijmegen, The Netherlands

R. H. J. Hornsveld et al. (eds.), *Assessment and Obligatory Treatment of Violent and Sexually Violent Offenders*, Advances in Preventing and Treating Violence and Aggression, https://doi.org/10.1007/978-3-030-27840-3_7

for behavior change. A general and comprehensive description of the principles of behavior change is presented in Bandura's self-regulation theory (SRT). According to SRT, the primary self-regulative mechanism operates through three principal subfunctions. They are: (1) self-monitoring of one's behavior, its determinants, and its effects, (2) judgment of one's behavior about personal standards and environmental circumstances, and (3) affective self-reaction. Thus, this self-regulative mechanism has a substantial impact on cognition, affect, action, and motivation. The self-monitoring function is influenced by (a) *self-diagnosis*, insight as a condition for a process of corrective change, and (b) *self-motivation*, the tendency of people to set themselves goals of progressive improvement. The judgmental function is determined by (a) *development of personal standards*, to be acquired through education as well as the evaluative reactions of others toward one's behavior, (b) *social referential comparisons*, the evaluation of one's performances in relation to the achievement of others, (c) *valuation of activities,* the relevance of one's performances for one's values and sense of personal adequacy, and (d) *perceived performance determinants*, whether one's accomplishments can be ascribed to one's abilities and efforts, or are the results of external supports. Finally, the self-reactive function relates to the use of self-incentives, self-satisfaction or tangible benefits conditional upon specific accomplishments. Thus, people who succeed in regulating their behavior and motivation, and achieve what they seek, differ from people who are unsuccessful in their regulatory efforts in the effective use of self-incentives.

Perceived self-efficacy is a judgment of one's ability to organize and execute given types of performances (Bandura, 1997). Self-beliefs of *efficacy* partly determine how the various subfunctions of a self-regulatory system operate. People who regard themselves as highly efficacious tend to ascribe their failures to insufficient effort, whereas those who see themselves as inefficacious view the cause of their failures as stemming from low ability. The more capable they judge themselves to be, the higher the goals they set for themselves and the more firmly committed they remain to them. Without aspirations and evaluative involvement in activities, people remain unmotivated, bored, uncertain about their capabilities, and dependent upon momentary external stimulation for their satisfaction. Many of the miseries people inflict upon themselves and others arise from dysfunctions in the self-regulatory system. For instance, depression is most likely to occur when personal standards of merit are set well above one's perceived self-efficacy to attain them (Bandura, 1991).

A somewhat different and elaborate description of self-regulated learning (SRL) is proposed by the social psychologist Zimmerman (2013). His cyclical model of SRL describes how proactive and reactive task-oriented students use self-regulation for the attainment of learning goals. According to his model, self-regulated learning comprises three self-regulatory phases: forethought, performance, and self-reflection. *Forethought* phase processes are used in preparation for efforts to learn and are intended to enhance that learning. *Performance* phase processes are employed during efforts to learn and are intended to facilitate self-control and self-monitoring of one's performance. *Self-reflection* phase processes occur after efforts to learn and are intended to optimize a person's reactions to his or her outcomes.

These self-reflections, in turn, influence forethought processes and beliefs regarding subsequent efforts to learn, thus completing a self-regulatory cycle.

The *Forethought phase* is composed of *task analysis,* which refers to a learner's efforts to break a learning task into crucial components, and *self-motivation beliefs.* Proactive learners can set specific, proximal, and challenging goals for themselves. While reactive students, because of their superficial task analyses, set vague, distal, or unchallenging goals for themselves. Therefore, proactive learners are motivated by higher self-efficacy beliefs, outcome expectancies, mastery of learning goals, and task interest or task valuing. In contrast, reactive learners display inferior forms of motivation and are as a result less self-motivated to analyze tasks, select goals, or plan strategically than proactive learners.

The *performance phase* comprises processes of *self-control,* which refers to the use of specific techniques to direct learning (e.g., self-instruction), and *self-observation.* During the self-control phase, proactive learners perform activities that are planned during the forethought phase, while reactive learners immerse themselves in a learning task without an explicit strategy to guide them. Furthermore, proactive learners rely on precise forms of self-observation to guide their efforts, such as metacognitive monitoring, which refers to the simple mental tracking of one's performances and outcomes, whereas their self-recording refers to creating formal records of performances and outcomes.

The *self-reflection phase* comprises two kinds of processes: *self-judgments* that include self-evaluations of the effectiveness of one's performance and attributions, and *self-reactions.* Proactive learners are guided by specific forethought phase goals and therefore their self-evaluation is based on the mastery of those goals. In contrast, reactive students lack specific forethought goals and often fail to self-evaluate because their comparisons yield less advantageous self-evaluations. Proactive students' self-evaluative judgments are linked closely to causal attributions about the results of learning efforts. Because reactive learners often rely on the outcomes of others to self-evaluate, they are prone to attribute their errors to a lack of competence, which is classified as an uncontrollable cause. Proactive students self-evaluate by self-chosen goals, and they typically attribute errors to ineffective strategies, which are classified as controllable causes. Attributions of one's results to personal control lead to a greater sense of satisfaction than attributions to external and uncontrollable causes. It is hypothesized that proactive students pursue courses of action that result in satisfaction and positive affect and avoid courses that produce dissatisfaction and negative affect. Reactive learners' attribution of errors to uncontrollable causes leads them to feel dissatisfied, which in turn discourages them from further efforts to learn.

Note that Zimmerman's model was designed to describe and explain the results of repeated efforts to learn, such as learning a new language, and needs empirical validation. Nonetheless, his elaborate description of the phases and processes may be of use in the assessment of skill deficits and the learning of self-management in offenders.

7.3 Self-Regulation and Sexual Offending

Deficits in self-regulation processes are suggested to underlie sexual offending. Ward and Gannon (2006) describe the function of self-regulation processes in the etiology of sexual offending. They claim that relapse in sexual offending cannot always be associated with a self-regulatory failure in the skills used to avoid sexual offending but sometimes is accompanied by careful and systematic planning and positive emotional states. In their Self-Regulating Model (SRM) some pathways are distinguished, representing different combinations of offense-related goals (to approach or avoid a sexual offense), and the use of distinct regulation styles concerning sexual offending (under-regulation, mis-regulation, or effective regulation). Each pathway is further divided into implicit and explicit sub-pathways, according to the varying degrees of awareness associated with decision-making strategies (passive, active, automatic, or explicit). The *avoidant-passive* pathway is characterized by the desire to avoid sexual offending, but the person lacks the coping skills to prevent it from happening (i.e., under-regulation). The *avoidant-active* pathway refers to mis-regulation, which implies a direct attempt to control deviant thoughts and fantasies but the use of ineffective or counterproductive strategies. The *approach-automatic* pathway is associated with under-regulation, the desire to sexually offend, and impulsive, poorly planned behavior. Finally, the *approach-explicit* pathway is marked by the desire to sexually offend, the use of careful planning to execute offenses, and the presence of harmful goals concerning sexual offending. According to Ward and Gannon (2006), strengths of the SRM are the way it highlights the role of agency and self-regulation in the offense process and its dynamic nature and assumption that the offense process can only be adequately understood in light of the interaction between individuals and their relevant circumstances. However, the greatest weakness of the SRM is the privileging of goals relating to behavioral control and subsequent failure to explicitly document the way human goals and their pursuit may be causally related to sexually offending. A further problem with the SRM is that although it describes the self-regulatory styles used by sex offenders in the commission of their offense well, it does not indicate the causal factors underlying these regulatory styles (Ward & Gannon, 2006).

According to Stinson, Becker, and McVay (2017), there are three limitations to the role of self-regulation in the offense process. To begin with, no research has supported the critical assumption of the model, namely that self-regulatory deficits underlie sexual offenses. Further, what is meant by self-regulation is not well defined, and finally the mechanism by which individuals develop self-regulatory deficits or acquire poor regulatory strategies is left unclear. Therefore, these authors proposed a new etiological theory, which focuses heavily on the individual's ability to self-regulate thoughts, emotions, and behaviors, and incorporates knowledge from developmental, cognitive, behavioral, and personality psychology to explain the development of sex-offending behaviors. Stinson, Becker, and Sales (2008) alleged that sex offenders use a variety of externalized strategies to cope with internal distress. These strategies may include behaviors that promise immediate gratification of desires and involve only little effort or short-term planning, such as substance use, antisocial or criminal behaviors, and sexual activity. Once these strategies have been selected and utilized by the individual, reinforcement contingencies largely determine which external regulatory strategies will be retained for later use and which will be abandoned as unsuccessful, too risky, or too complicated. A combination of effective reduction of distress or discomfort, consistent reinforcement, and lack of corrective action will ensure that the selected strategy will persist in future situations where self-regulation is necessary. A core feature of this concept is that self-regulatory deficits predispose these individuals to a variety of behaviors.

Deficits in adaptive functioning can arise in any or all of the four significant self-regulation categories: (a) emotion/mood regulation, (b) behavioral regulation, (c) cognitive regulation, and (d) interpersonal regulation. During development, individuals typically learn appropriate and adaptive means by which to regulate themselves in these four areas. However, some individuals have failed to internalize regulatory strategies and instead adopt maladaptive or dysfunctional strategies for self-regulation, which are likely to be those that are externally available, promise immediate relief from distress, and involve little effort. In their study of 95 sex offenders, Stinson, Becker and colleagues (2008) examined the validity of a proposed causal relationship between self-regulatory deficits, or dysregulation, and the development of sexually deviant behaviors. A self-regulatory deficit, as measured by affective instability or mood dysregulation, appeared to be a significant causal predictor of both sexual deviance and antisocial behaviors. This factor was even shown to be an underlying explanation for the shared variance between these two outcomes. This finding supported the assumptions posited in the self-regulation model of Ward and Hudson (2000) and the multimodal self-regulation theory of Stinson, Sales, and Becker (2008).

Stinson and Becker (2013) differentiated between four forms of regulation. Emotional regulation is broadly defined as the ability to identify, monitor, and modulate emotional responses. Cognitive regulation refers to the individual's ability to modulate and regulate thoughts. Interpersonal regulation is the ability to monitor interactions with others, integrate feedback, and regulate interpersonal behaviors. Finally, behavioral regulation describes the ability to control, inhibit, and express behavior. Based on the literature, these authors conclude that sex offenders demonstrate some degree of dysregulation in all these four domains. Sex offenders have been found being angry and hostile (Hanson & Morton-Bourgon, 2005), having poor problem-solving ability (Hanson, Harris, Scott, & Helmus, 2007), showing strong antisocial traits or psychopathy (Hanson & Morton-Bourgon, 2005), and engaging in frequent nonsexual aggressive behavior (e.g., Smallbone & Wortley, 2004), problematic substance abuse (Kraanen & Emmelkamp, 2017), and self-injurious behaviors (Pritchard & King, 2005). In a sample of 256 psychiatric inpatients with a history of illegal sexual behaviors, emotional, cognitive, and behavioral dysregulation, Stinson, Robbins, and Crow (2011) evaluated the relationships among self-regulatory deficits, dysregulation, and maladaptive behavior, including problematic sexual behavior. The results appeared to support their proposal that emotional and cognitive dysregulation are differentially predictive of different types of maladaptive behavior.

7.4 Summary of the Literature

The self-regulation models of the social psychologists Bandura and Zimmerman have in common that they regard an individual as someone who compares his knowledge or behavior with that of others, may decide to improve that knowledge or that behavior, carries out the necessary activities to address the desired result, and finally when the desired result is achieved is inclined to reward himself. Besides, Zimmerman emphasized the importance of choosing intermediate, achievable goals. However, both models refer to general human behavior and do not describe how an individual can learn to perform a step-by-step method with intermediate goals to achieve a final goal.

The self-management model of Ward and Hudson (2000) and Ward and Gannon (2006) for sexual offending may explain its development, but it has not led to a method for teaching sexual offenders' alternative behavior. One of the problems with the literature on self-regulation is that different definitions are provided of related concepts such as self-regulation, self-management, and self-control. In this book, self-regulation is defined as the ability to monitor and regulate our behavior, emotions, or thoughts, and altering them following our goals and the targets of the situation. Self-management is viewed as a method for behavior change, to be applied without the direct help of a therapist. The application of self-management methods in various situations is called self-control.

Self-management procedures are an essential supplement to treatment programs because with these procedures, behavior change is achieved without the direct support of relevant others. Self-management methods are specifically indicated when the problematic behavior stems from deficits in self-observation and self-evaluation (Kanfer & Gaelick-Buys, 1991). Moreover, self-management methods may enhance the transfer of treatment effects to offenders' real-life situations and probably strengthens their self-efficacy.

7.5 Self-Management Methods

The treatment programs for violent offenders and sexually violent offenders (Chap. 6) contain modules that focus on the learning of social skills, namely Prosocial Skills, Prosocial Network, Contact with Women, and Work and Leisure. Modeling and role-playing with the use of video equipment and an actress is an essential part of the modules. The video recording allows a participant to review his behavior and the actress enhances the realism of the training situations. After discussing the feedback from other participants and therapists, the role-play is rehearsed when necessary. For the performance of the modules, therapists have a manual at their disposal, and the participants a workbook for the completion of homework assignments. These homework assignments are meant for the maintenance and generalization of learned skills to new situations.

The self-management method that is used during the two programs is based on the Social Skills Training (SST) of Van Dam-Baggen and Kraaimaat (2014). Their approach to achieve self-control in new situations is feasible for both detained offenders who are about to go on leave and offenders in a community program. A combination of self-regulation procedures is used such as self-monitoring, self-directed use of graded practice, self-evaluation, and self-reinforcement together with problem-solving strategies. Procedures and strategies are meant to facilitate the generalization and transfer from the treatment situation to other social situations. The self-management method of Van Dam-Baggen and Kraaimaat (2014) learns offenders to distinguish between facts and thoughts, to set goals and subgoals, to monitor their behavior, to set adequate targets and criteria for their behavior, to adjust inadequate targets, to ask for and give feedback, to reinforce themselves, to work stepwise, and finally to generate alternative solutions for a problematic situation.

The self-management method of Van Dam-Baggen and Kraaimaat (2014) consists of the following components:

(a) Self-monitoring of performance (i.e., avoidance behavior)
(b) Self-directed use of graded practice of responses
(c) Self-evaluation of the performed response with the support of previously determined criteria
(d) Self-reinforcement
(e) Application of a problem-solving strategy by successively making use of components (a)–(d)

7.5.1 *Self-Monitoring*

By self-monitoring is meant the observing and registering by an offender of his or her problem behaviors. It helps to be aware of the nature and frequency of their behaviors and the situations in which they occur. It also serves as a measure of behavior change. The daily monitoring of avoidance or antisocial behavior enhances attention for their goals and facilitates the process of self-control. When a social skill is rehearsed within a session, the homework assignment is given to applying this skill in daily life situations (see for an example of a form to use to record a social skill Table 7.1). Afterward, the offender has to make a report of his or her performance of the social skill according to the elements of a behavioral chain and the guidelines given by the therapist.

Table 7.1 Example of a homework assignment

Describe the next week a situation where you have applied skill 1 (i.e., Complimenting someone) by answering the questions below:
• Who was it? *My colleague Rose.*
• Where were you? *At my work.*
• When was it? *During a coffee break.*
• About what? *Her preparation for today's job.*
• What did you say? *Hi Rose, great that you already did such a large job in preparing today's work; that helps a lot!*
• What said/did the other? *Yea isn't it great! You are welcome.*
• What did you think or feel? *I felt good and was pleased with her reaction.*
• What did you do well? *My compliment was direct and positive.*
• What would you like to improve? *To make more eye contact and to speak somewhat less loudly.*

Table 7.2 Example of a form for the recording of social skills

Ask yourself at the end of each day which social skills you have applied and how many times. Note each performance by "Yes" and when you did not perform while you could have by "No."

Social skill	Wednesday		Thursday		Friday		Saturday		Sunday		Monday		Tuesday	
	Yes	No	Yes	No	Yes	No	Yes	No	Yes	No	Yes	No	Yes	No
Complimenting someone	II	I	III		I	II	I		II		III	I	I	
Asking for help		I	I	II				I	I	I		I	I	
Responding to criticism		I	I	I			I		I		I		II	
Criticizing	II		III		II	I	III		II	II	I		III	

Self-monitoring of specific social skills is introduced not earlier than that skill has been rehearsed within a session, and monitoring of that skill is continued until the end of treatment. Other social skills follow the same procedure, which means that during each session the number of skills that should be monitored is extended with one. In Table 7.2, an example is presented of the monitoring of four skills that were exercised during the first four sessions of the module Prosocial Skills. Note that self-monitoring is limited because the registered behavior does not always correspond with the actual behavior. Self-monitoring often has reactive effects that fade out after some time. However, these limitations are negligible because in this case self-monitoring is not used for treatment evaluation purposes, but mainly has an informative function that facilitates the process of behavior change.

Self-monitoring also provides some general information about avoidance or antisocial behavior. For example, "not performed" may indicate that the situation did not occur, that the situation or skill was not recognized (e.g., in the case of asking for help: "It was a mess. But why should I ask for help."), but also that the skill or situation was avoided (e.g., "I did not return to the shop with the incomplete stuff.").

7.5.2 *Self-Directed Use of Graded– Practice of Responses*

Offenders learn to use a stepwise approach to achieve their final goals without a deadlock, for example, when their targets do not match their performance. Steps to the final goals are made explicit and practiced for a specific social skill. To make this possible, exercise situations have to be rank ordered according to the degree of difficulty.

Prerequisites for the use of graded exposure are that one is capable of observing himself and others and to formulate specific final- and sub-goals. Three steps are distinguished in the self-directed use of graded practice, namely rating situations according to the level of elicited discomfort/difficulty, the rank ordering of the situations to the level of discomfort/difficulty, and thinking of intermediate steps for the rank order of situations.

7.5.2.1 Rating of Situations According to the Level of Discomfort/ Difficulty

In the first session of this phase, the participants of a group treatment program are asked to rate the general practice situations of a particular social skill on discomfort/ difficulty with the help of a 10-point SUD-scale (from 0 = "not at all" to 10 = "highest discomfort/difficulty ever experienced"). The personal scores are collected with the help of a whiteboard or flip over. From these individual scores, a group hierarchy for that skill is derived. The situation with the least amount of discomfort/difficulty according to the group hierarchy will be the first exercise situation in the session. The participant with the lowest rating is the first to rehearse the skill within the session. The rehearsal takes place on the hand of each participant's situations. This procedure is aimed to prevent too high levels of discomfort/difficulty and probable sensitization. In the homework assignments, the participants start to exercise situations with the lowest ratings of discomfort/difficulty.

7.5.2.2 Rank Ordering of Situations to the Level of Discomfort/Difficulty

When participants can rate a situation on discomfort/difficulty, the next step is to learn to rank their exercise situations. After the participants have made a list of own exercise situations, they are asked to place at the head of the list the situation with the lowest amount of discomfort/difficulty, then the situation with the second lowest amount and so on, and at the bottom of the list the situation with the highest amount of discomfort/difficulty. In this way, a hierarchy of exercise situations is composed. An example of a homework assignment for rank ordering situations for "Complimenting someone" is presented in Table 7.3.

Once having learned to rank exercise situations, the participants have to follow the same procedure for all exercise situations that they introduce to the sessions.

Table 7.3 The rank order of situations for "Complimenting someone"

Consider five exercise situations for the skill "Complimenting someone" that may occur in the coming weeks. Write about each situation who it is and what you like to compliment. Write at the top the situation that gives you the least amount of discomfort/difficulty and at the bottom the situation that gives you the highest amount of discomfort/difficulty.	
1.	My mother for doing my laundry. *Thanks, mom for helping me!*
2.	My friend John for visiting me. *John, it's a pleasure to see you.*
3.	My colleague Mike for helping me with a difficult job. *Thanks, Mike with your help. I could not do this job without your help*
4.	A positive reaction of my boss to my request to leave an hour early. *Thanks a lot, boss.*
5.	Information of our administrator about some questions about my monthly payment. *That is very helpful. Now I understand how things were calculated.*

The ranking of situations before each session is a prerequisite for a rehearsal within the session in which only situations with a relatively low amount of discomfort/difficulty are exercised.

7.5.2.3 Intermediate Steps in the Rank Order of Exercise Situations

The steps between exercise situations in a rank order may vary in their amount of discomfort/difficulty. Sometimes a step between two following situations may be rather small (showing a relatively small difference in discomfort/difficulty), but sometimes such a step may be too difficult (showing a relatively great difference in discomfort/difficulty). To prevent that offenders rehearse too difficult situations, they are learned how to narrow or to enlarge the steps between two following situations. For example, narrowing is achieved by introducing an easier person with a similar easy subject, or a similar easy person with an easier subject. Making intermediate steps are practiced during a session when necessary. This strategy of graded practice cannot only be applied to social skills but on every other behavior that has to be increased or decreased. Ranking situations is an easy job for most offenders. Many people do have experience in daily life with graded practice, and this means that they do understand the principles and goals in due time. However, thinking of intermediate steps is a more difficult job, because it requires the comparison of different persons and subjects, especially for people with a limited ability to make abstractions. It sometimes helps to suggest that when keeping one variable unchanged (thus "same" instead of "similar"), the other variable can be varied (one step more difficult or easier). Note, that the different situations should be described concretely and accurately (to person and subject) because vague and general descriptions hinder the rating of discomfort and consequently the creating of intermediate steps.

7.5.3 Self-Evaluation

A crucial aspect of self-control is the ability to evaluate oneself and being independent of others (therapist, participants, partner, friends, and so on). Offenders are learning the following skills that are relevant for self-evaluation, namely to ask themselves which goals can be achieved in a particular situation or with a particular skill, to think of the criteria which have to be fulfilled in a specific situation and to compare their behavior with the criteria. These skills are rehearsed within the sessions and then gradually applied in the offenders' daily life situation with the help of the homework assignments. By directing the participants' attention to what they would like to achieve with a particular skill, what they did well and what might be improved, they are learned to produce solutions for future problem situations.

Goals for a social skill. Offenders learn to think about what they would like to achieve with a social skill, in other words, which goals want they achieve. This is the first step in the decision what to do with a situation or an action. Clarifying goals and intended outcomes will influence the motivation to perform the social skill. Before a social skill is rehearsed within a session, participants will get the homework assignment to produce all possible goals for that response and bring their report to the session. Within the session, all their goals will be listed. By this way, the participants are learned to make their goals explicit and to adjust them to the situation. Insufficiently explicitly named goals are often accompanied by dysfunctional cognitions which justify avoidance behavior, characterized by giving priority to the supposed goals of the other person and by being afraid for negative consequences on own behavior. By making the goals explicit, offenders and therapist get insight into the hidden meanings of offenders. For example: "On the one hand I do not like to help John this evening, but on the other hand I do not want to disappoint him." Therapist should stimulate participants to help each other in disclosing conflicted and unfeasible goals. To prevent that participants will write down their goals during the listing and in this way participate less actively in the group discussion, there are handouts for each skill with the most commonly occurring goals. The handouts may also be used in generating goals for other skills (see Table 7.4).

Criteria for effectively performing a social skill. Before a specific social skill is rehearsed within the session, the participants have to think about their ways of adequately performing the skill (criteria). By generating criteria (behavior features you would like to fulfill when refusing a request, standing up for yourself and so on), offenders will learn which features make social behavior effective and adequate. Using these criteria, they can choose for themselves whether their performance was adequate and which behavior features might be changed. Before a social response is rehearsed within a session, offenders will get the homework assignment to produce and write down essential criteria for the response next to the goals they did generate. Within the session, all criteria will be listed and afterward distributed to the offenders on a handout. In Table 7.4 an example is presented of the report of

Table 7.4 Generating goals and criteria: John's report for the coming session

The response that will be rehearsed in the next session is "Refusing a request." Write down what you would like to achieve by refusing a request. In other words, what goals do you want to achieve when refusing a request?
• Standing up for my rights.
• Being able to choose how to use my time.
• There are limits!
• Feeling more comfortable.
• Letting others know who I am.
(a) Write down which aspects of your behavior might be important in refusing a request. Take into account verbal as well as nonverbal aspects:
• Saying "no" in a clear way.
• Being friendly, do not use harsh words.
• Not apologizing for my refusal.
• Proposing another solution.
• Making eye contact.
• Saying "No" by shaking my head.

such a homework assignment with generating goals and criteria for the response "refusing a request." Within the sessions, the criteria will be used in the modeling and behavior rehearsal procedures. Using these criteria helps the offenders to identify which aspects of behavior are relevant. Besides, the criteria are essential in the evaluation of the rehearsed response using the feedback procedure.

Offenders are asked to produce the criteria for every skill, since the criteria may vary across skills. Make sure that the offenders choose for every response, which criteria they would like to fulfill in a particular practice situation.

Self-evaluation and self-reinforcement are assumed to have similar effects like external reinforcement. Positive self-reinforcement may be tangible (e.g., coffee) as well as a verbal-symbolic ("Good job," "Well done"). Applying negative consequences on behavior often consists of self-criticism, self-punishment, or the abstinence of positive reinforcement. Internal reinforcement compared with external reinforcement has the advantage that it leads to independence toward other persons. Bandura (1977) assumed a relationship between the standards or targets (goals) someone sets himself and the way he thinks about himself. Standards that are too high lead to negative self-statements, which, when frequently applied, may result in pathological reactions. Treatments directed toward concrete self-observations and realistic goals-setting foster positive self-reinforcement.

7.5.4 Self-Reinforcement

Problems in social interactions may lead to negative self-evaluations and vice versa. This downward spiral can be stopped, first, by improving and extending the skill repertoire. Second, by improving self-evaluation and positive self-reinforcement to maintain newly learned skills. Performance criteria will achieve positive consequences if they are adjusted at the performance level of that moment and in this part of the treatment program should not be higher than the current performance level of the offenders. First, the offenders learn to trace and, if needed, to readjust their performance criteria. Next, they learn to apply self-reinforcement either in the form of positive self-statements (e.g., "Well, I did that work very well.") or tangible reinforcers. In the introduction of self-evaluation and self-reinforcement, a brochure is used, called "Targets, activities, and evaluation" (see Appendix). Two steps are described in the brochure, namely identifying targets and adequate performance criteria, and tracing impeding performance criteria ("deadlocks").

7.5.4.1 Identifying Targets

The first step in this process is the identification of targets and performance criteria with the help of the brochure and the accompanying homework assignments. People often think that they do not set targets for themselves and are surprised to discover that they indeed do so. The identification of the targets starts with situations in which one is content with oneself. First, the offenders read the text concerning the relationship between these three aspects in the brochure (Appendix Sects. 1–3). Then, they describe an example of a situation in which they were content with their results. The aim of this assignment is that offenders identify and describe the targets and underlying performance criteria they set for that situation, including their positive self-statements. At this stage of the treatment, the assignment is not limited to social activities and may also concern all activities from everyday life. At first the offenders' targets may be rather global, later on, they become more precise and may converge with their specific performance criteria. When the offenders can identify their targets specifically for nonsocial activities, the next step is, preceding an activity, to set adequate targets with the aim to be content with the results. In Table 7.5, an example is given of an assignment in which John is asked to set the performance criteria beforehand, to evaluate his behavior, and to reinforce himself.

7.5.4.2 Identifying Impeding Targets or "Deadlocks"

The next step is that the offenders identify and readjust their impending targets. If targets are set higher than their actual performance, it is likely that one will not be content and that the targets should be readjusted. In this book, for the non-correspondence between target and performance, the term "deadlocks" is used. The distinction and relation between targets, activities, and evaluation should offenders give insight into why they discontinued performing some activities. The offenders should read the text concerning deadlocks in the brochure (Appendix Sects. 4 and 5). Also, they have to write down an example of such a deadlock and describing which target they set for themselves, which kind of deadlock was at stake, and how targets might be readjusted. Identifying targets, specifying performance criteria,

Table 7.5 John's application of self-evaluation and self-reinforcement while practicing the skill "Making a request"

Apply twice the skill "Making a request" and set the performance criteria preceding each situation.
• To whom did you direct your request? *My coach.*
• When? *Friday afternoon at 5 p.m.*
• Where? *In his office.*
• What about your request? *A day off.*
• Which criteria did you set? *I will be clear and to the point while saying what I would like.*
• How responded the other person? *"Okay, you have my permission. Are you going to enjoy yourself?"*
• Did you fulfill your criteria? *I am satisfied with my request: I was clear and to the point in what I would like to achieve.*
• Describe your positive self-statement. *"I am glad that I made my request, I finally do have my day off, and my coach showed interested in my plans."*
• Would you like to change something? *There is no need to change things because I fulfilled my criteria. I will repeat this behavior.*

Table 7.6 John's homework assignment on deadlocks

Read the Appendix Sects. 4 and 5 from the brochure "Targets, activities, and evaluation" and describe an activity in which you applied one of the deadlocks. It should concern an activity in which you discovered to have set too high targets. This does not mean that you intentionally applied such a deadlock.
• Describe your activity. *Improving my physical condition.*
• Which demand did you set? *Each day exercise for half an hour on the home-trainer.*
• What is your performance level until now? *Mostly, I exercised once a week.*
• How did you perform after setting the demand? *In the first week, I exercised three successive days and then stopped practicing because I was too tired.*
• Which deadlock did you apply? *My performance criterion was too high at the start.*
• What should you do to prevent discontinuing your activity? *Set a much lower demand, for instance, practicing the first week only 10 min daily.*

and readjusting sufficient and impeding targets will not be an easy task. Therefore, it is important that offenders not only read the brochure but also extensively discuss its content during the sessions. First, there is the opportunity to ask questions. Then, the offenders are asked to summarize the content in their own words, and finally every offender report what he or she has learned from reading it. It is essential to transfer and apply the content to daily life situations with the help of homework assignments. Examples from earlier participants will be helpful in performing the assignments of this part of the treatment (Table 7.6).

7.5.5 Problem-Solving Strategy

With the successive application of self-monitoring, graded practice, self-evaluation, and self-reinforcement the offenders learn a so-called problem-solving strategy (D'Zurilla & Nezu, 2010). The use of such a strategy is not restricted to social behaviors. It also teaches offenders the skills for the solution of present and future problem situations. The separate components of the self-control strategy are finally integrated into an individual plan. Using the brochure, every offender will make such a plan for a specific activity and then performs it. First, the offenders get the homework assignment to read the text concerning how to make plans (Appendix Sect. 6 and Table 7.7). Then, they are asked to make such a plan for a relatively simple nonsocial activity, such as weight lifting or reading a text. In the next session, this part of the brochure is discussed in the group, and every offender will read his or her report of the plan for a nonsocial activity. The therapist should be alert that this plan consists of a description of the activity, a division of the activity in steps, realistic and final goals, the actual performance level of the activity, and finally a target with specific criteria that are tailored to the actual performance level.

The participants should make this homework assignment concerning the plan for a nonsocial activity at least twice. The next step will be that the offenders make a plan for a social skill that has been rehearsed during the session. This plan should be finished before they exercise the skill to be used in their daily life situation. The plan is used as a guideline in daily life and contains also a description of the performance of the first step, the evaluation of this step, the next step in the case of a positive

Table 7.7 Rules or guidelines for an increase or improvement of activities

This approach is aimed at matching your targets with your activities and counteracting general and negative self-statements. Work step by step in the listed order!
• Make a description of the activity you want to improve (what, how often, time, etc.).
• Divide the activity into steps or components.
• Write down how the activity should look like at the end. What is your final result?
• What is your current performance? Examine this in everyday life and make a detailed report.
• Set your first demand not higher than your current performance. Write this demand down for your first exercise. Be specific and concrete. If necessary, transpose your targets as specific criteria (e.g., in such a way that a person who reads your demand can perform the activity).
• Perform the activity.
• Compare the execution of the activity with your demand. If the execution of the activity is lower/lesser than the demand goes back to rule 5.
• Prepare a new step by providing a new demand. Set your demand slightly higher than the actual performance of your activity. Write this down for your second exercise situation.
• Repeat the rules 6, 7 and 8, until you have reached your final goal.
You can increase the effectiveness of the above approach by a positive self-statement if the performance of the activity is equal to or better than your demand. Some examples of such statements that express a positive appraisal are: "I did well.", "Well done.", "This went well." or "Excellent."

Table 7.8 A session plan in the self-management phase

• During the *homework discussion,* one of the offenders reads aloud his plan for skill and reports on one of his exercise situations of the concerning skill. The homework discussion continues according to the previously described procedure.
• In this particular case, the *theme* of the session will be "positive self-statements." During the session, all possible goals for doing positive self-statements are listed. The same procedure will be executed concerning the performance criteria.
• In this phase of the treatment, the modeling by the therapist may be skipped. The alternative is to generate several reactions with the help of the performance criteria. After this procedure, every offender takes his turn in rehearsing the skill.
• The *homework assignment* is to re-evaluate the plan for positive self-statements that was made before the session and to readjust it eventually or to extend it. Also, offenders are assigned to exercise situations from this plan and make reports on their exercise.
• The *session evaluation* will take place as usual.

Table 7.9 Homework assignments for the self-management phase

1. Re-evaluate your plan for positive self-statements. If needed, add exercise situations to your rank order. Do positive self-statements in the two easiest situations of your rank. Describe the situations afterward with the help of the following cues (see also Table 7.5).
2. Mark your exercise as well as your avoidance behavior on the self-monitoring forms. Please deliver one of the forms next session and save a copy for yourself.
3. Continue practicing the skills that were already dealt with during the treatment program. Describe each exercise situation. If you like, you can deliver the described situations.

result, a readjusted first step in the case of a negative result, the next step and so on, until the final goal will be achieved. Afterward, offenders make a plan for a social skill before it is rehearsed within the session. They bring this plan to the session, and the situations in this plan will be rehearsed. Finally, during the last session of the treatment program, the homework assignments include making plans for social skills that will not be rehearsed anymore within the treatment program.

Making plans with the help of the brochure "Targets, activities, and evaluation" asks a lot of the offenders. The therapist should be aware of the differential cognitive capacities of the offenders. Some offenders are soon able to make well-elaborated plans. For others, the only achievement is that they can set a final goal, divide the activity into steps, and adjust their first step to their actual performance level. With the help of the therapist, the other offenders, and much repetition, offenders with limited mental capacities could also learn to apply these principles. Note that acquiring the principles is the primary goal and not making excellent plans. During all steps of learning to make plans, examples are provided from homework reports of previous offenders. In Table 7.8, an example of a session plan in the self-management phase of the treatment is given. The complete set of homework assignments are described in Table 7.9.

7.5.6 Termination of a Treatment Program

The transition from the offenders' weekly therapy meetings to their more or less independent life in the community is rather unexplored territory in literature. A good organization of such a transition is especially crucial for offenders in closed institutions who must or can return to the community at a particular moment. However, for detainees, it is only partly possible to prepare for high-risk situations in the community because of the structure and control within the institution, although the use of Virtual Reality seems to offer new possibilities (Hornsveld, Kraaimaat, Zwets, & Kanters, 2017). To date, an offender goes on escorted or unaccompanied leave to assess whether he or she can maintain himself or herself in the community, what additional interventions are necessary to achieve this in the short term, or whether a more extended stay and return in the institution is required.

During the leave, a therapist checks whether an offender can apply recently learned skills in new situations (the generalization of skills). Also, the offender learns to execute their plans without the help of the therapist and to acquire new necessary skills with the aid of a step-by-step plan (self-management). Therefore, a treatment program and the learning of new behaviors does not end when a detainee goes on leave or with discharge. To facilitate the detainee's gain in self-control further coaching from a community program with the maintenance of self-control is highly recommended.

Community programs have the advantage that a delinquent can practice risk situations during treatment in a natural environment. A gradual termination of the program is possible by having the group treatment meetings take place at increasingly larger intervals and to use booster sessions. Specifically, in the last part of the treatment, the therapist fades his interventions more and more with the aim to demand an increasing responsibility from the offenders. This strategy promotes a shift from external to internal control as well as a shift from the offender's practicing skills within sessions to practicing between sessions. Furthermore, it is also necessary that offenders continue to practice the learned behaviors in new situations and apply self-management methods with the help of an individual step-by-step plan after the end of the treatment. In addition to the maintenance of coping skills which are acquired during treatment, further attention is needed to relapse prevention.

7.6 Relapse Prevention

Notwithstanding the effectiveness of cognitive-behavioral treatment, it is known from the literature that a substantial percentage of offenders relapse to their prior antisocial behavior. At the end of the therapy and specifically in the follow-up sessions, it is recommended that each offender with the help of the therapist construct a tailor-made relapse prevention plan or relapse roadmap (Larimer, Palmer, & Marlatt, 1999). Such a plan comprises a cognitive-behavioral analysis of high-risk situations that emphasize the different choices available for coping or avoiding these situations as well as their consequences. The additional value of a relapse prevention plan is its focus on dealing with future and probable high-risk situations as well as with an increase of cognitive, emotional, and behavioral risk factors associated with the offender's problem behavior. Relapse prevention plans stem from the literature on addiction that assumes that dealing with an addiction is a lifelong process. The same might hold for the sexual urges and cravings of a substantial number of rapist and child sexual abusers.

Appendix: Targets, Activities, and Evaluation

Introduction

You start with a new activity or start improving an already ongoing activity. However, after a few times practice, you cease doing so. Self-regrets prevail, and you say to yourself "I am no good at all," "I am a sissy," "I lack motivation," "I am good at nothing," and so on. Despite your good intentions and investments, you do not reach your ultimate goal and give up. What happened? In the following text, we will try to give you some answers.

1. Activities and Their Consequences

What we undertake, postpone, or avoid is determined mainly by its consequences. In case we reach a pleasant or desired result with an activity, then we are inclined to undertake this activity also in the future. However, an activity with an unpleasant, embarrassing, or unwanted outcome will be undertaken less frequently. As a general rule, one can say that consequences influence activities.

An important consequence of our activities is the appraisal of others or ourselves. Evaluation by ourselves or others has a high influence on the frequency at which our activities will take place. Often, we are not aware of the impact of our assessment of our activities. In the case of a mostly negative appraisal of our activities, we tend to stop, while we continue activities in the event of primarily positive evaluation.

2. How Is the Evaluation of Activities Accomplished?

We speak of targets in case of specific goals for a particular activity. Our appraisal is never isolated but always related to the targets we have to meet with ourselves and during the actual course of the activity. In the case of evaluation, we compare the actual course of action with our targets. This can result in a negative appraisal or a positive one. We achieve a:

- Negative evaluation, if the performance of the activity is less good than planned
- Positive evaluation, if the performance of the activity matches the target
- Positive evaluation, if the performance of the activity is better than the target
- The general rule for the more frequent or better performance of an activity is: Make sure that its execution leads to positive results. People often make the mistake to set a too high target when they start with an activity. If that is the case, they can be sure to achieve a negative evaluation. For instance, someone who smokes an average of 20 cigarettes a day and has a target to quit smoking quickly, disappoints him of herself. Even if he or she should smoke only ten cigarettes in the first days after his decision, failure prevails.

3. Self-Statements

Comments about ourselves frequently accompany an evaluation. We tend to make negative self-statements after failures to meet challenging targets. Some examples of negative self-statements:

- "I cannot stop smoking (or drinking, stuttering, shouting, etc.)."
- "I forget the meaning of this word always."
- "My writing is terrible."

A problem with negative self-statements is that they are often exaggerations. Most of the time they are a too general and a too negative evaluation of our activity. In this way, the features of the activity that did correspond to someone's target will also be evaluated negatively. So is the statement: "My writing is terrible" definitely too generally formulated. Without question, there were words, which were written readable. The use of words such as "always," "never," "any," "all," or "something" is characteristic of too general formulations of self-statements. Some examples of negative public self-statements:

- "There must be *something* wrong with me."
- "Why can I *never* act spontaneously?"
- "*Nobody* likes me."
- "I will *never* understand calculating."
- "I *always* say stupid things."

With negative self-statements, we achieve the opposite of what we want: we want to undertake activities or to improve them, but the result is that we stop doing them.

4. What Happens If We Stop at an Early Stage with an Activity?

If you cease with an activity before you have reached your ultimate goal, you have applied a failure rule or a deadlock.

(a) You did not match your targets with how you can perform the activity. The target you have set is much higher than the actual performance of the activity. Create easier targets, specify the criteria of your performance, and try to meet the final target in several and small steps.
(b) You have increased your targets during the execution of the activity. In the final evaluation, you feel downtrodden: you are dissatisfied with your performance because your specific requirements were too high.
(c) You exercise the same action several times, but each time you set the same target:
    - In case of a target that is too difficult, you give up the activity.
    - When the target was met initially, you stopped the activity because you have reached this requirement. However, your end goal is not achieved.
(d) You have not described your target in concrete terms (i.e., specific criteria) so that the actual execution of the activity cannot be compared with your target. This may lead to an under- or over-estimation of the result. To tackle this obstacle, make a description of the activity to be performed in such a concrete and step-by-step way that anyone who reads it knows what he or she must do.

5. Examples of the Application of Failure Rules or Deadlocks

Time Walking

Dick was seriously hurt in a car accident. After a 2-month stay in a hospital, he was sent home to revalidate further. At this moment he hardly left his home and wanted to improve his walking. At this time, he walked about 8 min to and from the shopping center where he buys a newspaper every day. He was tired and his legs hurt when he walked longer than 8 min. In the first exercise, he set the target to walk a quarter of an hour in his neighborhood. The course of his daily exercises looks like this:

Exercise Target Performance Evaluation

• First exercise: Target 15 min; performance 8 min; evaluation negative
• Second exercise: Target 15 min; performance 9 min; evaluation negative
• Third exercise: Target 15 min; performance 7 min; evaluation negative
• Fourth exercise. Dick gives up. He says to himself: "I have no stamina at all," "This does not work," "What has become of me?"

Task:

- Write down what failure rule or deadlock Dick applied.
- Change his targets for the first and second exercise.

Stuttering

Peter stutters when he calls on others. Sometimes he stutters as much as that he discontinues the conversation. He does not succeed in speaking on the phone like others.

To practice, Peter decided to inquire by phone about the price of a new laptop. His ultimate goal was to stutter only once per phone call. He examined how often he stutters before he formulated his first goal. He stuttered 20 times during the try-out conversation. His exercises were as follows.

Exercise Target Performance Evaluation

• First exercise: Target 20 stutters; performance 19 stutters; evaluation positive.
• Second exercise: Target 18 stutters, performance 14 stutters; evaluation positive.
• Third exercise: Target 15 stutters; performance 10 stutters; evaluation positive.
• Fourth exercise: Target 7 stutters; performance 10 stutters; evaluation negative.
• Fifth exercise: Target 7 stutters; performance 11 stutters; evaluation negative.
• Sixth exercise: Target 0 stutters; performance 17 stutters; evaluation negative.
• Seventh exercise: Peter stops practicing. He was very disappointed and tense.

Task:

- Please write down the failure rules or deadlocks Peter applied and when he did so.
- If necessary, adjust the targets for Peter.

In the following part, we present a different approach than that of Dick or Peter with more chances for success.

6. Rules or Guidelines for an Increase or Improvement of Activities

This approach is aimed at matching your targets with your activities and counteracting general and negative self-statements. Work step by step in the listed order!

1. Make a description of the activity you want to improve (what, how often, time, etc.).
2. Divide the activity into steps or components.
3. Write down how the activity should look like in the end. (What is your final result?).
4. What is your current performance? Examine this in everyday life and make a detailed report.
5. Set your target not higher than your current performance. Write this target down for your first exercise. Be specific and concrete. If necessary, write your targets as specific criteria in such a way that a person who reads your target can perform the activity.

6. Perform the activity.
7. Compare the execution of the activity with your target. If the performance of the activity is lower/lesser than the target goes back to rule 5.
8. Prepare a new step by providing a new target. Set your target slightly higher than the actual performance of your activity. Write this down for your second exercise situation.
9. Repeat the rules 6, 7, and 8, until you have reached your final goal.

You can increase the effectiveness of the above approach by a positive self-statement if the performance of the activity is equal to or better than your target. Some examples of such statements that express a positive appraisal are:

- "I did well."
- "Well done."
- "This went well."
- "Excellent!"

An example of the application of the rules mentioned above:

Two months ago, John was discharged from a forensic institute and lives now in a new area in the city. He has just started a new job as a junior mechanic in a garage. John finds it very difficult to make a request. He says to himself: "You must not bother others," "People might think I'm stupid." He avoids doing so whenever possible.

1. Description of the activity namely "Making a request." This included:
   (a) The person you would like to ask something ordered from easy to difficult. This was his girlfriend, his neighbors, his colleagues, and officials respectively.
   (b) The nature of the request. He found it difficult to make a request that costs the other person extra time or energy.
2. Divide the activity into intermediate steps taking the person and the nature of the request into account.
   (a) Ask his girlfriend to bring the laundry to the cleaning lady.
   (b) Ask his neighbor Carl to lend him a hammer.
   (c) Ask his neighbor Renate when she goes to the store to bring vegetables for him.
   (d) During the break in a computer course, ask another offender for an explanation of the meaning of a particular instruction.
   (e) Ask a colleague for a ride to the station.
   (f) Ask the financial administrator of the garage for information about some items on the slip of his monthly salary.
3. His ultimate goal was after 3 months of exercise: On important occasions, to make a request to known as well as unknown persons, even if these requests cost the other person additional time or energy.

4. At present, John seldom made a request. If he does so, he speaks hesitantly and avoids eye contact.
5. His first step was to ask his girlfriend for help with some jobs (e.g., bringing his laundry to the cleaning lady, take his bicycle to the repair shop). He sets as a target to speak loud and clearly and to keep eye contact. He wrote these criteria down.
6. He performed this activity. He said to his girlfriend: "Judy, could you take my laundry to the cleaning shop for me?" He spoke loud and clear and looked at her.
7. John compared his performance with his target. He did ask his girlfriend to take the laundry to the cleaning shop, and spoke clearly and kept eye contact. He was satisfied and said to himself "well done."
8. Next, he wrote down the targets for his second request: Ask his neighbor Carl to lend him a hammer (with a clear voice, direct eye contact, what he wants to ask, etc.).
9. He rehearsed the rules 6, 7, and 8 until he reached his ultimate target, etc.

References

Bandura, A. (1977). *Social learning theory*. Englewood Cliffs, NJ: Prentice Hall.

Bandura, A. (1991). Social cognitive theory of self-regulation. *Organizational Behavior and Human Decision Processes, 50*, 248–287.

Bandura, A. (1997). *Self-efficacy: The exercise of control*. New York: Freeman.

Bandura, A. (2001). Social cognitive theory: An agentic perspective. *Annual Review of Psychology, 52*, 1–26.

D'Zurilla, T. J., & Nezu, A. M. (2010). Problem-solving therapy. In K. S. Dobson (Ed.), *Handbook of cognitive-behavioral therapies* (pp. 197–225). New York: Guilford.

Hanson, R. K., Harris, A. J. R., Scott, T., & Helmus, L. (2007). *Assessing the risk of sexual offenders on community supervision: The Dynamic Supervision Project*. Corrections Research User Report No. 2007-05. Ottawa: Public Safety Canada.

Hanson, R. K., & Morton-Bourgon, K. E. (2005). The characteristics of persistent sexual offenders: A meta-analysis of recidivism studies. *Journal of Consulting and Clinical Psychology, 73*, 1153–1163. https://doi.org/10.1037/0022-006X.73.6.1154

Hornsveld, R. H. J., Kraaimaat, F. W., Zwets, A. J., & Kanters, T. (2017). Beyond Aggression Replacement Training: Cognitive-behavioral programs for Dutch (sexually) violent forensic psychiatric inpatients, Chapter 82. In P. Sturmey (Ed.), *Handbook of violence and aggression*. Chichester: Wiley-Blackwell.

Kanfer, F. H., & Gaelick-Buys, L. (1991). Self-management methods. In F. H. Kanfer & A. P. Goldstein (Eds.), *Helping people change: A textbook of methods* (Pergamon general psychology series) (Vol. 52, pp. 305–360). Elmsford, NY: Pergamon.

Kraanen, F. L., & Emmelkamp, P. M. G. (2017). Alcohol and drugs in relation to sexual offending. In T. Sanders (Ed.), *The Oxford handbook of sex offences and sex offenders* (pp. 143–162). New York: Oxford University Press.

Larimer, M. E., Palmer, R. S., & Marlatt, G. A. (1999). Relapse prevention: An overview of Marlatt's Cognitive-Behavioral Model. *Alcohol, Research & Health, 23*(2), 151–160.

Pritchard, C., & King, E. (2005). Differential suicide rates in typologies of child sex offenders in a 6-year consecutive cohort of male suicides. *Archives of Suicide Research, 9*, 35–43. https://doi.org/10.1080/13811110590512903

Smallbone, S., & Wortley, R. K. (2004). Criminal diversity and paraphilic interests among males convicted of sexual offenses against children. *International Journal of Offender Therapy and Comparative Criminology, 48*, 175–188. https://doi.org/10.1177/0306624X03258477

Stinson, J. D., & Becker, J. V. (2013). *Treating sex offenders. An evidence-based manual.* New York: Guilford.

Stinson, J. D., Becker, J. V., & McVay, L. A. (2017). Treatment progress and behavior following 2 years of inpatient sex offender treatment: A pilot investigation of safe offender strategies. *Sexual Abuse: A Journal of Research and Treatment, 29*, 3–27. https://doi.org/10.1177/1079063215570756

Stinson, J. D., Becker, J. V., & Sales, B. D. (2008). Self-regulation and the etiology of sexual deviance: Evaluating causal theory. *Violence and Victims, 23*, 35–51. https://doi.org/10.1891/0886-6708.23.1.35

Stinson, J. D., Robbins, S. B., & Crow, C. W. (2011). Self-regulatory deficits as predictors of sexual, aggressive, and self-harm behaviors in a psychiatric sex offender population. *Criminal Justice and Behavior, 38*, 885–895.

Stinson, J. D., Sales, B. D., & Becker, J. V. (2008). *Sexual offending: Causal theory and its implications for research, prevention, and treatment.* Washington, DC: American Psychological Association.

Van Dam-Baggen, R., & Kraaimaat, F. (2014). *Cognitive-behavioral group therapy for social anxiety and social incompetence: A social skills perspective.* Maarn/Nijmegen. Open Access book: http://www.floriskraaimaat.nl/pdfiles/sstjune2014.pdf

Ward, T., & Gannon, T. A. (2006). Rehabilitation, etiology, and self-regulation: The comprehensive good lives model of treatment for sex offenders. *Aggression and Violent Behavior, 11*, 77–94. https://doi.org/10.1016/j.avb.2005.06.001

Ward, T., & Hudson, S. M. (2000). A self-regulation model of relapse prevention. In D. R. Laws, S. M. Hudson, & T. Ward (Eds.), *Remaking relapse prevention with sex offenders: A sourcebook* (pp. 79–101). Thousand Oaks, CA: Sage.

Zimmerman, B. J. (2013). From cognitive modeling to self-regulation: A social cognitive career path. *Educational Psychologist, 48*, 135–147. https://doi.org/10.1080/00461520.2013.794676

Chapter 8
Facilitating Treatment Integrity in Penitentiary and Forensic Psychiatric Institutions

Floris W. Kraaimaat and Ruud H. J. Hornsveld

8.1 Introduction

Treatment integrity (also called treatment fidelity, fidelity of implementation, intervention integrity, and treatment adherence) may be defined as the extent to which an intervention is intended, initially designed, or implemented as planned (Perepletchikova, Treat, & Kazdin, 2007; Sanetti & Kratochwill, 2009; Sanetti, Kratochwill, & Long, 2013). While evidence-based practice in psychology (EBPP) (American Psychological Association, 2002; American Psychological Association Presidential Task Force on Evidence-Based Practice, 2006) is strongly advocated, how interventions are applied is often overlooked in research as well as in clinical practice. However, only when the level of treatment integrity is sufficient, can a positive, negative, or absence of a change in an individual's performance be reasonably attributed to the intervention. Also, for the interpretation of the effect of an intervention study one needs to have some assurance that the treatment was carried out as it was designed. Therapists may implement all of the procedures specified in the treatment protocol, some of them or none of them, or may supplement prescribed tasks with procedures from other interventions. Compromised treatment integrity in research might lead to unjustified conclusions regarding treatment effectiveness. It might produce outcomes suggesting that effective procedures are ineffective and vice versa. In the clinical practice in judicial institutions, deviating from the protocol of an evidence-based intervention without substantive arguments or careless application of procedures can hinder the offender's recovery and is ethically questionable.

F. W. Kraaimaat
Radboud University Nijmegen, Nijmegen, The Netherlands

R. H. J. Hornsveld (✉)
Erasmus University Medical Center, Rotterdam, The Netherlands
e-mail: ruud.hornsveld@ziggo.nl

R. H. J. Hornsveld et al. (eds.), *Assessment and Obligatory Treatment of Violent and Sexually Violent Offenders*, Advances in Preventing and Treating Violence and Aggression, https://doi.org/10.1007/978-3-030-27840-3_8

8.2 How to Facilitate Treatment Integrity?

Treatment integrity is a multifaceted construct with aspects that refer to the design of treatment programs; the knowledge and experience of therapists and supervising clinicians; and the material and administrative facilities available in an institution. Treatment integrity data show to what extent an intervention has been implemented, what steps were omitted, and what barriers were met by the implementation, performance, and maintenance of the therapy.

8.2.1 Treatment

In the treatment programs as described in Chap. 6, the findings of two lines of research come together. Namely, cognitive-behavioral treatment programs are currently the first choice for offender programs (Cooke & Philip, 2001; Walton & Chou, 2015; Wilson, Bouffard, & MacKenzie, 2005) and these programs should focus on the reduction of dynamic criminogenic risk factors (Bonta & Andrews, 2007) and the strengthening of protective factors (Ward, 2002). The advantage of cognitive-behavioral treatment programs is that the different procedures and phases in the treatment are described in concrete terms and that critical aspects are distinguished (Kazdin, 1986). They are often accompanied by a treatment manual that is an operationalization of the treatment program by describing instructions, procedures, and activities in detail. As a result, both the therapist and the offender remain focused on the crucial factors that reinforce or weaken the behavior that is the subject of the module in question. Group treatment also offers the possibility to observe the interpersonal behavior of the participants and to change it if necessary. In this way, a manual as described in Chaps. 10 and 11 reduces the variability in the implementation and performance of treatment, thereby increasing the treatment integrity and indirectly the effectiveness of the treatment.

The aims and exercises of a manual-based group treatment program have to connect with the functional analysis or case formulation of an individual offender. Therefore, there has to be a match between an offender's specific treatment plan and the general aims and targets of the group treatment. However, it will be clear that a manual is not a cookbook and that sometimes improvisations have to be made depending on the needs of the participants, cultural differences, or logistical limitations. The therapist's skills and knowledge of the offender's functional analysis or case formulation enable him or her to tune specific therapeutic instructions and procedures to the needs and particular circumstances of the offender in question. However, therapists may deviate from a specific procedure or instruction if small adjustments are sufficient to facilitate the engagement or understanding of the participants, but in general, they should follow the program manual as much as possible to prevent so-called 'therapy drift'.

8.2.2 Therapists

According to Perepletchikova et al. (2007), treatment integrity encompasses three aspects: (a) therapist treatment adherence, the degree to which the therapist utilizes prescribed procedures and avoids proscribed procedures; (b) therapist competence, the level of the therapist's skills and judgments; and (c) treatment differentiation, whether treatments differ from each other along critical dimensions. The internal validity of EBPP (American Psychological Association Presidential Task Force on Evidence-Based Practice, 2006) may be threatened as therapists become less adherent to the treatment protocol. Therefore, applying manual-based treatment programs requires well-educated and well-trained therapists. On the one hand, he or she must be able to fit his or her activities within the framework of the manual, while on the other hand he or she must be able to improvise within its limits. Doing this requires experience with the problem behaviors or symptoms to be treated, with their theoretical context, and with the various modules of the treatment program. Therefore, modifications that depart from the patient's needs are not justified (Sanetti & Kratochwill, 2009). Particular attention should be given to skills which are needed to motivate participants and to deal with participants in a group format. Consequently, training is recommended in which a group of therapists in training follows the manual under the guidance of an experienced therapist who sometimes role-plays the therapist and sometimes role-plays the delinquent. Afterwards, the therapists are assessed on knowledge and competence. The competence of the therapist is further promoted by supervision of the entire treatment program by an experienced clinician with expertise in such treatment programs (Kazdin, 2003). To prevent gradual deviation from and alteration of the treatment manual (therapy drift), ongoing evaluations and regular meetings are provided in which therapists and clinical staff jointly correct deviations from treatment goals and procedures.

8.2.3 Offenders Adherence to the Treatment

The performance of the treatment and the associated treatment adherence of the offenders both contribute to the result of the treatment. The responsivity principle of Andrews and Bonta (2010) determines that treatment interventions are most effective when they are adapted to the abilities, skills, and learning styles of the offender. A treatment program that takes account of this principle leads to maximum engagement of the participants. Engagement may also be facilitated when participants have a more or less similar social background. Another condition for engagement in treatment is that the problems are addressed with an emphasis on role-play, rehearsal, feedback, and other active exercises. Fernandez, Shingler, and Marshall (2006) argued that a better balance between cognitive and behavioral change techniques will facilitate the achievement of treatment goals and will offer therapists strategies for handling group interactions. It is also essential that the participants agree with the instructions of the workbook, understand them and use the trained skills (Hollin, 1999). Specifically, when treatment is mandated there is a risk of deliberate failure to engage (Long, Dolley, & Hollin, 2013).

Monitoring the adherence of participants to a treatment program, their investments in the different activities and the quality of their homework assignments are essential feedback for participants as well as therapists. For example, giving feedback about their behavior after a role-play or during the homework assignments are opportunities to promote the engagement of the participants. Also, these activities provide the therapist with information about the feasibility of the offered interventions. They are also intended to increase the participants' interest in behavior change and must be rewarding to promote a therapeutic alliance. Only in the context of positive feedback and a climate of safety participants' compliance will improve.

8.2.4 The Organization of a Penitentiary or Forensic Psychiatric Institute

8.2.4.1 Facilities

The need for treatment integrity makes many demands on the infrastructure of institutions that aim to offer safety to society and treatment to offenders. Hollin (1999) stated that as institutions strive toward delivering more effective treatment services, three areas stand out as demanding attention, all of which are prerequisites for treatment integrity. These areas are (a) the need for an organizational structure that values and facilitates treatment; (b) the need to train staff to deliver programs; and (c) the need for management systems that monitor the design, implementation, and progress of treatment programs.

The institution has to provide the necessary facilities such as group treatment rooms, audio/video equipment, and administrative support. Moreover, it is essential that the general objective of treatment is widely presented in the various units of the institution. Norms, values, and beliefs about treatment need to be shared among all members of the staff. An entirely confusing and counterproductive situation might arise when for instance some members of the team promote the expression of aggression from altogether different theoretical perspectives such as gestalt or psychodynamic orientations (Hollin, 1995). Further, the organization provides the offenders an opportunity to implement their learned behaviors within and as far as possible outside the institution. While residential treatments can be useful, they should be linked structurally with community-based interventions (Hollin, 1999).

8.2.4.2 Quality of Staff

The turnover of personnel offers opportunities for quality improvement through selection and training. Therefore, the management finances and facilitates education and training for new staff members who are involved in the rehabilitation or treatment programs. A management system is also required that monitors the design, implementation, and progress of the treatment programs (Gendreau, 1996). Thus, the management stimulates competence and high quality. Evaluation of efficacy, effectiveness, and integrity is carried out at different levels of the organization. In this way, an account can be taken of the treatment programs for staff, patients, administrators, and financial contributing institutions.

8.2.4.3 Governmental Policies

In most Western countries, governments have made in recent years a policy change from restrictive to more humane values and attitudes. However, under pressure from institutions, ministries, and other stakeholders, the focus of treatment programs will shift to mainly administrative and financial goals (Hollin, 1999). Monitoring of economic costs usually features high on the agenda of many managers. It is conceivable that with a changing policy, shrinking budgets, and large staff turnover, the supporting infrastructure and, in particular, the professional quality of the treatment staff can be jeopardized. A negative spiral can occur when integrity assessments are abused for controlling and limiting the efforts of therapists and clinical staff. Most mental health practitioners start with the intention to help and serve others, so intrinsic motivation is present, but it may be frustrated by a lack of support from the institution (Midgley, 2009).

8.3 Assessment of Treatment Integrity

8.3.1 Methods

Essential to the measurement of treatment integrity is that the intervention can be delineated into a series of steps, components, or actions that allow for an appraisal in quantifiable terms (Sanetti & Kratochwill, 2009). Various tools can be used to evaluate the way a treatment program is implemented and to clarify any obstacles to the implementation of components or procedures. The data obtained can provide an estimate of the extent to which the implemented interventions approach the intended interventions. For example, quantitative data can be collected by registering the frequency of a particular activity in a given situation during a specified period.

One method is the use of rating scales. Assessments using these scales can be performed by therapists, patients, staff members on the ward, managers, or professionals from external institutions. Assessments are more proximal in the case of activities, interventions, or components of a treatment program and more distal when it concerns a whole care unit or an entire institute, the latter two, for example, for the benefit of accreditation. One or more of the following methods can be used for the assessments: observation, self-report, and permanent products (for a detailed overview see Haynes & O'Brien, 2000).

A second method is direct observation which measures the availability and quality of the applied interventions, as well as adherence to treatment. However, this method requires trained observers and can be quite time-consuming. An observation scale includes at least the definitions of the different components of the intervention with corresponding actions and the possibility to record the occurrence of each component or action. If possible, several observers must be involved in the assessments, using the same criteria. However, therapists and offenders may react differently in the presence of an observer. This problem does not occur if sessions are recorded on video, but a disadvantage of video recording is that not all components of an intervention may be recorded.

A third method is *s*elf-report with the aid of a checklist or a validated questionnaire which is a quick way to assess treatment integrity after a session and can indicate the extent to which a planned intervention has been implemented and conducted. A disadvantage of this method is that the validity of the scores depends on the skills and interpretations of the observers (see also Chap. 3). Discussing observed differences between ratings of therapists, patients, and supervisors can be used for treatment or training purposes. Scoring by therapists themselves can also help them to implement forgotten components of an intervention in subsequent sessions.

Finally, permanent products, such as finished homework assignments and recording of attendance during treatment sessions, are less likely to be affected by the reactivity of therapists and patients. An advantage is also that no observer needs to be present. However, the information obtained is limited to only a few aspects of the treatment.

8.3.2 Data Collection

Preferably a database can be created in which all integrity data of the treatment programs are collected accurately and systematically. The file contains data about the methods used, by whom and in what situation. On a calendar, one can see who has to do which assessments at what time. The advantages and disadvantages of each method must be considered when formulating a final judgment. These final judgments can be used to manage the application of an intervention and to guarantee its quality. The results of an integrity assessment indicate what was successful and what needs to be improved. Assessment of the efficacy and integrity of treatment programs is part of the implementation and application of EBPP (American Psychological Association Presidential Task Force on Evidence-Based Practice, 2006) and essential for the evaluation of the treatment programs. A checklist is presented in Table 8.1 with 13 features of treatment integrity and three dimensions of evaluation.

Assessing the integrity of the treatment can be time-consuming and when using external consultants even quite expensive. However, much can be done at an early stage of implementation of a program by building integrity facilitating features in

Table 8.1 Main features of treatment integrity and dimensions of evaluation

	Availability		Adherence				Quality of implementation			
	Y	N	0	1	2	3	0	1	2	3
Treatment										
Treatment manual for therapists	O	O	O	O	O	O	O	O	O	O
Workbook for offenders	O	O	O	O	O	O	O	O	O	O
Therapist										
Knowledge	O	O	O	O	O	O	O	O	O	O
Competence	O	O	O	O	O	O	O	O	O	O
Training	O	O	O	O	O	O	O	O	O	O
Supervision	O	O	O	O	O	O	O	O	O	O
Offenders										
Adherence of sessions	O	O	O	O	O	O	O	O	O	O
Homework assignments	O	O	O	O	O	O	O	O	O	O
Institution										
Spatial and financial facilities	O	O	O	O	O	O	O	O	O	O
Focus on reducing recidivism risk	O	O	O	O	O	O	O	O	O	O
Education and training	O	O	O	O	O	O	O	O	O	O
Maintenance infrastructure	O	O	O	O	O	O	O	O	O	O

Note. Availability is scored as yes or no. *Adherence* is the degree to which the specific intervention steps are implemented as planned (0 = no information, 1 = some, 2 = moderate, 3 = high). *Quality of implementation* (0 = no information, 1 = poor, 2 = moderate, 3 = high)

the design of the program and the conditions under which the treatment is provided. Also, a treatment manual for the therapist and a workbook for the offender may guide and prompt adherence.

8.3.3 Assessment of Integrity on Different Levels

Treatment integrity may be assessed at several levels (e.g., therapist, offenders, team, unit, institution) with proximal as well as distal data and in a rather specific or global way. An example of a proximal and specific method of assessing treatment integrity is asking offenders for the forthcoming week to rate daily the frequency of instructed exercises or activities. Each exercise is presented in a checklist and has to be rated on a five-point scale (1 = almost never; 2 = occasionally; 3 = regular; 4 = often; 5 = very often). The results of this kind of assessment may be used in the treatment sessions. Similarly, at the end of a treatment session offenders may be asked to rate on a five-point scale with statements such as "I actively participated in the session," and "I learned a lot by practicing responses."

Perepletchikova et al. (2007) used the Implementation of Treatment Integrity Procedures Scale (ITIPS) to evaluate the degree to which treatment integrity procedures were addressed in journal articles on the evaluation of treatments. The ITIPS addresses several domains of treatment integrity (establishing, assessing, evaluating, and reporting) and the main aspects of therapist adherence and competence. The ITIPS consists of 22 items, each rated on a four-point scale (www.treatmentintegrity.com).

Sometimes, an assessment of effectiveness is requested for the accreditation of services offered by the institution or by order of legal or governmental organizations which supervise judicial institutions. Adaptations of the Correctional Program Evaluation Inventory (Gendreau & Andrews, 1991) resulted in the Correctional Programs Checklist (CPC) (University of Cincinnati, 2008). The CPC was designed to evaluate the extent to which correctional intervention programs adhere to the principles of effective intervention. Different versions of the CPC have been created for use in different types of correctional services. The CPC-Group Assessment (CPC-GA) has been validated and is geared to offender-based treatment groups (e.g., Aggression Replacement Training). The CPC is divided into two primary areas: Capacity and Content. The *Capacity area* is designed to measure whether a correctional treatment delivers evidence-based interventions and services for offenders. There are three domains: (1) Leadership and Development; (2) Staff Characteristics; and (3) Quality Assurance. The *Content area* focuses on the substantive domains of (1) Offender Assessment and (2) Treatment Characteristics. In total there are seventy-seven indicators. Each area and all domains are scored and rated as either highly effective, effective, needs improvement, or ineffective. The scores in all five domains are totaled, and the same scale is used for the overall assessment score.

8.3.4 Psychometric Qualities and Ethical Issues

Because treatment integrity is a multidimensional construct, integrity data are associated with issues such as reliability, validity, and representativeness. When comparing studies on the evaluations of treatment programs, in our opinion standardized measurement instruments such as ITIPS should be used. Therefore, an assessment of treatment integrity is recommended during the implementation of empirically assisted treatment programs, such as the treatment programs in this book (Chap. 6). The information obtained informs clinicians about the extent to which the implementation and performance of a treatment program correspond with the original design. Because it is advisable to use for this purpose internationally accepted instruments, current instruments may need to be adapted for the application in specific components of treatment programs. Then irrevocably the question of the psychometric quality of these measurement instruments comes into play (Perepletchikova, 2014).

Internet and smartphones are increasingly used in healthcare, but the use of this technology is only possible to a limited extent in the forensic community because of security and confidentiality problems. This problem is less an issue for offenders who follow community programs, and therefore data provided via the internet can play a role in assessing the treatment integrity of such treatment programs (Andersson, 2009). Privacy and ethical guidelines require professionals to request permission from offenders before proceeding with an assessment of treatment integrity. An exception may be when the assessment is performed as a routine activity for educational, institutional, or organizational purposes (American Psychological Association, 2002). Therefore, it is recommended that integrity assessment is a standard procedure embedded in manuals for therapists and offenders. In all other cases, professionals must decide whether they are ethically obliged to request permission (McGivern & Walter, 2014).

8.4 Maintenance of Treatment Integrity

A maintenance plan is required to maintain the integrity of a treatment program for the long term, for example, 2–5 years. The maintenance activities include the different levels of the organization, namely treatment program, manual, therapists, care unit, and institution. Preferably, discussions about this plan are carried out by the relevant personnel in the context of a problem-solving and pleasant atmosphere, not as negative criticism. Reflection and evaluation of oneself and performance of others require a safe environment within the institution.

When multiple groups of offenders are treated, and sufficient integrity data are collected, evaluative analyses can be made. The results obtained may indicate that some adjustments are needed concerning the content of the treatment program, the manual, the competence of therapists, the selection of offenders, the level of support of the staff, and the budget provided. Treatment programs can be seen as work in progress, and the timing of the individual maintenance activities depends on the number of offenders and groups, available staff, administrative support, policy of the institute, and available budget. The provision of a research assistant who is involved in the planning, delivery, and evaluation of the treatment programs is strongly recommended.

The cycle of evaluation and adjustment of treatment programs can be complicated if it involves a relatively small number of offenders and therapists and a limited budget is available. Notably, this may happen when it concerns treatment programs intended for a small, specific group of offenders. In that case, cooperation with other institutions seems to be necessary. This cooperation is also apparent if only limited budgets are available for education, training, and supervision of therapists. A recent development in this context is the foundation of internet platforms by universities and professional organizations to support professionals and promote the dissemination of treatment programs. The evident outcomes of cooperation in the area of treatment programs, workshops, training courses, and publications may improve the notion of treatment to policymakers, and the general public.

8.5 Conclusions and Recommendations

The integrity of treatment programs is of great importance for practitioners and support staff at the different levels of an institution. Measurements of integrity indicate the extent to which a designed treatment program has actually been implemented and conducted. Much can be done at an early stage to promote the integrity of treatment programs by substantively complying with the criteria for EBPP, investing in education and training of therapists, and creating the necessary material and financial conditions.

Treatment programs must be regularly evaluated to be adjusted and improved if necessary. Unfortunately, to date, the assessment of treatment integrity is not part of the regulations, neither for judicial institutions nor for professional organizations. At an institutional level, promoting treatment integrity can lead to dilemmas. On the one hand, one wants to guarantee a high quality of treatment for society and offenders, on the other hand, there are the material and financial limitations that institutions receive from the government. All sorts of measures that institutions must implement to ensure the safety of society, as well as offenders, are sometimes contrary to the aim of optimal treatment integrity. To be able to handle these conflicting interests, professional and competent leadership is required at all levels of an institution.

References

American Psychological Association. (2002). Ethical principles of psychologists and code of conduct. *American Psychologist, 57*, 1060–1073. https://doi.org/10.1037/0003-066X.557.12.1060

American Psychological Association, Presidential Task Force on Evidence-Based Practice. (2006). Evidence-based practice in psychology. *American Psychologist, 61*, 271–285. https://doi.org/10.1037/0003-066X.61.4.271

Andersson, G. (2009). Using the internet to provide cognitive behaviour therapy. *Behavior Research and Therapy, 47*, 175–180.

Andrews, D. A., & Bonta, J. (2010). *The psychology of criminal conduct* (5th ed.). New Providence, NJ: Matthew Bender & Company.

Bonta, J., & Andrews, D. A. (2007). *Risk-need responsivity model for offender assessment and rehabilitation.* Ottawa: Public Safety Canada.

Cooke, D. J., & Philip, L. (2001). To treat or not to treat? An empirical perspective. In C. R. Hollin (Ed.), *Handbook of offender assessment and treatment* (pp. 17–34). Chichester: Wiley.

Fernandez, Y. M., Shingler, J., & Marshall, W. L. (2006). Putting "behavior" back into cognitive-behavioral treatment of sexual offenders. In W. L. Marshall, Y. M. Fernandez, L. E. Marshall, & G. A. Serran (Eds.), *Sexual offender treatment. Controversial issues* (pp. 211–224). Chichester: Wiley.

Gendreau, P. (1996). Offender rehabilitation: What we know and what needs to be done. *Criminal Justice and Behavior, 23*, 144–161.

Gendreau, P., & Andrews, D. A. (1991). *Correctional program evaluation inventory* (2nd ed.). St. John: University of New Brunswick.

Haynes, S. N., & O'Brien, W. H. (2000). *Principles and practice of behavioral assessment.* New York: Plenum.

Hollin, C. R. (1995). The meaning and implications of "treatment integrity". In J. McGuire (Ed.), *What works: Reducing reoffending-guidelines from research and practice* (pp. 195–208). Chichester: Wiley.

Hollin, C. R. (1999). Treatment therapies for offenders. Meta-analysis, "What works" and beyond. *International Journal of Law and Psychiatry, 22*(3–4), 361–372.

Kazdin, A. E. (1986). Comparative outcome studies of psychotherapy: Methodological issues and strategies. *Journal of Consulting and Clinical Psychology, 54*, 95–105. https://doi.org/10.1037/0022-006X.54.1.95

Kazdin, A. E. (2003). *Research design in clinical psychology* (4th ed.). Boston, MA: Allyn & Bacon.

Long, C. G., Dolley, O., & Hollin, C. (2013). Engagement in psychosocial treatment: Its relationship to outcome and care pathway progress for women in medium-secure settings. *Criminal Behavior and Mental Health, 22*, 336–349.

McGivern, J. E., & Walter, M. J. (2014). Legal and ethical issues related to treatment integrity in psychology and education. In H. L. M. Sanetti & T. R. Kratochwill (Eds.), *Treatment integrity: A foundation for evidence-based practice in applied psychology*. Washington, DC: American Psychological Association.

Midgley, N. (2009). Editorial: Improvers, adapters and rejectors: The link between "evidence-based practice" and "evidence-based practitioners". *Clinical Journal of Child Psychology and Psychiatry, 14*, 323–327. https://doi.org/10.1177/1359104509104045

Perepletchikova, F. (2014). Assessment of treatment integrity in psychotherapy research, Chapter 6. In L. M. Hagermoser Sanetti & T. R. Kratochwill (Eds.), *Treatment integrity: A foundation for evidence-based practice in applied psychology*. Washington, DC: American Psychological Association.

Perepletchikova, F., Treat, T. A., & Kazdin, A. E. (2007). Treatment integrity in psychotherapy research: Analysis of the studies and examination of the associated factors. *Journal of Consulting and Clinical Psychology, 75*, 829–841.

Sanetti, L. M. H., & Kratochwill, T. R. (2009). Toward developing a science of treatment integrity: Introduction of the special school series. *School Psychology Review, 38*, 445–459.

Sanetti, L. M. H., Kratochwill, T. R., & Long, A. C. J. (2013). Applying adult behavior change theory to support mediator-based intervention implementation. *School Psychology Quarterly, 28*, 47–62. https://doi.org/10.1037/spq0000007

University of Cincinnati. (2008). *Evidence-based Correctional Program Checklist (CPC) training protocol*. Cincinnati, OH: The University of Cincinnati Corrections Institute, University of Cincinnati. Retrieved from http://www.uc.edu/criminaljustice

Walton, J. S., & Chou, S. (2015). The effectiveness of psychological treatment for reducing recidivism in child molesters: A systematic review of randomized and nonrandomized studies. *Trauma, Violence, & Abuse, 16*, 401–417. https://doi.org/10.1177/15248380145379

Ward, T. (2002). Good lives and the rehabilitation of offenders: Promises and problems. *Aggression and Violent Behavior, 7*, 513–528. https://doi.org/10.1016/S1359-1789(01)00076-3

Wilson, D. B., Bouffard, L. A., & Mackenzie, D. L. (2005). A quantitative review of structured, group-oriented, cognitive-behavioral programs for offenders. *Criminal Justice and Behavior, 32*, 172–204. https://doi.org/10.1177/0093854804272889

Chapter 9
Reflections and Future Directions

Floris W. Kraaimaat and Ruud H. J. Hornsveld

9.1 Introduction: a Case Study

If the recommendations are followed as they were made in Chaps. 1–8, then an assessment and treatment trajectory for an individual offender in a penitentiary or forensic psychiatric institution, in this case, the Dutch high-risk violent offender John, looks like as described below. In describing this ideal trajectory, it should be realized that the professionals who deal with violent offenders do serve two customers: the offender and the society that must be protected against him. The description of John's progress is elaborated following the cognitive-behavioral principles we advocated in this book.

John was sentenced to an obligatory treatment in a specialized maximum-security forensic psychiatric hospital because he had committed manslaughter but was not held fully accountable by the court for the committed offense. The court made that decision on the basis of an extensive psychiatric and psychological evaluation in a special forensic assessment organization that established a relation between a severe antisocial personality disorder and the committed offense. In the hospital (patient to staff ratio 1:1.8; an average length of stay is 9 years), John stayed at a high-security ward with 11 patients. During a period of approximately 4 months after admission, John's problems, deficits, and resources were inventoried. Assessment, including risk assessment, comprised record review, structured interviews, and psychological tests, but also the observation of his behavior by the staff on the ward. All these assessment procedures resulted in a functional analysis of his dynamic criminogenic needs that became the basis of an individual treatment

F. W. Kraaimaat
Radboud University Nijmegen, Nijmegen, The Netherlands

R. H. J. Hornsveld (✉)
Erasmus University Medical Center, Rotterdam, The Netherlands
e-mail: ruud.hornsveld@ziggo.nl

R. H. J. Hornsveld et al. (eds.), *Assessment and Obligatory Treatment of Violent and Sexually Violent Offenders*, Advances in Preventing and Treating Violence and Aggression, https://doi.org/10.1007/978-3-030-27840-3_9

plan for the short and long term. That plan described the specialized educational, vocational, and group treatment programs, and additional individual treatments that John had to follow.

The group treatment programs and individual treatments for which John was indicated were evidence-based and were conducted by well-trained and experienced trainers. For his participation in the group treatment programs, John received a workbook with information on (sexual) behavior, homework assignments, and self-monitoring instruments. During regular meetings of the treatment team, mostly in the presence of John, therapists, trainers, and staff on the ward discussed the progress of the treatment. Then, the team worked with John about the next steps to be taken. Unexpected lack of progress in the realization of the treatment plan sometimes led to additional assessment and adjustments of the plan.

Recidivism risk was estimated every 2 years by means of a standardized set of risk assessment instruments. Based on these risk assessments the court decided if treatment should be prolonged or that resocialization could start. After 8 years, John's recidivism risk was reduced to such an extent that he could leave the hospital for a few hours, first under the protection and supervision of staff members. When that turned out to go well over a more extended period, John could gradually go longer and more often on leave, and under less and less supervision. He had to demonstrate that he knew to behave adequately in new situations by using self-management skills.

When the leave period was successfully completed, John was transferred to a rehabilitation facility in the center of the city and lived there under the supervision of the outpatient forensic psychiatric clinic. However, if John had made too little progress during the treatment, for example, because the formulated treatment goals proved to be too difficult, then the treatment plan had to be thoroughly revised, probably after additional assessment. If it turned out that John could not return to the community without risk, a more permanent solution might be found, for example, in the form of a long-stay setting.

The results of all assessment procedures of the offenders are stored in a standard and secure database. These data can be used to determine the progress of the treatment for each offender, but the data of groups of offenders can also be used to measure the effectiveness of individual and group treatments. The database is managed by a research assistant and is accessible to a professional involved in the treatment of an individual offender, provided that he or she be authorized to do so.

9.2 Reflections and Suggestions

Looking at the ideal trajectory of John described above, the question arises to what extent further progress can be made in the assessment and treatment of violent offenders, such that the effectiveness of admission to a penitentiary or forensic psychiatric institution can be increased.

9.2.1 Emotion Regulation

The theoretical foundations of current treatments for violent offenders might benefit from theories about emotions (Gunst, Watson, Desmet, & Willemsen, 2017; Roberton, Daffern, & Bucks, 2012). In dual-process models of emotional regulation, antecedent-focused (automatic) and response-focused (strategic) emotional regulation are regarded as endpoints of a continuum (Frijda, 1986, 1988; Gross, 1998, 2007, 2015). Automatic emotional regulation is generated by sensory input, which in turn activates implicit cognitive structures (schemas, scripts, concepts) that do not require attentional resources and therefore no voluntary control. Automatic emotion regulation manifests itself in impulsive and rapid responding with interconnected patterns of physiological, motor, and verbal responses. Strategic emotional regulation, on the other hand, requires attentional resources, is voluntary, and is driven by explicit goals. Strategic emotional regulation manifests itself in longer response times and deliberate patterns of physiological, cognitive, and motor reactions. At this point, it is important to note that complex behavior, such as driving, playing the piano, or exhibiting social behavior, is only automatically triggered by overlearning and frequent rehearsals. It is overlearning that reduces the role of cognitive and motor control in the execution of complex behavior, and that facilitates automation. Following the dual-process models of emotional regulation, reactive and proactive aggression can also be conceptualized as endpoints of the continuum of emotional regulation. Such a continuum has been supported, among others, by a study of Cima, Raine, Meesters, and Popma (2013) who found that in a sample of 845 offenders and non-offenders reactive and proactive aggression, as measured with the Dutch Reactive-Proactive Questionnaire (RPQ), showed that reactive aggression correlated significantly positive with impulsiveness, while proactive aggression correlated significantly positive with callousness. From this perspective, two issues require more attention in treatment, namely the role of impulsivity in reactive aggression and the role of overlearning prosocial skills in proactive aggression. The last issue is about replacing automatic antisocial emotions with automatic prosocial emotions.

9.2.2 Impulsivity

Impulsivity can be defined as the failure of cognitive and motor inhibitions due to deficits in executive functions. Impulsivity has proven to be a predictor of antisocial behavior in several prospective studies (Moffitt, Caspi, Rutter, & Silva, 2003; Tremblay, Pihl, Vitaro, & Dobkin, 1994). Today, however, most treatments often focus on conscious cognitive control and are therefore less suitable for offenders with deficits in executive functions. Therefore, it seems necessary to recognize this subpopulation early, for example, using self-report questionnaires for impulsivity such as the Barratt Impulsiveness Scale (BIS-11, Patton, Stanford, & Barratt, 1995; Stanford et al., 2009) or neuropsychological tests such as the Go No-Go Task (Fillmore, 2003). Offenders with high scores on impulsiveness may benefit from a treatment, in which frequency and duration of the sessions, instructions, and exercises are tuned to their functioning (Olver & Wong, 2009), analogous to the developed group interventions for people with intellectual disabilities who show sexually misconduct (Malovic, Rossiter, & Murphy, 2018). Also, a possibility may be a psychopharmacological treatment, alone or in combination with behavioral interventions (Braquehais, Ramos-Quiroga, & Sher, 2010; Markovitz, 1995). Evaluation studies have to show what the effect is of each intervention separately or all interventions together.

In social interactions, there is often hardly any time to think about the situation that has arisen and rapid response is required. New complex behaviors such as social skills are only automatically displayed after repeated applications. Overlearning ensures that an individual is resistant to stress and distraction (resilience). Resilience is necessary because the newly acquired behavior must compete with the repertoire of existing skills. A problem with current treatments may be that due to the multitude of objectives, there is too little attention and time for overlearning so that the therapist's efforts and time on treatment may be in vain. For this reason, it is therefore essential that treatment programs for offenders are conducted by experienced therapists who, if needed, can pay attention to the overlearning of prosocial skills, for example, by involving previously exercised skills in the learning of new skills.

9.2.3 Motivation for Change

Failure to comply with obligatory treatment makes it impossible to reduce recidivism risk in offenders (Nunes, Cortoni, & Serin, 2010). Offenders with many psychopathic traits appear to be more resistant to treatment than offenders with few psychopathic traits. Offenders who drop out prematurely or are excluded from treatment have a higher recidivism risk, and are less motivated for treatment than offenders who complete treatment (Nunes & Cortoni, 2006). A meta-analysis of 139 studies by Parhar, Wormith, Derkzen, and Beauregard (2008) suggested that obligatory treatment is less effective than voluntary treatment because some offenders assume that recognizing problems leads to a more extended stay in the closed institution (Wheatley, 1998). However, Polaschek and Skeem (2018) concluded from a large number of studies that there are insufficient reasons to exclude offenders with psychopathic traits from treatment, but that further research is badly needed to treatment programs for high-risk offenders. They raise a number of questions to investigate in future evaluation studies such as whether treatments designed to reduce antisocial behavior have an effect on core psychopathic traits.

Prochaska, DiClemente, and Norcross (1992) distinguished five stages in the process of change. These were precontemplation (no intention to change behavior), contemplation (awareness of a problem but no commitment to act), preparation (intention to act and address the problem), action (modification of behavior, experiences, or environment in order to overcome the problem), and maintenance (to prevent relapse and consolidate the gains attained during action). With an absent or low motivation to change, it cannot be expected that offenders will commit themselves to address their problematic behavior. The first stages of treatment are therefore crucial for increasing their intention to address their problems. Through role-play and other active exercises, it is possible to confront offenders with their deficits and excesses, as a result of which their awareness of problems may increase. Maintaining newly acquired behavior and problem-solving skills depends on a successful shift from external to internal motivation, for example, through the acquisition of self-management skills. Therefore, the assessment of the motivation for treatment is essential when drawing up a treatment plan so that counterproductive interventions can be prevented.

9.2.4 A New Model of Sexual Deviance

Most existing etiological models describe sexual offending behavior as a variant of offending behavior and mostly include factors referring to disinhibition and sexual deviance (Smid & Wever, 2019). However, according to these authors, there is additional value in describing sexual offending behavior as sexual behavior in terms of an incentive model of sexual motivation. From the perception of a competent stimulus to the actual engagement in sexual interaction and the achievement of gratification, the motivational cycle of liking, wanting, and disinhibition is repeated multiple times. Consequently, Smid and Wever (2019) regard sexual offending behavior primarily as a variant of sexual behavior and not (only) as a variant of offending behavior and therefore their Incentive Model of Sexual Motivation (IMM) emphasizes the development of deviant sexual interests and preferences. Because sexual arousal itself is an emotion, there is a bidirectional relationship between sexual self-regulation and emotional self-regulation. Not only can sex be used to regulate emotional states (i.e., sexual coping), emotions can also be used, consciously or automatically, to regulate sexual arousal (i.e., sexual deviance).

Unfortunately, there is no actual empirical evidence for the IMM available yet, and subsequent empirical studies will have to test whether the model has real empirical adequacy. That the model is relatively complicated is not so much due to the different assumptions but rather to the inclusion of phenomena like circularity, reciprocity, and multicausality. Note that the problem behavior the model describes is complex and multifaceted, and therefore must not be oversimplified (Smid & Wever, 2019).

9.2.5 Virtual Reality

The structured and controlled environment of a penitentiary institution or forensic psychiatric hospital hinders the generalization of newly acquired behaviors. Often there is a disbalance in the gender ratio of offenders and clinical staff, situations eliciting problem behaviors are mainly absent or artificial, and there is limited exposure to typical social interactions. Realistic situations are essential conditions for the generalizability and maintenance of newly acquired behaviors. One way to bring the outside world into the treatment room is by making use of actors or volunteers trained in role-playing and exhibiting problem behaviors. A new development is the use of virtual reality applications in treatment. Promising results were obtained by virtual reality exposure, in which participants were confronted with a computer-generated, virtual environment (Parsons & Rizzo, 2008; Powers & Emmelkamp, 2008). Within a virtual world, it is possible to systematically present situations beyond those that are available with traditional methods. However, Virtual Reality applications are costly, development requires specific expertise, implementation requires joint actions across institutions, and additional funding is needed for evaluation and research. To promote generalization and to maintain the obtained effects after discharge from the prison or hospital, the treatment has to be continued in the community. Then, internet applications and assisted guidance may facilitate the generalizability and maintenance of results.

9.3 Policies and Cooperation

9.3.1 Institutional Policies

The mission of a penitentiary or forensic psychiatric institution is reflected in the range of therapeutic, educational, recreational, and other activities that the offenders are offered. In most countries, this range is broader for forensic psychiatric patients than for offenders in a penitentiary institution. However, in both cases, the offer should include theoretically founded and empirically proven activities that match the (dynamic criminogenic) needs of the offenders or patients. Guidelines from professional and health organizations prescribe that evidence-based practice in psychology (EBPP) is obligatory (American Psychological Association Presidential Task Force on Evidence-Based Practice, 2006). Notwithstanding this, the current state of affairs is that, mostly for practical or ethical reasons, treatment evaluations rarely or never meet the strict standards of random-controlled trials and that only a small number of treatments have been empirically investigated in one way or another (see also Chap. 5).

Notwithstanding these difficulties, a hierarchy of levels in support may determine the choice of treatment, ranging from 1 ("weak support") to 6 ("strong support"). Level 1 means that antecedents and determinants of specific deviant behavior were examined in the literature and are the targets of the treatment. At level 2 a guideline or treatment manual for therapists and trainers is available. Level 3 means that the methods for behavioral change on which the treatments are based are found to be effective in other problem behaviors. Level 4 is related to pre-post evaluations of the treatment that show statistical and clinical improvement. At level 5 the pre-post evaluations contrast with comparative samples from offenders and the results support statistically or clinically significant effectiveness. Finally, level 6 implies that there is supporting evidence of which offenders with specific characteristics gain on the outcomes of the treatment, directly after the end of treatment but also after a period of several years.

A therapy or a treatment program is usually part of a wide range of activities such as milieu therapy, professional therapies, professional and other education, recreation, sports, and other types of activities. Unfortunately, in many institutions, the question is not answered to what extent these activities fit within the mission of penitentiary or forensic psychiatric institutions and even more important to what extent they fit in the functional analysis-based treatment plans of the individual offenders (Zwets et al., 2016). Much profit can be gained by selecting sharply in the selection of the activities to be offered. Extra gain can also be obtained if the management of an institution chooses treatment integrity as a top priority (see also Chap. 8).

9.3.2 Cooperation with Universities

Penitentiary and forensic psychiatric institutions may highly profit from the well-established infrastructure of academic education and research programs. The partnership of these institutions with a university facilitates the accreditation and the promotion of funding opportunities and the continuation of education activities. In most instances, the budget for research and development activities of a prison or a forensic psychiatric institution is limited or even absent. A partnership with a university is often a win-win situation for both parties: The institution has offenders and training opportunities for students, while a research program and researchers are available from the university. Meetings with clinical and research staff provide a forum for the exchange of scientific information and the promotion of treatment manuals built on the best available evidence. Note that all these activities serve the benefit of offenders, professionals, and society in general.

9.4 Two Suggestions for Future Research

Two concrete suggestions are made for future studies. The first study would be on the question of whether making individual functional analyses resulting in a detailed treatment plan or case formulation contributes to more significant effects of an obliged to follow treatment program. The second study is on the question to what extent cognitive behavioral interventions, pharmacological interventions, or a combination of both contributes to a decrease in recidivism in sexually violent offenders.

9.4.1 Case Formulation

As indicated in Chap. 6, the main objectives of treatment for violent offenders are influencing dynamic risk factors. If a group of offenders has many objectives in common, then in our view a group treatment is often indicated. Specific treatment goals can be addressed in individual treatments. Offenders may also have problems that cannot be considered as dynamic criminogenic factors, for example, depression.

Humanitarian considerations should lead to the treatment of such problems being added to the treatment plan. A treatment plan on the basis of case formulation is often called "tailor-made." Over the past 10 years, more and more publications have appeared internationally that argue for a precise case formulation (Craig & Rettenberger, 2018; Eells & Lombart, 2011; Kuyken, Padesky, & Dudley, 2008; Persons, 2008, 2013; Persons & Tompkins, 2007; Tarrier, 2006).

The cognitive behavioral therapeutic process implies that the formulation of a treatment plan is preceded by an extensive assessment and the drawing up of so-called functional analyses of the different problem behaviors. The therapist who formulates the treatment plan must realize that the information from interviews, self-report questionnaires, and observation scales can be strongly colored (see Chap. 3). Questions from structured interviews and self-report questionnaires may be socially desirable answered, and observation scales require a staff on the ward that is trained in behavioral observation, and that is not always available.

Involving the offender when formulating the treatment plan presupposes that this increases the motivation of the person involved in implementing the plan. Such a method was advocated by Miller and Rollnick (2002) in the form of motivational interviewing. Moreover, a tailor-made treatment may result in a better treatment result than a standard treatment protocol. Ghaderi (2011), however, believed from the literature that the relationship between the different forms of case formulation and treatment results is unclear, given the limited number of studies with both positive and negative findings. Also, these studies showed various methodological shortcomings. In a study into the reliability and quality of case formulation, Kuyken, Fothergill, Musa, and Chadwick (2005) found that both are related to the clinical experience of the assessors and their accreditation status. Corresponding results were found by Dudley, Ingham, Sowerby, and Freeston (2015) in their study into the methods of cognitive behavioral therapists, namely that case formulation can help to make decisions about effective treatments and that experienced therapists can more effectively prepare a case formulation than less experienced therapists.

Further research into the relationship between case formulation and the effect of cognitive-behavioral therapeutic interventions is worthwhile. Then, it may also be possible to examine whether the training and experience of assessors influence the quality of their functional analyses and thus indirectly on the effect of their treatments.

9.4.2 Cognitive-Behavioral and Pharmacological Interventions for Sex Offenders

The study into the effect of treatment programs for sexually violent offenders appears to be stagnating in several Western countries due to the lack of national and international agreement on the composition of a treatment program and the design of an effect study. This lack of agreement is, to a great extent, the result of a particular competition between institutions, so that, for example, manuals for programs are not published.

9.4.2.1 Cognitive-Behavioral Programs

As described in Chap. 5, international meta-analyses have consistently demonstrated that treatment for sex offenders result in a significant but modest reduction in both general and sexual recidivism (De Ruiter, Veen, & Greeven, 2008; Gannon, Olver, Mallion, & James, in press; Grossman, Martis, & Fichtner, 1999; Lösel & Schmucker, 2005), for which cognitive-behavioral interventions produced the most substantial decrease in recidivism. These interventions for sexual offenders are among others inspired by the Self-Regulation Model of the sexual offense (Ward, Hudson, & Keenan, 1998), which distinguishes four hypothesized pathways that lead to sexual offending. Hanson (2000), however, stated that treatment interventions should focus on risk factors that initiate sexual offenses and factors that could prevent relapse rather than strategies that could lead to sexual offenses.

Examining the treatment effects of interventions is difficult because of the relatively low base rate of sexual recidivism. Hanson and Bussière (1998) found that the average rate of observed sexual recidivism among previously convicted sexual offenders was only 13.4% (18.9% for rapists and 12.7% for child sexual abusers) after a follow-up period of 5 years. Additionally, effect studies hardly report on the issue of treatment integrity, except for Friendship, Mann, and Beech (2003). Therefore, to demonstrate significant effects, treatment interventions need to be powerful and include a large number of participants (Hanson, 2014; Prentky, 2003). Further, treatment should be conducted by trained and supervised professionals following a manual (Mann, 2009).

9.4.2.2 Pharmacological Treatment

In order to reduce deviant sexual interest, hormonal and psychopharmacological treatments can be used in sexually violent offenders (Gijs & Gooren, 1996; Holoyda & Kellaher, 2016; Thibaut et al., 2010; Turner & Briken, 2018). Hormonal treatments include both the antiandrogens medroxyprogesterone acetate (MPA) and cyproterone acetate (CPA), and luteinizing hormone-releasing hormone agonists (LHRH agonists). By lowering the amount of testosterone in the blood to a prepubertal level, these drugs are supposed to result in a reduced intensity of sexual interest. However, side effects can be significant, such as severe bone loss, weight gain, and breast formation in men (Gooren, 2011).

As an alternative, selective serotonin reuptake inhibitors (SSRIs) are used in this population because of the desired side effect, namely loss of sexual interest (Briken & Kafka, 2007). The treatment does not, like the hormonal treatments, have the negative connotation of "chemical castration" and is, therefore, more readily accepted by patients (De Kogel, 2008). However, there may also be undesired side effects when using SSRIs, such as erectile dysfunction and delayed ejaculation. In some uncontrolled studies, the intensity of deviant sexual fantasies was found to be reduced by treatment with SSRIs (Adi et al., 2002). Anti-psychotic medication is sometimes prescribed to reduce the intensity of deviant sexual interest, although these drugs are not registered for this purpose, just like SSRIs, and outcome research is lacking (Goethals & Van Zessen, 2018). In practice, the choice of pharmacological treatment is also determined by factors such as medical history, patient cooperation, the intensity of deviant sexual interests, and the risk of new sexual violence (Assumpção, Garcia, Garcia, Bradford, & Thibaut, 2014). However, Khan et al. (2015) concluded from some older studies that there is hardly any evidence for the effectiveness of drug-based interventions on recidivism percentages. To date, there is a lack of recent and controlled research into the effects of drug treatment on sexual violent offenders (Briken, Hill, & Berner, 2014). Society and forensic psychiatric institutions seem to oppose controlled research into the effectiveness of hormonal treatments for sex offending behavior (Briken et al., 2018).

In clinical practice, drug treatment seems to be indicated for hypersexual and offenders with paraphilic disorders who have great difficulty in keeping their deviant sexual impulses under control (Thibaut et al., 2010; Turner, Petermann, Harrison, Krueger, & Briken, 2017). SSRIs would be particularly suitable for sex offenders with a low to average recidivism risk and hormonal treatments for sex offenders with an average to high recidivism risk (Briken et al., 2014). The latter often relapse if they also have a high score on psychopathy (Hawes, Boccaccini, & Murrie, 2013).

Unfortunately, little is known about when and how decisions are made about stopping or lowering the doses of testosterone-lowering medications (Briken et al., 2018), in part because outcome research is lacking. Therefore, there is an urgent need for better research on the use and effects of pharmacological interventions in the treatment of sex offenders.

9.4.2.3 Treatments Compared

In several studies, the results of both medical and psychological programs for sexually violent offenders were investigated. Lösel and Schmucker (2005) found, for example, that medical interventions such as castration and hormonal treatments were more effective than psychological interventions. Långström et al. (2013) investigated pharmacological, psychological, and psychoeducational interventions in child sexual abusers and found in all three cases evidence for a decrease in recidivism risk. Various authors, therefore, advocated the integration of cognitive-behavioral therapy with pharmacological interventions (Assumpção et al., 2014; Briken & Kafka, 2007; Saleh & Guidry, 2003; Schmucker & Lösel, 2015). However, to date, no solid research has been conducted on the results of both interventions separately and in combination.

De Ruiter et al. (2008) described the results of five American and Canadian psychological treatment programs. They mentioned that during only one program, the Clearwater Sexual Offender Treatment Program, pharmacotherapy could be used if necessary. Three of the five programs, together with an Australian program, are discussed in a study by Olver and Wong (2013), which in four out of five cases did not mention pharmacological interventions. This seeming absence of medication as part of a program is remarkable given the findings of McGrath, Cumming,

Burchard, Zeoli, and Ellerby (2010), who found that in 2009, 89% of the American and 75% of the Canadian sexual offenders were given medication in residential settings. This finding seems to indicate that in most studies on the effect of cognitive-behavioral interventions the influence of simultaneous pharmacological interventions has not been discounted.

9.4.2.4 Research

Therefore, studies are advocated into the effect of a treatment program for rapists and child sexual abusers, for instance as described in Chap. 6, in combination with pharmacological interventions according to the algorithm as described by the World Association of Societies of Biological Psychiatry (Thibaut et al., 2010; Turner & Briken, 2018). According to this algorithm, the medication has to be adjusted in a number of steps to the intensity of the deviant sexual interest and the risk of recidivism. This research should deal with three conditions: only the cognitive-behavioral interventions, only the pharmacological interventions, and finally the entire program including both interventions. For sufficient participants in the study, it is necessary that several countries with relatively few sexually violent offenders agree on the content of the program and the design of the research. Control by the various Ministries of Justice is in our opinion inevitable.

9.5 Conclusions and Recommendations

Are spectacular new developments to be expected in the treatment of violent and sexually violent offenders? Except for Virtual Reality, we do not think so. Future neuropsychological research may result in more insight into the efficacy of the different areas in the brain, but this insight will not lead to new treatments for violent offenders since they refuse medication in the vast majority of cases. A fundamental problem that seems unsolvable for the time being is that the angle of approach in assessment and treatment of offenders is always the kind of offense for which an offender has been convicted and not his or her neurobiological and psychological makeup. Nevertheless, there is still a lot to be gained, for example, by reaching international consensus on the form and content of a treatment program for violent and sexually violent offenders and publishing a corresponding manual translated into multiple languages. The effectiveness of treatments will improve through a thorough education and training of assessors and trainers in the cognitive-behavioral therapeutic frame of reference. On the quality of the staff on the ward, international training and experience requirements may be formulated. Finally, it seems to us that the involvement of the management of institutions with the development and implementation of the treatment policy sometimes needs improvement. To conclude, much progress can be made by a decisive and concerted action of all participants in making use of the available evidence-based instruments, treatments, and procedures.

References

Adi, Y., Ashcroft, D., Browne, K., Beech, A., Fry-Smith, A., & Hyde, C. (2002). Clinical effectiveness and cost-consequences of selective serotonin reuptake inhibitors in the treatment of sex offenders. *Health Technology Assessment, 6*, 28.

American Psychological Association, Presidential Task Force on Evidence-Based Practice. (2006). Evidence-based practice in psychology. *American Psychologist, 61*, 271–285. https://doi.org/10.1037/0003-066X.61.4.271

Assumpção, A. A., Garcia, F. D., Garcia, H. D., Bradford, J. M. W., & Thibaut, F. (2014). Pharmacologic treatment of paraphilias. *Psychiatric Clinics of North America, 37*, 173–181. https://doi.org/10.1016/j.psc.2014.03.002

Braquehais, M. D., Ramos-Quiroga, J. A., & Sher, L. (2010). Impulsivity: Current and future trends in pharmacological treatment. *Expert Review of Neurotherapeutics, 10*, 1367–1369. https://doi.org/10.1586/ern.10.100

Briken, P., Hill, A., & Berner, W. (2014). Pharmacotherapy of sexual offenders and men who are at risk of sexual offending. In D. P. Boer, R. Eher, L. A. Craig, M. H. Miner, & F. Pfäfflin (Eds.), *International perspectives on the assessment and treatment of sexual offenders* (pp. 437–449). Chichester: Wiley-Blackwell.

Briken, P., & Kafka, M. P. (2007). Pharmacological treatments for paraphilic patients and sexual offenders. *Current Opinion in Psychiatry, 20*, 609–613.

Briken, P., Müller, J. L., Berner, W., Bödeker, R. H., Vollman, J., Kasperk, C., et al. (2018). Failure of a study in forensic psychiatric hospitals: Clinical trial to investigate the additive effect of triptorelin on the efficacy of psychotherapy. *Der Nervenarzt, 88*, 480–485. https://doi.org/10.1007/s00115-017-0301-7

Cima, M. J., Raine, A., Meesters, C., & Popma, A. (2013). Validation of the Dutch Reactive Proactive Questionnaire (RPQ): Differential correlates of reactive and proactive aggression from childhood to adulthood. *Aggressive Behavior, 39*, 99–113. https://doi.org/10.1002/ab.21458

Craig, L. A., & Rettenberger, M. (2018). An etiological approach to sexual offender assessment: CAse Formulation Incorporating Risk Assessment (CAFIRA*). Current Psychiatry Reports, 20*, 43.

De Kogel, C. H. (2008). *The brain in the picture. Neurobiological research and issues in the field of explanation, reduction, and prevention of crime*. The Hague: WODC.

De Ruiter, C., Veen, V., & Greeven, P. (2008). De effectiviteit van psychologische behandeling bij volwassen verkrachters: bevindingen van een meta-analyse [The effectiveness of psychological treatment in adult rapists: Findings from a meta-analysis]. *Tijdschrift voor Seksuologie [Dutch Journal of Sexology], 32*, 28–41.

Dudley, R., Ingham, B., Sowerby, K., & Freeston, M. (2015). The utility of case formulation in treatment decision making; the effect of experience and expertise. *Journal of Behavior Therapy and Experimental Psychiatry, 48*, 66–74. https://doi.org/10.1016/j.jbtep.2015.01.009

Eells, T. D., & Lombart, K. G. (2011). Theoretical and evidence-based approaches to case formulation. In P. Sturmey & M. McMurran (Eds.), *Forensic case formulation* (pp. 3–32). Chichester: Wiley.

Fillmore, M. T. (2003). Drug abuse as a problem of impaired control: Current approaches and findings. *Behavioral & Cognitive Neuroscience Reviews, 2*, 179–197. https://doi.org/10.1177/1534582303257007

Friendship, C., Mann, R. E., & Beech, A. R. (2003). Evaluation of a national prison-based treatment program for sexual offenders in England and Wales. *Journal of Interpersonal Violence, 18*, 744–759.

Frijda, N. H. (1986). *The emotions*. Cambridge: University Press.

Frijda, N. H. (1988). The laws of emotion. *American Psychologist, 43*, 349–358.

Gannon, T.A., Olver, M.E., Mallion, J.S., & James, M. (in press). Does pecialized psychological treatment for offending reduce recidivism? A meta-analysis examining staff and program variables as predictors of treatment effectiveness. Clinical Psychology Review

Ghaderi, A. (2011). Does case formulation make a difference in treatment outcome? In P. Sturmey & M. McMurran (Eds.), *Forensic case formulation* (pp. 61–79). Chichester: Wiley.

Gijs, L., & Gooren, L. (1996). Hormonal and psychopharmacological interventions in the treatment of paraphilias: An update. *The Journal of Sex Research, 33*, 273–290.

Goethals, K., & Van Zessen, G. (2018). Hyperseksualiteit [Hypersexuality]. In L. Gijs, L. Aerts, M. Dewitte, P. Enzlin, J. Georgiadis, B. Kreukels, & E. Meuleman (Eds.), *Leerboek Seksuologie [Textbook on Sexology]* (3rd Rev. ed., pp. 479–491). Houten: Bohn Stafleu Van Loghum.

Gooren, L. J. (2011). Ethical and medical considerations of Androgen Deprivation Treatment of sex offenders. *Journal of Clinical Endocrinology & Metabolism, 96*, 3628–3637. https://doi.org/10.1210/jc.2011-1540

Gross, J. J. (1998). The emerging field of emotion regulation: An integrative review. *Review of General Psychology, 2*, 271–299.

Gross, J. J. (2007). *Handbook of emotion regulation*. New York: Guilford.

Gross, J. J. (2015). Emotion regulation: Current status and future prospects. *Psychological Inquiry, 26*, 1–26. https://doi.org/10.1080/1047840X.2014.940781

Grossman, L. S., Martis, B., & Fichtner, M. D. (1999). Are sex offenders treatable? A research overview. *Psychiatric Services, 50*, 349–361.

Gunst, E., Watson, J. C., Desmet, M., & Willemsen, J. (2017). Affect regulation as a factor in sex offenders. *Aggression and Violent Behavior, 37*, 210–219. https://doi.org/10.1016/j.avb.2017.10.007

Hanson, R. K. (2000). Treatment outcome and evaluation problems (and solutions). In D. R. Laws, S. M. Hudson, & T. Ward (Eds.), *Remaking relapse prevention with sex offenders: A sourcebook* (pp. 485–499). Thousand Oaks, CA: Sage.

Hanson, R. K. (2014). Treating sexual offenders: How did we get here and where are we headed? *Journal of Sexual Aggression, 20*, 3–8. https://doi.org/10.1080/13552600.2013.861524

Hanson, R. K., & Bussière, M. T. (1998). Predicting relapse: A meta-analysis of sexual offender recidivism studies. *Journal of Consulting and Clinical Psychology, 66*, 348–362. https://doi.org/10.1037/0022-006X.66.2.348

Hawes, S. W., Boccaccini, M. T., & Murrie, D. C. (2013). Psychopathy and the combination of psychopathy and sexual deviance as predictors of sexual recidivism: Meta-analytic findings using the Psychopathy Checklist-Revised. *Psychological Assessment, 25*, 233–243.

Holoyda, B. J., & Kellaher, D. C. (2016). The biological treatment of paraphilic disorders: An updated review. *Current Psychiatry Reports, 18*, 19. https://doi.org/10.1007/s11920-015-0649-y

Khan, O., Ferriter, M., Huband, N., Powney, M. J., Dennis, J. A., & Duggan, C. (2015). Pharmacological interventions for those who have sexually offended or are at risk of offending (Review). *The Cochrane Library.* Chichester: Wiley.

Kuyken, W., Fothergill, C. D., Musa, M., & Chadwick, P. (2005). The reliability and quality of cognitive case formulation. *Behaviour Research and Therapy, 43*, 1187–1201. https://doi.org/10.1016/j.brat.2004.08.007

Kuyken, W., Padesky, C. A., & Dudley, R. (2008). The science and practice of case conceptualization. *Behavioural and Cognitive Psychotherapy, 2008*, 757–768. https://doi.org/10.1017/S1352465808004815

Långström, N., Enebrink, P., Laurén, E., Lindblom, J., Werkö, S., & Hanson, R. K. (2013). Preventing sexual abusers of children from reoffending: Systematic review of medical and psychological interventions. *British Medical Journal, 347*, f4630. https://doi.org/10.1136/bmj.f4630

Lösel, F., & Schmucker, M. (2005). The effectiveness of treatment for sexual offenders: A comprehensive meta-analysis. *Journal of Experimental Criminology, 1*, 117–146.

Malovic, A., Rossiter, R., & Murphy, G. H. (2018). Keep safe: The development of a manualized group CBT intervention for adolescents with ID who display harmful sexual behaviours. *Journal of Intellectual Disabilities and Offending Behaviour, 9*, 49–58. https://doi.org/10.1108/JIDOB-10-2017-0023

Mann, R. E. (2009). Sex offender treatment: The case for manualization. *Journal of Sexual Aggression, 15*, 121–131. https://doi.org/10.1080/13552600902907288

Markovitz, P. J. (1995). Pharmacotherapy of impulsivity, aggression and related disorders. In E. Hollander & D. Stein (Eds.), *Impulsivity and aggression* (pp. 263–287). New York: Wiley.

McGrath, R. J., Cumming, G. F., Burchard, B. L., Zeoli, S., & Ellerby, L. (2010). *Current practices and emerging trends in sexual abuser management: The Safer Society 2009 North American survey*. Brandon, VT: Safer Society Press.

Miller, W. R., & Rollnick, S. (2002). *Motivational interviewing. Preparing people for change* (2nd ed.). New York: Guilford.

Moffitt, T. E., Caspi, A., Rutter, M., & Silva, P. A. (2003). *Sex differences in antisocial behavior. Conduct disorder, delinquency and violence in the Dunedin Longitudinal Study*. Cambridge: University Press.

Nunes, K. L., & Cortoni, F. (2006). *Heterogeneity of treatment non-completers*. Research Report No. R-176. Ottawa: Correctional Service of Canada, Research Branch.

Nunes, K. L., Cortoni, F., & Serin, R. C. (2010). Screening offenders for risk of dropout and expulsion from correctional programs. *Legal and Criminological Psychology, 15*, 341–356.

Olver, M. E., & Wong, S. C. P. (2009). Therapeutic responses of psychopathic sexual offenders: Treatment attrition, therapeutic change, and long-term recidivism. *Journal of Consulting and Clinical Psychology, 77*, 328–336. https://doi.org/10.1037/a0015001

Olver, M. E., & Wong, S. C. P. (2013). A description and research review of the Clearwater Sex Offender Treatment Programme. *Psychology, Crime & Law, 19*, 477–492. https://doi.org/10.1080/1068316X.2013.758983

Parhar, K. K., Wormith, J. S., Derkzen, D. M., & Beauregard, A. M. (2008). Offender coercion in treatment. A meta-analysis of effectiveness. *Criminal Justice and Behavior, 35*, 1109–1135. https://doi.org/10.1177/0093854808320169

Parsons, T. D., & Rizzo, A. A. (2008). Affective outcomes of virtual reality exposure therapy for anxiety and specific phobias: A meta-analysis. *Journal of Behavior Therapy and Experimental Psychiatry, 39*, 250–261. https://doi.org/10.1016/j.jbtep.2007.07.007

Patton, J. H., Stanford, M. S., & Barratt, E. S. (1995). Factor structure of the Barratt impulsiveness scale. *Journal of Clinical Psychology, 6*, 768–774.

Persons, J. B. (2008). *The case formulation approach to cognitive-behavior therapy*. New York: Guilford.

Persons, J. B. (2013). Who needs a case formulation and why: Clinicians use the case formulation to guide decision-making. *Pragmatic Case Studies in Psychotherapy, 9*, 448–456.

Persons, J. B., & Tompkins, M. A. (2007). Cognitive-behavioral case formulation. In T. D. Eells (Ed.), *Handbook of psychotherapy case formulation* (2nd ed., pp. 290–316). New York: Guilford.

Polaschek, D. L. L., & Skeem, J. L. (2018). Treatment of adults and juveniles with psychopathy. In C. Patrick (Ed.), *Handbook of psychopathy* (pp. 710–731). New York: Guilford.

Powers, M. B., & Emmelkamp, P. M. G. (2008). Virtual reality exposure therapy for anxiety disorders: A meta-analysis. *Journal of Anxiety Disorders, 22*, 561–569. https://doi.org/10.1016/j.janxdis.2007.04.006

Prentky, R. A. (2003). A 15-year retrospective on sexual coercion: Advances and projections. *Annals of the New York Academy of Sciences, 989*, 13–32. https://doi.org/10.1111/j.1749-6632.2003.tb07291.x

Prochaska, J. O., DiClemente, C. C., & Norcross, J. C. (1992). In search of how people change. *American Psychologist, 47*, 1102–1114.

Roberton, T., Daffern, M., & Bucks, R. S. (2012). Emotion regulation and aggression. *Aggression and Violent Behavior, 17*, 72–82. https://doi.org/10.1016/j.avb.2011.09.006

Saleh, F. M., & Guidry, L. L. (2003). Psychosocial and biological treatment considerations for the paraphilic and nonparaphilic sex offender. *The Journal of the American Academy of Psychiatry and Law, 31*, 486–493.

Schmucker, M., & Lösel, F. (2015). The effects of sexual offender treatment on recidivism: An international meta-analysis of sound quality studies. *Journal of Experimental Criminology, 11*, 597–630. https://doi.org/10.1007/s11292-015-9241-z

Smid, W. J., & Wever, E. C. (2019). Mixed emotions: An incentive motivational model of sexual deviance. *Sexual Abuse, 31,* 731 - 764. https://doi.org/10.1177/1079063218775972

Stanford, M. S., Mathias, C. W., Dougherty, D. M., Lake, S. L., Anderson, N. E., & Patton, J. H. (2009). Fifty years of the Barratt Impulsiveness Scale: An update and review. *Personality and Individual Differences, 47,* 385–395. https://doi.org/10.1016/j.paid.2009.04.008

Tarrier, N. (Ed.). (2006). *Case formulation in cognitive behaviour therapy*. Hove: Routledge.

Thibaut, F., De la Barra, F., Gordon, H. M., Cosyns, P., Bradford, J., & WFSBP Task Force on Sexual Disorders. (2010). The World Federation of Societies of Biological Psychiatry (WFSBP) guidelines for the biological treatment of paraphilias. *World Journal of Biological Psychiatry, 11,* 604–655.

Tremblay, R. E., Pihl, R. O., Vitaro, F., & Dobkin, P. L. (1994). Predicting early onset of male antisocial behavior from preschool behavior. *Archives of General Psychiatry, 51,* 732–739.

Turner, D., & Briken, P. (2018). Treatment of paraphilic disorders in sexual offenders or men with a risk of sexual offending with Luteinizing-Hormone-Releasing- Hormone-Agonists: An updated systematic review. *The Journal of Sexual Medicine, 15,* 77–93. https://doi.org/10.1016/j.jsxm.2017.11.013

Turner, D., Petermann, J., Harrison, K., Krueger, R., & Briken, P. (2017). Pharmacological treatment of patients with paraphilic disorders and risk of sexual offending: An international perspective. *The World Journal of Biological Psychiatry, 17,* 1–10. https://doi.org/10.1080/15622975.2017.1395069

Ward, T., Hudson, S. M., & Keenan, T. R. (1998). A self-regulation model of the sexual offense process. *Sexual Abuse: A Journal of Research and Treatment, 10,* 141–157. https://doi.org/10.1023/A:1022071516644

Wheatley, M. (1998). The prevalence and relevance of substance use in detained schizophrenic patients. *Journal of Forensic Psychiatry, 9,* 114–129.

Zwets, A. J., Hornsveld, R. H. J., Muris, P., Kanters, T., Langstraat, E., & Van Marle, H. J. C. (2016). Psychomotor therapy as an additive intervention for violent forensic psychiatric inpatients: A pilot study. *International Journal of Forensic Mental Health, 15,* 222–234. https://doi.org/10.1080/14999013.2016.1152613

Part III
Manuals

Chapter 10
Treatment Modules for Violent Offenders

Ruud H. J. Hornsveld and Floris W. Kraaimaat

10.1 Introduction

The modules described in this chapter can be part of a treatment program according to the needs of the participants. However, we recommend that the modules Anger Management and Moral Reasoning, each with at least five sessions, are performed as described. For the module Prosocial Skills, we provide the session plan for only one session, because the other session plans are identical. Trainers can decide for themselves whether they want to devote five or more sessions to this subject. For each module of the Extended Program, the plan for the first session has only been described. Additional information is given for a maximum of four other sessions per module. Almost all modules include exercises and homework assignments. Also, reference is made in many cases to information brochures (Appendices 1–5). It is advisable to compose a workbook for the participants in which these exercises, assignments, and brochures are included.

Trainers have to be prepared that the implementation of a program is often difficult. Violent offenders often find that in some situations violence is justified. Therefore, trainers must schedule direct confrontations in such a way that the continuity of the group is not jeopardized. For some participants, participation in the group will hardly lead to further insight into their problems or any behavior change.

R. H. J. Hornsveld (✉)
Erasmus University Medical Center, Rotterdam, The Netherlands
e-mail: ruud.hornsveld@ziggo.nl

F. W. Kraaimaat
Radboud University Nijmegen, Nijmegen, The Netherlands

R. H. J. Hornsveld et al. (eds.), *Assessment and Obligatory Treatment of Violent and Sexually Violent Offenders*, Advances in Preventing and Treating Violence and Aggression, https://doi.org/10.1007/978-3-030-27840-3_10

10.2 Basic Program: Anger Management

Plan of Session 1

Goals

- Welcoming the participants
- Announcing the module Anger Management
- Learning to distinguish between interpretations and observations
- Explaining new homework assignments

Agenda

0:00	Opening
0:05	Making acquaintance
0:35	Appointments and introduction of portfolio
0:40	Announcing the module Anger Management
0:45	Observation exercise 1: Distinction between observations and interpretations
1:00	Observation exercise 2: State only observations/facts
1:15	Explaining new homework assignments
1:20	Evaluation of the session
1:30	Closing

Course

Opening

- Welcoming the participants
- Brief discussion of the session plan

Making Acquaintance

- Each participant briefly tells something about himself, to begin with, some biographical data ("What is your profession? Do you have a family? What are your plans for the future?"). Then the trainer asks each participant why he has to follow the program ("What is the latest offense for which you have been convicted? What punishment have you received?"), which problems he has with managing emotions like anger, and in what way these emotions are now verbally and nonverbally expressed.
- The trainer explains what is understood by aggressive and violent behavior. Aggressive behavior is, for example, scolding or threatening. Violence is physically aggressive behavior. Aggressive behavior can also be nonverbal, by talking loudly, looking long at someone, ignoring someone, and the like.

Appointments and Portfolio

- The trainer discusses the goal and method of the program, confidentiality during the sessions, consequences of absence, and reporting the referrer.
- The trainer gives a portfolio to each participant. The participants are asked to bring along this portfolio every session.

Announcing the Module Anger Management

- The trainer explains the goal of the Anger Management module.

Observation Exercise 1

- The trainer explains the purpose of the exercise: Learning to look and listen to the behavior of others and yourself and to describe this behavior concretely. Both goals are conditions for accomplishing behavior change. This will be exercised with a role-play.
- The trainer instructs the participants about the role-play "in the subway." The trainer intends that the participants watch what happens and then write it down. The trainer will indicate the start and end of the role-play. Trainer "makes a subway" by facing two chairs.
- Situation: The trainer sits down in one of the chairs and is reading a magazine. Seeks extensively in his pockets, cannot find it, and grumbles "Where have I left it, that's too crazy? I just had it," without saying what he is looking for. Finally, he mutters: "I do not understand anything" and continues reading.
- The trainer asks the participants to write down what has happened and gives them the time to do so. Trainer asks the participants their explanation of the situation and writes this using bullet points on a blackboard in two columns. Next, the trainer asks the participants what the difference is between both columns. If the participants do not notice it, the trainer helps. Then, the columns are labeled as observations (facts) and interpretations (impressions, conclusions).
- The trainer asks the participants what the purpose of the exercise might be: Making a distinction between what you see or hear and what you think it means.

Observation Exercise 2

- The trainer performs a second role-play with a similar instruction. After the end of the role-play, the participants have to record only observations (facts).
- Situation: The trainer is waiting on the street and shows nonverbally impatient behavior, walks back and forth, looks up his watch, looks into the distance, and murmurs: "I am on time, am I in the wrong place?", without to say who or what

he is waiting for. The trainer looks in his diary and decides finally to leave, muttering: "Well, that's it."

- The trainer gives participants the opportunity to write down observations, which are then discussed one by one and tested for observation versus interpretation.

Homework Assignments

- The trainer explains the homework assignments and the information in the portfolio. The homework assignments are:
  - (a) Read the information in the brochure Observing (Appendix 1) and do the exercises.
  - (b) Observe someone in the next week and make a report of your observations and interpretations.
  - (c) Do the same exercise again.

Evaluation

- The trainer asks each participant what he has learned from the session.

For the Participants

Exercise

- Observation exercise 1
  In the subway. What is happening?..
- Observation exercise 2
  Walking on the street. What do you observe? ....

Homework Assignments

(a) Read the information in the brochure Observing (Appendix 1). Underline on the last page in the four situations the sentences that are observations or facts.
(b) Observe someone you know in the next week without that person noticing that you are observing him or her. You only have to be brief looking at him or her, for example, at most a half minute. When you have done that, you write down what you saw and what you heard, by asking the questions below.

- Who did you look at (first name)? ....
- Where was it that you looked at him or her them? ....
- Which day was it? ....

- What did the other person do while you looked at him or her (facts/observations)?..
- What did the other person say? ....
- What conclusion did you draw while you looked at the other person (conclusions/interpretations)? ....

(c) Do the same exercise again. Write down what you saw and what you heard by answering the questions below.

- Who did you look at (first name)? ....
- Where was it that you looked at the other person? ....
- Which day was it? ....
- What did the other person do while you looked at him or her (facts/observations)? ....
- What did the other person say? ....
- What conclusion did you draw while you looked at the other person? (conclusions/interpretations)? ....

Plan of Session 2

Goals

- Discussing homework assignments
- Learning to consider alternative interpretations
- Learning to recognize observations/interpretations in case of irritation eliciting situations and thinking of alternative interpretations
- Discussing the behavior chain
- Explaining new homework assignments

Agenda

0:00	Opening
0:05	Discussing homework assignments
0:35	Thoughts exercise 1: Considering alternative explanations
0:55	Thoughts exercise 2: Considering alternative explanations in irritation eliciting situations
1:10	Discussing behavior chain: Antecedents
1:15	Explaining new homework assignments
1:20	Evaluation of the session
1:30	Closing

Course

Opening

- Brief discussion of the session plan.

Homework Assignments

- The trainer discusses the information in Observing as follows:
  * Invites participants to ask questions or to make comments
  * Asks participants to summarize what matters briefly
  * Discusses one of the exercise situations through short discussions per sentence: Observation or interpretation?
- The trainer asks one participant to read his report of the situation in which he briefly observed someone.
- The trainer asks all participants what they learned from the exercises.
- The trainer records the reports.

Thought Exercise 1

- The trainer reconsiders the distinction between observations and interpretations by emphasizing that interpretations are conclusions that you may draw from the situation and the behavior of the other person. This means that in the same situation often more than one interpretation is possible. The trainer explains this using a situation reported by a participant of a personal situation.
- The trainer asks the participants for each of the following situations to think of which different conclusions are possible.

  * Situation 1: You receive a gift voucher as a birthday present. You think: "Ugh, what a boring gift! He/she has no interest in me."
  * Situation 2: A family member makes you a compliment. You think: "What does he/she want from me?"
  * Situation 3: An acquaintance criticizes your clothes. You think: "He/she is teasing me."

Thought Exercise 2

- The trainer tells about an own situation in which he/she felt irritated and asks the participants to think about the possible interpretations by their questions about the observations.
- The trainer asks all participants to consider aloud a situation in which they felt annoyed and to write it down regarding observations and interpretations. A few situations are discussed for which different interpretations can be made.

Discussing the Behavior Chain

- The trainer asks the participants what may be the importance of the exercises and then discusses the behavior chain Antecedent → Thoughts → Behavior.
- The trainer gives an example of himself or herself.

New Homework Assignments

(a) Read the information in Anger Management (Appendix 2) through Thoughts (paragraph 3).
(b) Describe next week a situation where you felt irritated with the aid of the previously mentioned behavioral chain and consider alternative interpretations/conclusions.
(c) Describe a second situation in the next week where you feel annoyed.

Evaluation

- The trainer asks each participant what he has learned from the session.

For the Participants

Thought Exercise 1

- Situation 1: You receive a gift voucher as a birthday present. You think: "Ugh, what a boring gift. He/she has no interest in me."
- Situation 2: A family member makes you a compliment. You think: "What does he/she want from me?"
- Situation 3: An acquaintance criticizes your clothes. You think: "He/she is teasing me."

Thought Exercise 2

Antecedent

- Who was it? ……………………………………………………………………
- Where were you? ……………………………………………………………
- What day was it? ……………………………………………………………
- What did the other person say and do? …………………………………

Thoughts

- What conclusion did you draw? …………………………………………
- What else could you have thought? ………………………………………
- What more could you have thought? ……………………………………

Behavior

- What did you say and do? ………………………………………………

New Homework Assignments

(a) Read the information in Anger Management (Appendix 2) through Thoughts (paragraph 3).
(b) Describe next week a situation where you felt irritated by answering the questions below:

Antecedent

- Who was it? ………………………………………………………………………..
- Where were you? ………………………………………………………………
- What day was it? ………………………………………………………………..
- What did the other person say and do (observations)? …………………………

Thoughts

- What conclusion did you draw? …………………………………………………
- What else could you have thought? ……………………………………………..
- What more could you have thought? ……………………………………………..

Behavior

- What did you say and do? ……………………………………………………..

(c) Describe a second situation in the next week where you felt irritated by answering the questions below:

Antecedent

- Who was it? ……………………………………………………………………
- Where were you? ………………………………………………………………
- What day was it? ………………………………………………………………..
- What did the other person say and do (observations)? …………………………

Thoughts

- What conclusion did you draw? …………………………………………………
- What else could you have thought? ……………………………………………..
- What more could you have thought? ……………………………………………

Behavior

- What said/did you? ……………………………………………………………

Plan of Session 3

Goals

- Discussing homework assignments.
- Announcing the theme for the session: Lowering physical tension in anger-eliciting situations.
- Discussing the behavior chain.
- Explaining new homework assignments.

Agenda

0:00	Opening
0:05	Discussing homework assignments
0:35	Discrimination exercise 1: Ways to lower physical tension
0:55	Discrimination exercise 2: Lowering physical tension in anger-eliciting situations
1:10	Discussing the behavior chain: Physical tension
1:15	Explaining new homework assignments
1:25	Evaluation of the session
1:30	Closing

Course

Opening

- Brief discussion of the session plan.

Homework Assignments

- The trainer asks if there are any questions or comments on the brochure Anger Management (Appendix 2). The trainer asks the participants to give a summary of this.
- The trainer asks all participants what they have learned from the exercises.
- The trainer records the reports.

Discrimination Exercise 1

- The trainer explains the purpose of the exercise: Lowering physical tension. By lowering your physical tension under challenging situations, you get a better overview of that situation, and you can think of a better solution. There are many ways to reduce physical tension.

- An inventory is made of which ways participants and trainers lower their physical tension. Possibilities are:
  * Breathing deeply
  * Counting backwards
  * Doing relaxation exercises
  * Thinking about a pleasant image
  * Joking
  * Getting the facts strait
  * Walking away
  * Counting to ten
- The trainer then briefly discusses with the participants which way is most effective: When to apply a strategy, what do you think of it and what is in it for you? The trainer ensures, among other things, that the participants do not have too high goals to themselves.

Discrimination Exercise 2

- The trainer asks all participants to recall aloud a situation in which they felt angry and to write it down. Some specific situations are discussed, while the participants are asked how they have lowered their physical tension in that situation.
- The trainer does a role-play in which he or she shows how in a situation of their own he or she has lowered his physical tension. Then he or she asks some participants to exercise this situation. The trainer ensures that the participants use a situation that is appealing to them.

Discussing the Behavior Chain

- The trainer asks the participants what the importance of the exercise may be and then discusses the behavior chain Antecedent → Thoughts → Physical tension → Behavior.
- The trainer gives an example of himself of herself.

New Homework Assignments

(a) Read the information in Anger Management (Appendix 2) through Tension (paragraph 4).
(b) Next week, describe a situation where you were irritated or felt angry with the help of the behavior chain. Apply the best way for you to relax physically.
(c) Describe a second situation where you felt angry.

Evaluation

- The trainer asks each participant what he has learned from the session.

For the Participants

Discrimination Exercise 2

Antecedent

- Who was it? ....
- Where were you? ....
- What day was it? ....
- What did the other person say or do (observations)? ....

Thoughts

- What conclusion did you draw? ....

Tension

- How physically tense did you feel? ....

Behavior

- What did you say or do? ....

New Homework Assignments

(a) Read the information in Anger Management (Appendix 2) through Tension (paragraph 4).

(b) Next week, describe a situation where you were irritated or felt angry by answering the questions below:

Antecedent

- Who was it? ....
- Where were you? ....
- What day was it? ....
- What did the other person say or do (observations)? ....

Thoughts

- What conclusion did you draw? ....

Tension

- How physically tense did you feel? ……………………………………………
- How did you lower your physical tension? ……………………………………
- What was the result? ……………………………………………………………

Behavior

- What did you say or do afterwards? ……………………………………………

(c) Describe a second situation where you felt angry by answering the questions below:

Antecedent

- Who was it? ………………………………………………………………………
- Where were you? …………………………………………………………………
- What day was it? …………………………………………………………………
- What did the other person say or do (observations)? ……………………………

Thoughts

- What conclusion did you draw? …………………………………………………

Tension

- How physically tense did you feel? ……………………………………………
- How did you lower your physical tension? ……………………………………
- What was the result? ……………………………………………………………

Behavior

- What did you say or do afterwards? ……………………………………………

Plan of Session 4

Goals

- Discussing homework assignments.
- Learning to recognize emotions in anger-eliciting situations.
- Discussing the behavior chain.
- Provide instructions for the choice of five social skills to be exercised.
- Explaining new homework assignments.

Agenda

0:00	Opening
0:05	Discussing homework assignments
0:35	Emotion exercise 1: Recognizing emotions
0:55	Emotion exercise 2: Recognizing emotions in anger-eliciting situations
1:10	Discussing the behavior chain
1:15	Explaining new homework assignments
1:20	Evaluation of the session
1:30	Closing

Course

Opening

- Brief discussion of the session plan.

Homework Assignments

- The trainer asks two participants to report on the homework assignments.
- The trainer asks all participants what they have learned from the homework assignments.
- The trainer records the reports.

Emotion Exercise 1

- The trainer draws two dimensions (positive vs. negative and strong vs. weak) on the blackboard in the form of a cross. Then, with the aid of the pictures on the card with emotions, the participants are asked to indicate where that emotion should be placed in the four quarters of the cross. The trainer is taking care that

both positive and negative and both moderate and extreme emotions are mentioned.
- The trainer returns to some situations of the participants as mentioned earlier and asks to the possible emotions in these situations.

Emotion Exercise 2

- The trainer asks all participants to recall aloud a situation in which they felt angry and to write this situation down. Some situations are discussed, in which the participants are asked what the different emotions are those that can be distinguished.
- The trainer gives examples of different emotions in his or her own situation.

Discussing the Behavior Chain

- The trainer asks the participants what may be the importance of the exercises and then discusses the behavior chain Antecedent → Thoughts → Physical tension → Emotion → Behavior.
- The trainer gives an example from himself or herself.

New Homework Assignments

(a) Read the information in Anger Management (Appendix 2) to Emotions (paragraph 5).
(b) Describe the next week a situation where you were irritated, angry, or furious with the help of the discussed behavior chain. Be aware of other emotions.
(c) In the next module Prosocial Skills, we can exercise five skills. To choose those five behaviors, we ask you the following: In your portfolio, you will find a list of random ordered 12 so-called social behaviors or social skills. Put the behavior you want to exercise first at number 1, the behavior that you would like exercise second at number 2, and so on until you have finished all 12 skills.

Evaluation

- The trainer asks each participant what he has learned from the session.

For the Participants

Emotion Exercise 1

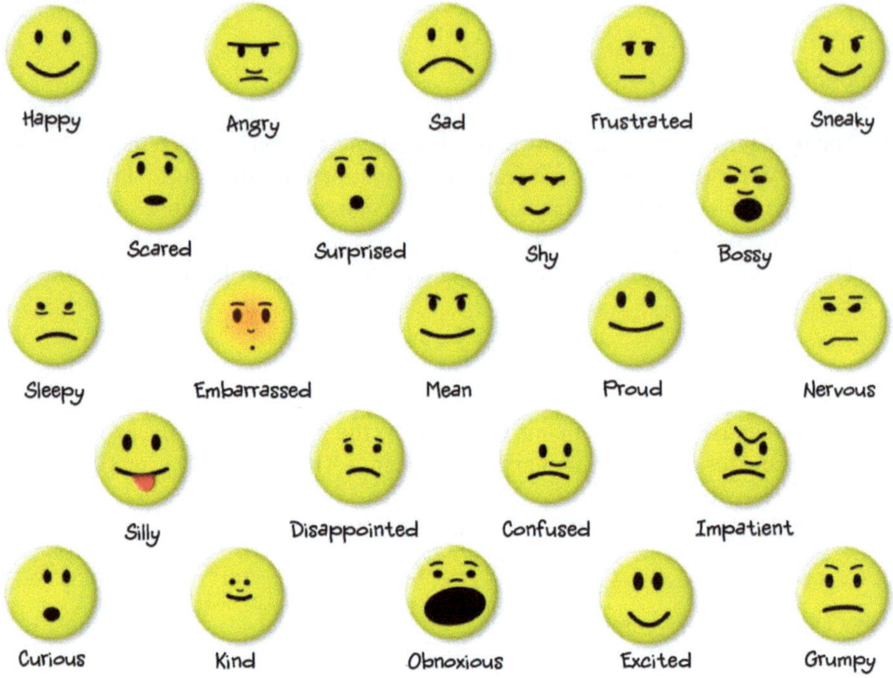

This emotion cart is a Tinycard from Duolingo.

Emotion Exercise 2

Antecedent

- Who was it? ....
- Where were you? ....
- What day was it? ....
- What did the other person say/do (observations)? ....

Thoughts

- What conclusion did you draw? ....

Tension

- How did you lower your physical tension? ....
- What was the result? ....

Emotion

- How did you feel at that moment? ....

Behavior

- What did you say or do? ....

New Homework Assignments

(a) Read the information in Anger Management (Appendix 2) through Emotion (paragraph 5).
(b) Next week, describe a situation where you were irritated or felt angry by answering the questions below:

Antecedent

- Who was it? ....
- Where were you? ....
- What day was it? ....
- What did the other person say or do? ....

Thoughts

- What conclusion did you draw? ....

Tension

- How did you lower your physical tension? ....
- What was the result? ....

Emotion

- How did you feel at that moment? ....
- Were there other emotions? ....

Behavior

- What did you say or do afterwards? ....

(c) Below you see a list of 12 so-called social behaviors or social skills. These are mentioned under each other in the left column. Put the five skills you want to exercise in the right order. The most important you give five points, the skill that you find something less important four points and so on to the least important, which will have one point.

Twelve social skills

	Skill	Example	Exercise sequence
1	Making and maintaining a contact	You have been to the film with a girl at work, and afterwards, you ask her whether she wants to go out again.	....
2	Ending a situation	You have a difference of opinion with the teacher at school and want to think about what he has said.	....
3	Asking for help	You ask your mate whether he wants to help you with repairing your car.	....
4	Refusing	Your mate asks if he may borrow your cell phone, but you do not want to do that.	....
5	Responding to a refusal	Your girlfriend says she does not want to go to the disco with you.	....
6	Criticizing	You say to your boss that he never gives you a compliment, even when you hear from others that he is satisfied with your work.	....
7	Responding on criticism	Your mother says your music is too loud.	....
8	Giving your opinion	You say in the classroom or at your work what you think of traffic jams.	....
9	Standing up for yourself	You ask your trainer why he did not put you in the football team	....
10	Complimenting someone	You tell your mother/wife/girlfriend that the dinner she made tastes good.	....
11	Complimenting yourself	You tell your mother/wife/girlfriend that you passed the exam.	....
12	Responding to a compliment	Your brother/mate says that he is proud that you have scored a goal.	....

Plan of Session 5

Goals

- Discussing homework assignments
- Learning to recognize short term and long-term consequences in anger-eliciting situations
- Discussing the extension of the behavior chain
- Explaining new homework assignments

Agenda

0:00	Opening
0:05	Discussing homework assignments
0:35	Consequence exercise 1: Recognizing the consequences of behavior in the short and long term
0:55	Consequence exercise 2: Recognizing consequences in the short and long term in anger-eliciting situations
1:10	Discussing the behavior chain
1:15	Explaining new homework assignments
1:20	Evaluation of the session
1:30	Closing

Course

Opening

- Brief discussion of the session plan.

Homework Assignments

- The trainer asks two participants to report on the homework assignments.
- The trainer asks all participants what they have learned from the homework assignments.
- The trainer records the reports.

Consequence Exercise 1

- The trainer does a role-play by a situation of himself or herself, in which the protagonist is subassertive or assertive, or exhibits aggressive behavior. The participants will then be asked to consider possible short- and long-term consequences of this behavior from three problem situations. The trainer lists these consequences in two columns on the blackboard.
- The trainer recalls some situations of the participants as mentioned earlier and asks what consequences the displayed behavior may have in the short and long term.

Consequence Exercise 2

- The trainer mentions situations of himself or herself and asks participants to think about different consequences.
- The trainer asks all participants to consider aloud a situation in which they felt aggressive and to write this situation down. Some situations are discussed, where the participants are asked for possible consequences in the short and long term.

Discussing the Behavior Chain

- The trainer asks the participants what the importance of this exercise for them and then discusses the behavior chain Antecedent → Thoughts → Tension → Emotion → Behavior → Consequences.

New Homework Assignments

(a) Read the information in Anger Management (Appendix 2) through Consequences (paragraph 6).
(b) Describe a situation in the next week where you were irritated, angry, furious, or aggressive with the help of the mentioned behavior chain. Consider the short- and long-term consequences.
(c) Describe a second situation where you felt annoyed, angry, furious, or aggressive.

Evaluation

- The trainer asks each participant what he has learned from the session.

For the Participants

Consequence Exercise 1

Problem Situation 1

Sean is 32 years old and works at a plastic factory. First, he has spent some time with a girlfriend, but now he lives alone on a flat, and that is not easy. Recently, he learned from his boss at the factory that he has made a mistake. He finds this is unfair because his boss is responsible too. When he comes home, he finds a letter from the housing association that he must pay the overdue rent immediately otherwise, he will be expelled from the flat. Sean's reaction is:

(a) *Subassertive:* He has taken the letter from the housing association hard and puts him in a big pile. He does not say anything at work either. He becomes more and more depressed and starts drinking.
(b) *Assertive:* Sean calls the housing association and explains that he has forgotten the rent because he was very busy. At work, he will discuss the conflict with his boss.
(c) *Aggressive:* Sean becomes extremely angry, calls housing association and yells at the operator. When the next morning the boss asks him something, he says: "Do it yourself, you can go to hell."

Problem Situation 2

Miranda and Nancy, two sisters of 18 and 20 years old, go to a party where later in the evening cocaine is used. Miranda has not used it for some time and does not want to use it any more. When her sister, who still uses, offers her something, her response is:

(a) *Subassertive:* Miranda reminds her sister that she does not want to take it anymore. But after a lot of urging from her sister, she takes the coke anyway, because she wants to be part of the group.
(b) *Assertive:* Miranda refuses the coke. She explains that she is not using any more and that she does not want to start again. She stands up immediately and goes home.
(c) *Aggressive:* Miranda gets enraged that her sister brought her to a party with a group of users, and that she tries to persuade her to use. Miranda scolds her sister and says she will never go with her again to a party.

Problem Situation 3

Rob always has to get up early in the morning, because he wants to be at work on time. In the evening when it is time to go to bed, the neighbor begins to play loud music and Rob cannot come to sleep. The music continues throughout the evening. Rob does the following:

(a) *Subassertive:* Rob goes to sleep on the couch in the living room so that he has less trouble with the music. He says nothing to the neighbor.
(b) *Assertive:* Rob goes to the neighbor's house and tells the neighbor he has to get up early. He asks if the music which can be softer. Together they find a solution.
(c) *Aggressive:* Furious Rob calls the police. He demands that they make sure that his neighbor immediately plays the music softer. The neighbors blame for Rob that he did not warn them first.

Consequence Exercise 2

Antecedent

- Who was it? ....
- Where were you? ....
- What day was it? ....
- What did the other person say or do (observations)? ....

Thoughts

- What conclusion did you draw? ....

Tension

- How did you lower your physical tension? ....

Emotion

- How did you feel at that moment? ....

Behavior

- What did you say or do? ....

Consequences

- What were the consequences in the short term? ....
- What were the consequences in the long term? ....

New Homework Assignments

(a) Read the information in Anger Management (Appendix 2) through Consequences (paragraph 6).
(b) Describe in the next week a situation where you were irritated, angry, furious, or aggressive by answering the questions below:

Antecedent

- Who was it? ....
- Where were you? ....
- What day was it? ....
- What did the other person say or do (observations)? ....

Thoughts

- What conclusion did you draw? ....

Tension

- How did you lower your physical tension? ....
- What was the result? ....

Emotion

- How did you feel at that moment? ....

Behavior

- What did you say or do afterwards? ....

Consequences

- What were the consequences in the short term? ....
- What were the consequences in the long term? ....

(c) Describe a second situation where you felt annoyed, angry, furious, or aggressive.

Antecedent

- Who was it? ....
- Where were you? ....
- What day was it? ....
- What did the other person say or do (observations)? ....

Thoughts

- What conclusion did you draw? ....

Tension

- How did you lower your physical tension? ....
- What was the result? ....

Emotion

- How did you feel at that moment? ....

Behavior

- What did you say or do afterward? ……………………………………………

Consequences

- What were the consequences in the short term? ……………………………
- What were the consequences in the long term? ……………………………

10.3 Basic Program: Prosocial Skills

Plan of Session 6

Goals

- Discussing homework assignments
- Announcing module Prosocial Skills
- Distributing calculation of ranking
- Practicing social skills 1
- Explaining new homework assignments

Agenda

0:00	Opening
0:05	Discussing homework assignments
0:25	Announcing the module Prosocial Skills
0:30	Distribution of social skills ranking
0:35	Practicing social skill 1
1:15	Explaining new homework assignments
1:20	Evaluation of the session
1:30	Closing

Course

Opening

- Brief discussion of the session plan.

Homework Assignments

- The trainer asks two participants to report on the homework assignments.
- The trainer asks if there are any questions/comments on the brochure Anger Management (Appendix 2) up to and including “Consequences” (paragraph 6). He or she asks the participants to give a summary.
- The trainer asks all participants what they have learned from the homework assignments.
- The trainer records the reports.

Announcing the Module Prosocial Skills

- The trainer explains the goal of the Prosocial Skills module.

Distribution of Social Skills Ranking

- The trainer shares the calculation of the social skills ranking and indicates in which order the five skills will be exercised during upcoming sessions. The calculation is carried out as follows: (1) ask each participant the ranking of his five most important social skills; (2) give the main skill 5 points, the skill then four points and so on up to and including the least important skill, which gets 1 point; (3) add up the scores each other in the column. Total and determine the group ranking.

Social Skill 1

- The trainer shares a list of five exercise situations for skill 1 and a list of goals (what do you want to achieve?) and criteria (what do you pay attention to?). The participants are asked to indicate the difficulty they have with every situation on a three-point scale. The scores are inventoried, after which the group hierarchy is composed. Then the participants are asked to choose the easiest general situation, and to turn it into an own exercise situation. This is modeled by the trainer.
- The trainer gives an example of a similar situation that he or she has experienced. First, goals and criteria are determined (Appendix 3), then the trainer will demonstrate the situation. The situation will be evaluated in the follow-up discussion on the basis of goals and criteria.
- Finally, all participants exercise with their own situation, followed by feedback from the participants and trainers on both goals and criteria.

New Homework Assignments

(a) Describe a situation coming up next week where you will apply skill 1. The trainer discusses a possible exercise situation with each participant.
(b) Do the same exercise again.
(c) Discuss five exercise situations for skill 2, including goals and criteria.

Evaluation

- Trainer asks each participant what he has learned from the session.

Calculating social skills ranking

	Social skill	Ranking for each participant								Group ranking	
		Name	Name	Name	Name	Name	Name	Name	Name	Total	Ranking
1	Making and maintaining a contact	……	…….	…….	…….	…….	…….	…….	…….	…….	…….
2	Ending a situation	……	…….	…….	…….	…….	…….	…….	…….	……	……
3	Asking for help	……	…….	…….	…….	…….	…….	…….	…….	……	……
4	Refusing	……	…….	…….	…….	…….	…….	…….	…….	……	……
5	Responding to a refusal	……	…….	…….	…….	…….	…….	…….	…….	……	……
6	Criticizing	…….	…….	…….	…….	…….	…….	…….	…….	……	……
7	Responding on criticism	…….	…….	…….	…….	…….	…….	…….	…….	……	……
8	Giving your opinion	…….	…….	…….	…….	…….	…….	…….	…….	……	……
9	Standing up for yourself	…….	…….	…….	…….	…….	…….	…….	…….	……	……
10	Complimenting someone	…….	…….	…….	…….	…….	…….	…….	…….	……	……
11	Complimenting yourself	…….	…….	…….	…….	…….	…….	…….	…….	……	……
12	Responding to a compliment	…….	…….	…….	…….	…….	…….	…….	…….	……	……

Chosen ranking of social skills

1	…………………………………………………………………………………………
2	…………………………………………………………………………………………
3	…………………………………………………………………………………………
4	…………………………………………………………………………………………
5	…………………………………………………………………………………………
6	…………………………………………………………………………………………
7	…………………………………………………………………………………………
8	…………………………………………………………………………………………
9	…………………………………………………………………………………………
10	…………………………………………………………………………………………
11	…………………………………………………………………………………………
12	…………………………………………………………………………………………

In some cases, it is recommended to depart from the group ranking of the skills to be exercised. For instance, it is better not to start with difficult skills such as "responding to criticism" or "criticizing," but a less difficult skill such as "complimenting someone." Also, it is advisable to first teach "criticizing" and then "responding on criticism" and similarly teach "refusing" followed by "responding to a refusal."

Social skills to be exercised

1	....
2	....
3	....
4	....
5	....

For the Participants

Exercise Situations for Skill 1

Below are five exercise situations for skill 1. Indicate how difficult you find those situations: "Difficult," "Average," or "Easy."

	Situation	Judgment	
1	....	O	Difficult
	....	O	Average
	....	O	Easy
2	....	O	Difficult
	....	O	Average
	....	O	Easy
3	....	O	Difficult
	....	O	Average
	....	O	Easy
4	....	O	Difficult
	....	O	Average
	....	O	Easy
5	....	O	Difficult
	....	O	Average
	....	O	Easy

What do we want to achieve in those situations (goals)?

1	....
2	....
3	....
4	....
5	....

What do we take into account in our behavior (criteria)?

1	....
2	....
3	....
4	....
5	....

New Homework Assignments

(a) Describe the next week a situation where you have applied skill 1 by answering the questions below:

- Who was it? ....
- Where were you? ....
- What day was it? ....
- What did the other person say or do? ....
- What did you do well? ....
- What else could you improve? ....

(b) Describe the next week a second situation where you have applied skill 1 by answering the questions below:

- Who was it? ....
- Where were you? ....
- What day was it? ....
- What did the other person say or do? ....
- What did you do well? ....
- What else could you improve? ....

(c) Consider five exercise situations for skill 2, which might occur in the next few weeks. Write about each situation who it is and what it is about. Write at the top the situation that gives you the least tension and at the bottom the situation that gives you the most tension.

	Who	What about
1	……………………………	…………………………………………………………………………
2	……………………………	…………………………………………………………………………
3	……………………………	…………………………………………………………………………
4	……………………………	…………………………………………………………………………
5	……………………………	…………………………………………………………………………

What do we want to achieve in those situations (goals)?

1	…………………………………………………………………………………………………
2	…………………………………………………………………………………………………
3	…………………………………………………………………………………………………
4	…………………………………………………………………………………………………
5	…………………………………………………………………………………………………

What do we consider in our behavior (criteria)?

1	…………………………………………………………………………………………………
2	…………………………………………………………………………………………………
3	…………………………………………………………………………………………………
4	…………………………………………………………………………………………………
5	…………………………………………………………………………………………………

Plan of Sessions 7, 8, 9, and 10

Goals

- Discussing homework assignments
- Practicing social skills 2/3/4/5
- Explaining new homework assignments

Agenda

0:00	Opening
0:05	Discussing homework assignments
0:25	Practicing social skill 2/3/4/5
1:15	Explaining new homework assignments
1:20	Evaluation of the session
1:30	Closing

Course

Opening

- Brief discussion of the session plan.

Homework Assignments

- The trainer asks two participants to report on the homework assignments.
- The trainer asks all participants what they have learned from the homework assignments.
- The trainer records the reports.

Social Skill 2/3/4/5

- The trainer shares a list with five exercise situations for skill 2/3/4/5 and a list of goals (what do you want to achieve?) and criteria (what do you pay attention to?). The participants are asked to indicate the difficulty they have with every situation on a three-point scale. The scores are inventoried, after which the group hierarchy is put together. Then the participants are asked to choose the easiest general situation, and to turn it into an own exercise situation. This is modeled by the trainer.

- Trainer gives an example of a similar situation that he or she has experienced. First, the goals and criteria are determined, and then the trainer will model the situation. The situation will be evaluated in the follow-up discussion by goals and criteria.
- Finally, all participants exercise with their own situation, followed by feedback from the participants and trainers concerning both goals and criteria.

New Homework Assignments

(a) Describe the next week a situation where you have applied skill 2/3/4/5. The trainer discusses a possible exercise situation with each participant.
(b) Do the same exercise again.
(c) Consider five exercise situations for skill 3/4/5, including goals and criteria.

Evaluation

- The trainer asks each participant what he has learned from the session.

For the Participants

Exercise Situations for Skill 2/3/4/5

Below are five exercise situations for skill 2/3/4/5. Indicate how difficult you find those situations: "Difficult," "Average," or "Easy."

	Situation	Judgment	
1	....	O O O	Difficult Average Easy
2	....	O O O	Difficult Average Easy
3	....	O O O	Difficult Average Easy
4	....	O O O	Difficult Average Easy
5	....	O O O	Difficult Average Easy

What do we want to achieve in those situations (goals)?

1	....
2	....
3	....
4	....
5	....

What do we take into account in our behavior (criteria)?

1	....
2	....
3	....
4	....
5	....

New Homework Assignments

(a) Describe the next week a situation where you have applied skill 2/3/4/5 by answering the questions below:

- Who was it? ....
- Where were you? ....
- What day was it? ....
- What did the other person say or do? ....
- What did you do well? ....
- What else could you improve? ....

(b) Describe the next week a second situation where you have applied skill 2/3/4/5 by answering the questions below:

- Who was it? ....
- Where were you? ....
- What day was it? ....
- What did the other person say or do? ....
- What did you do well? ....
- What else could you improve? ....

(c) Consider five exercise situations for skill 3/4/5, which might occur in the next week. Write about each situation, who it is and what it is about. Write at the top the situation that gives you the least tension and at the bottom the situation that gives you the most tension.

	Who	What about
1	....	....
2	....	....
3	....	....
4	....	....
5	....	....

What do we want to achieve in those situations (goals)?

1	....
2	....
3	....
4	....
5	....

What do we take into account in our behavior (criteria)?

1	....
2	....
3	....
4	....
5	....

10.4 Basic Program: Moral Reasoning

Plan of Session 11

Goals

- Discussing homework assignments
- Announcing module Moral reasoning
- Practicing Jason's problem situation
- Explaining new homework assignments

Agenda

0:00	Opening
0:05	Discussing homework assignments
0:35	Announcing the module Moral Reasoning
0:40	Practicing Jason's problem situation
1:15	Explaining new homework assignments
1:20	Evaluation of the session
1:30	Closing

Course

Opening

- Brief discussion of the session plan.

Homework Assignments

- The trainer asks two participants to report on the homework assignments.
- The trainer asks all participants what they have learned from the homework assignments.
- The trainer records the reports.

Announcing the Module Moral Reasoning

- The trainer explains the goal of the Moral Reasoning.

Jason's Problem Situation

- The trainer asks all participants to read the text about Jason's problem situation. Then the questions about this will be discussed, and one situation is exercised in role-play. The trainer emphasizes that this exercise is not about good or bad reactions.

> Jason's problem situation is mainly about the importance of trust in friendly relationships. Participants are generally inclined to the view that [1] Jason says that the CD player is his, [2] Jason cannot trust that David will not steal from him, [3] that David is not allowed to steal the CD player, even if it is intended for Jason's birthday, and [4] that the latter also counts as the CD player belongs to a stranger.
>
> More pragmatic participants will argue that Jason does not tell Kevin "because then you will be without a birthday present" and that David will get angry when he realizes this. These participants will also claim that a friend who steals can be trusted not to steal from you. They will say that they have such friends. Therefore, there is a chance of a divided opinion on question 2.
>
> However, the most controversial question is whether or not Jason has to tell David. Often opinions are divided. Participants who believe that Jason should tell, emphasize the risk that David took and that if Jason does not tell then he gets involved in David's theft. Participants who feel that Jason should not tell, emphasize that David is also a friend and that you never let a friend down.
>
> Sometimes a participant claims that it is not bad that David has stolen the CD player if it's not from one of his friends' cars. It is not bad if it is one of a stranger.

New Homework Assignments

(a) Answer the questions at Gary's problem situation.
(b) Describe how you have solved a moral problem that you had to face.
(c) Describe the next week a situation where you have applied skill 1, 2, 3, 4, or 5.

Evaluation

- Trainer asks each participant what he has learned from the session.

For the Participants

Exercise

Jason's Problem Situation[1]

Jason and David are friends. Jim, who almost has his birthday, tells David that he would like to have a CD player in his van so that he can listen to music while driving. David steals a CD player from a car and gives this to Jason for his birthday. Jason, who does not know that the gift is stolen, is very happy with it. The next day, Jason meets another friend, Kevin. Because Kevin is good at electronics, Jason asks him to help with the assembly of the CD player he received for his birthday. "Of course," Kevin says with a sigh. "What do you look grumpy Kevin, what's going on?" "Yes, I've been robbed," Kevin says. "Yeah, what did they take?" Jason asks. "My CD player," Kevin says and names the brand. Later, Jason thinks that it is a coincidence that the Kevin's CD player is stolen and that David gave him one with the same brand shortly after. Jason becomes distrustful and calls David. David immediately admits that he has stolen the CD player from Kevin's car. After a while, Kevin calls Jason to help him with mounting the CD player. Will Kevin probably recognize the CD player?

What could Jason say or do?

1. Must Jason tell Kevin that David has stolen his CD player?

   yes | no | no opinion [circle your answer]

2. What kind of friend is David? Can Jason trust that David will not steal anything from him?

   yes | no | no opinion [circle your answer]

3. David has stolen the CD player for a good cause (Jason's birthday). Would David therefore be allowed to steal the CD player?

   yes | no | no opinion [circle your answer]

4. What if David had not stolen the CD player from Kevin's car? What if David had stolen the CD player from a stranger's car? Would David be allowed to steal the CD player for Jason's birthday from a stranger?

   yes | no |no opinion [circle your answer]

New Homework Assignments

(a) Answer the questions at Gary's problem situation[2]

---

[1] This problem situation is an adaptation of Jim's problem situation as it has been published in Gibbs, Potter, and Goldstein (1995) and in Goldstein, Glick, and Gibbs (1998).

[2] This problem situation is an adaptation of Jerry's problem situation as it has been published in Gibbs et al. (1995) and in Goldstein et al. (1998).

Gary had just changed jobs and felt pretty lonely when one day Brandon introduced himself to him. "Hey Gary, my name is Brandon. I heard from the boss that you were new. If you have nothing to do after work, come along for some football." Gary and Brandon soon became good friends. One day, when Gary was playing football on his own, a football coach saw him. He invited him to play in his team. Gary joined the team and trained every day after working hours. After training, Gary and his teammates were eating together more and more often. On weekends they sometimes went out together for a day. Gary spent more and more time with his team and his old friend Brandon he saw less and less. One day Gary is called by Brandon: "Say, I'm celebrating my thirtieth birthday. Do you have time to come? You can eat with me that evening." Gary answers Brandon that he will try to come on his birthday but during the training on that Thursday Gary hears that they will all go to McDonald's afterwards.

What could Gary say or do?

1. Should Gary go with the team?

   yes | no | no opinion [circle your answer]

2. What if Gary calls Brandon from his work and says that he is sorry that something has happened and that he has cannot come on closer inspection? Should Gary join the team?

   yes | no | no opinion [circle your answer]

3. What if Gary thinks his teammates will find it weird when he does not agree, and that they will find him not such a good friend? Should Gary go along with the team?

   yes | no | no opinion [circle your answer]

4. What if Gary thinks that Brandon helped him when he felt alone? Should Gary then be able to go along with the team?

   yes | no | no opinion [circle your answer]

5. Let's change the situation a bit. Let's say that before Brandon asks Gary to come by, the teammates have Gary asked whether he will join them on Thursday. Gary says that he will think about it. Then Brandon asks Gary to come. Could Gary then go along with the team?

   yes | no | no opinion [circle your answer]

6. What is more important: one good friend or a whole group of superficial friends?

   a good friend | a group of superficial friends | no opinion [circle your answer]

7. Let's change the situation again. What if Gary and Brandon are not such good friends but only mutual acquaintances? Should Gary then go with the team?

   yes | no | no opinion [circle your answer]

(b) Describe how you have solved a moral problem that you had to face:

- What did the problem situation look like [where, when, with whom]? …………
………………………………………………………………………………………
- Between which two options did you have to choose?

  1. ………………………………………………………………………………
  2. ………………………………………………………………………………

- Which option did you choose and why? ………………………………………
- How did you finally solve the problem? ………………………………………
- Were you satisfied with your solution and why? …………………………………

(c) Describe the next week a situation where you have applied skill 1, 2, 3, 4, or 5.

- Who was it? ………………………………………………………………………
- Where were you? …………………………………………………………………
- What day was it? …………………………………………………………………
- What did the other person say or do? ………………………………………………
- What did you do well? ……………………………………………………………
- What else could you improve? ……………………………………………………

Plan of Session 12

Goals

- Discussing homework assignments
- Practicing Melvin's problem situation
- Explaining new homework assignments

Agenda

0:00	Opening
0:05	Discussing homework assignments
0:35	Practicing Melvin's problem situation
1:15	Explaining new homework assignments
1:20	Evaluation of the session
1:30	Closing

Course

Opening

- Brief discussion of the session plan.

Homework Assignments

- Trainer asks two participants to report on the homework assignments.

Gary's problem situation is about feelings of friendship and loyalty. Generally, participants think that Gary has to go to Brandon's birthday. Gary and Brandon were good friends and the birthday offers an opportunity to renew that friendship. Most participants will say that Gary will feel bad when he goes with the team.

Participants sometimes also think from a pragmatic point of view that Gary should go to Brandon's birthday: "Gary is already doing a lot with the team, but birthdays are there only once a year" or "Maybe Gary wants to do something different than always going out with the team."

Question 6 tackles the heart of the matter. The choice for a good friend is often unanimous. Participants who argue that Gary should go along with the team are often opportunists: "With the team, Gary will have more fun." They

(continued)

are inclined to minimize the damage to Brandon. Usually, these participants can be persuaded to a different position.

In question 7, the participants often opt for "going along with the team" because in that question, Gary and Brandon are no longer friends but acquaintances.

- The trainer asks all participants what they have learned from the homework assignments.
- The trainer records the reports.

Melvin's Problem Situation

- The trainer asks all participants to read the text about Melvin's problem situation. Then the questions about this will be discussed and one situation is exercised in role-play. The trainer emphasizes that this exercise is not about good or bad reactions.

Melvin's problem situation focuses on the problem of how to end a relationship that has no future. The importance of this problem situation for moral judgment has to do with the last question, which is about revenge.

The majority of participants will opt for positive reactions: Melvin has to tell the reason for the termination of the relationship [1] and not tell fibs [2] or make dates with other women [3]. An abrupt change occurs in question 5 when Melvin and Rita are life partners and have two children. Most participants are then inclined to choose for not breaking the relationship because Melvin is responsible for raising his children.

Most participants also have a positive attitude towards the questions about revenge. The majority is against revenge by Rita [6] or by Melvin [7] as the roles are turned around. However, be aware that there are group members who advocate revenge, especially by Melvin on Rita. Sometimes it makes sense to ask the group what is meant by "revenge." Although most participants will disapprove revenge by Melvin or Rita, they would probably practice it in real-life situations. What participants claim they might do is often in stark contrast to the exercise.

New Homework Assignments

(a) Answer the questions at Nicky's problem situation.
(b) Describe how you have solved a moral problem that you had to face.
(c) Describe the next week a situation where you have applied skill 1, 2, 3, 4, or 5.

Evaluation

- Trainer asks each participant what he has learned from the session.

For the Participants

Exercise

Melvin's Problem Situation[3]

Melvin has been dating Rita for about 2 months. At first, they had a lot of fun together, but the relationship is gradually becoming more of a grind. Melvin would sometimes want to go out with other women. Melvin meets Rita in the mall.

What could Melvin say or do?

1. Should Melvin avoid the subject, so Rita would not become hurt?

   yes | no |no opinion [circle your answer]

2. Must Melvin apologize with "I have it so busy the last time," and cut off the contact?

   yes | no |no opinion [circle your answer]

3. Just let Melvin go out with other women so that Rita hears about it at some moment?

   yes | no | no opinion [circle your answer]

4. How could he deal the Rita's feelings? ....
5. Let's change the situation a bit. What if Melvin and Rita lived together for several years and now have two small children? Would Melvin then still be allowed to break up with Rita?

   yes | no | no opinion [circle your answer]

6. Let us go back to the original situation. This is what happens: Melvin breaks up with Rita. He lets her know how he feels and starts dating with another woman. Rita feels hurt and jealous. She wants to take revenge on Melvin. Should Rita do this?

   yes | no | no opinion [circle your answer]

7. What if the roles were reversed and Rita did the same to Melvin? Should Melvin take revenge on Rita?

   yes | no | no opinion [circle your answer]

[3] This problem situation is an adaptation of Mark's problem situation as it has been published in Gibbs et al. (1995) and in Goldstein et al. (1998).

New Homework Assignments

(a) Answer the questions at Nicky's problem situation[4]

One day, Jeff, Nicky's older brother, tells Nicky a secret: Jeff deals drugs. Nicky and Jeff both know that the drug that Jeff is dealing is very addictive and causes lung and brain injury. It can even be fatal. Nicky asks his brother to stop dealing. But the family is poor, and Jeff says he only does it because of the financial problems of the family. Jeff asks his younger brother not to tell about it anymore.

What could Nicky say or do?

1. Must Nicky promise to keep it quiet and not to betray his brother??

   yes | no | no opinion [circle your answer]

2. What if Jeff tells Nicky that dealing is nothing special and that many of Jeff's friends do the same? Must Nicky keep his mouth shut?

   yes | no | no opinion [circle your answer]

3. What if Nicky discovers that Jeff is dealing drugs to 10-year-olds? Should Nicky keep his mouth shut?

   yes | no | no opinion [circle your answer]

4. What if Jeff does not use himself because he knows how addictive and harmful the stuff is? Should Nicky keep his mouth shut?

   yes | no | no opinion [circle your answer]

5. What if Nicky discovers that Jeff does not help the family at all with the money earned, but instead spends it on liquor and other things for himself? Should Nicky keep his mouth shut?

   yes | no | no opinion [circle your answer]

6. Can it be right to betray someone?

   sometimes | never | no opinion [circle your answer]

7. Who is the culprit in this situation?

   Nicky | Jeff | others | no opinion [circle your answer]

(b) Describe how you have solved a moral problem that you had to face:

- What did the problem situation look like [where, when, with whom]? ....
  ....
- Between which two options did you have to choose?

  1. ....
  2. ....

---

[4]This problem situation is an adaptation of George's problem situation as it has been published in Gibbs et al. (1995) and in Goldstein et al. (1998).

- Which option did you choose and why? ....
- How did you finally solve the problem? ....
- Were you satisfied with your solution and why? ....

(c) Describe the next week a situation where you have applied skill 1, 2, 3, 4, or 5.

- Who was it? ....
- Where were you? ....
- What day was it? ....
- What did the other person say or do? ....
- What did you do well? ....
- What else could you improve? ....

Plan of Session 13

Goals

- Discussing homework assignments
- Practicing Lesley's problem situation
- Explaining new homework assignments

Agenda

0:00	Opening
0:05	Discussing homework assignments
0:35	Practicing Lesley's problem situation
1:15	Explaining new homework assignments
1:20	Evaluation of the session
1:30	Closing

Course

Opening

- Brief discussion of the session plan.

Homework Assignments

- The trainer asks two participants to report on the homework assignments.

There is a lot at stake in Nicky's problem situation and it is all about how to deal with an irresponsible friend or relative. The ones who are buying drugs from Nicky's brother, Jeff, can be in danger. Again, most participants will respond positively. Nicky has to tell his brother's secret [1–5 included] because it is sometimes right to tell someone's secret [6]. Jeff is the culprit in this situation [7], and it is very important that judges send drug dealers to jail [8]. There is a lot of worry about the fact that Jeff sells a drug that can be deadly, and it is particularly objectionable that he sells it to children [3]. Nicky's problem situation, however, is controversial. The majority of participants came into contact with drugs or have dealt drugs and therefore identify themselves with Jeff.

- The trainer asks all participants what they have learned from the homework assignments.
- The trainer records the reports.

Lesley's Problem Situation

- The trainer asks all participants to read the text about Lesley's problem situation. Then the questions about this will be discussed and one situation is exercised in role-play. The trainer emphasizes that this exercise is not about good or bad reactions.

> Lesley's situation also concerns a problematic friend. Lesley's friend is planning to escape. Most participants will be responsible. Lesley has to tell about Bruce' plans [1, 2, 3, 6 and 7], it is Lesley's problem what Bruce does [4]. It is sometimes right to betray someone when a life is at stake [5], and it is essential that other people do not get hurt. This is especially true as the group leader is a distant relative of Lesley [6] and when Bruce is an acquaintance of Lesley's parents [7].

New Homework Assignments

(a) Answer the questions at Sam's problem situation.
(b) Describe how you have solved a moral problem that you had to face.
(c) Describe the next week a situation where you have applied skill 1, 2, 3, 4, or 5.

Evaluation

- The trainer asks each participant what he has learned from the session.

For the Participants

Exercise

Lesley's Problem Situation[5]

Right after Lesley arrived in prison, he tried to escape. The result was that he had to stay in prison longer. It took almost 4 months before the staff trusted Lesley again. Lesley now thinks he was stupid to try to escape. Bruce, a friend of Lesley, tells

[5] This problem situation is an adaptation of Leon's problem situation as it has been published in Gibbs et al. (1995) and in Goldstein et al. (1998).

Lesley that he is planning to escape that night. "I have it all figured out" says Bruce. I hit the group leader on his head with an iron bar and then take away his keys. Lesley tries to persuade Bruce to change his mind, but Bruce does not want to listen.

What could Lesley say or do?

1. Must Lesley tell the staff that Bruce is planning to escape?

   yes | no | no opinion [circle your answer]

2. What if Bruce is a violent person and Lesley thinks that Bruce could seriously injure the group leader? Should Lesley inform the staff?

   yes | no | no opinion [circle your answer]

3. What if everyone hates the group leader? Should Lesley inform the staff?

   yes | no | no opinion [circle your answer]

4. Is it Lesley's concern what Bruce does?

   yes | no |no opinion [circle your answer])

5. Is it sometimes right to betray someone?

   yes | no | no opinion [circle your answer]

6. Let's change the situation a bit. Let's say that the group leader is a distant relative of Lesley. Should Lesley inform the staff?

   yes | no | no opinion [circle your answer]

7. Let's change the situation again. Let's say Bruce is a friend of Lesley's parents. Must Lesley then inform the staff?

   yes | no | no opinion [circle your answer]

8. What is the most important?

   do not betray your friend | ensure that other people are not injured | mind your own business [circle your answer]

New Homework Assignments

(a) Answer the questions at Sam's problem situation[6]

Sam and his friend John are shopping in a sports shop. Sam has insisted on going to the store. John picks up a pair of sports shoes that he wants to have and quickly puts it in his backpack. After giving Sam a sign, John runs out of the store. But Sam does not pay attention to John. A moment later the shop owner and a security officer

[6] This problem situation is an adaptation of Sam's problem situation as it has been published in Gibbs et al. (1995) and in Goldstein et al. (1998).

come to Sam. The store owner says to the security officer: "That's one of the boys who stole the shoes!" The security officer searches Sam's backpack, but does not find sports shoes. "Okay, you can go, but who was the guy who was with you?" asks the security officer to Sam. "I am almost bankrupt due to shoplifting," says the owner. "I cannot let this happen."

What should Sam say or do?

1. Must Sam keep his mouth shut and refuse to give John's name to the security officer?

   yes | no | no opinion [circle your answer]

2. What should Sam do from the perspective of the store owner? Should Sam then give John's name?

   yes | no | no opinion [circle your answer]

3. What if the owner is a nice man, sometimes buys DVDs or CDs for children, even when he does not have enough money? Should Sam then give John's name?

   yes | no | no opinion [circle your answer]

4. What if the store owner is Sam's father? Should Sam then give John's name?

   yes | no | no opinion [circle your answer]

5. Is it sometimes right to betray someone?

   yes | no | no opinion [circle your answer]

6. Who is guilty in this situation?

   Sam | John | store owner | others | no opinion [circle your answer]

7. How important is it for the shop owner that shoplifters are prosecuted?

   very important | important | not important [circle your answer]

(b) Describe how you have solved a moral problem that you had to face:

- What did the problem situation look like [where, when, with whom]? ....
- Between which two options did you have to choose?

  1. ....
  2. ....

- Which option did you choose and why? ....
- How did you finally solve the problem? ....
- Were you satisfied with your solution and why? ....

(c) Describe the next week a situation where you have applied skill 1, 2, 3, 4, or 5.

- Who was it? ....
- Where were you? ....

- What day was it? ……………………………………………………………....
- What did they say or do? ………………..…………………………………………
- What did you do well? ……………………………………………………..……
- What else could you improve? ……………………………………………..….

Plan of Session 14

Goals

- Discussing homework assignments
- Practicing Raymond's problem situation
- Explaining new homework assignments

Agenda

0:00	Opening
0:05	Discussing homework assignments
0:35	Practicing Raymond's problem situation
1:15	Explaining new homework assignments
1:20	Evaluation of the session
1:30	Closing

Course

Opening

- Brief discussion of the session plan

Homework Assignments

- The trainer asks two participants to report on the homework assignments.

> The majority position in the case of Sam's problem situation as follows: Sam must give the security officer John's name [1 to 4 included] because it is sometimes right just to betray someone [5]. John is the culprit in this situation [6]. It is very important not to commit theft from stores [7] and it is very important for shop owners to report shoplifters [8]. Some participants will blame the store owner because he did not check backpacks before the customers enter the store. That is how he may prove later that the sports shoes have been stolen.

- The trainer asks all participants what they have learned from the homework assignments.
- The trainer records the reports.

Raymond's Problem Situation

- The trainer asks all participants to read the text about Raymond's problem situation. Then the questions about this will be discussed and one situation is exercised in role-play. The trainer emphasizes that this exercise is not about good or bad reactions.

> Raymond's problem situation is not so much about pressure from peers but from parents. Another difference is that peers often have a negative or irresponsible goal and, in any case, Raymond's mother has good intentions.
>
> The situation is problematic for the participants until question 3. From that question onwards, the majority finds that Raymond has to tell his mother what he knows. The majority is also inclined to opt for "doing the best for the family" as the most important consideration in Raymond's decision [4]. In question 5 it is considered important to tell the truth.
>
> Some participants will say that it is wrong of Raymond's mother to involve Raymond [2] and that as a result, too heavy a burden is placed upon him as a child. Raymond might feel guilty as his revelation would result in a separation. They will suggest that Raymond can help by having a separate conversation with his father. As Raymond would tell his secret to his mother, there is a chance that his father will beat him. However, the participants will not attach too much importance to the father's drinking a beer on his way home.

New Homework Assignments

(a) Answer the questions at Andrew's problem situation.
(b) Describe how you have solved a moral problem that you had to face.
(c) Describe the next week another situation where you have applied skill 1, 2, 3, 4, or 5.

Evaluation

- The trainer asks each participant what he has learned from the session.

For the Participants

Exercise

Raymond's Problem Situation[7]

"Your father is late again," says Raymond's mother to Raymond during dinner. Raymond knows why: on the road from his work home, he saw his father's car parked in front of a bar. Raymond's mother and father often had quarreled about his father's visit to the bar. After the last quarrel, his father had promised never to do it again. "I wonder why your father is so late," says Raymond's mother. "Do you think that I can trust him and that he is stopped drinking? Or do you think that he went back to the bar?" Raymond's mother asks him. What could Raymond say or do?

1. Must Raymond cover up for his father by lying to his mother?

   yes | no | no opinion [circle your answer]

2. Was it right that Raymond's mother involved Raymond to the issue by asking him a question about his father?

   yes | no | no opinion [circle your answer]

3. What if Raymond's father drinks a lot when he visits the bar and then comes home to beat Raymond's mother and sometimes even Raymond? Should Raymond then tell the truth?

   yes | no | no opinion [circle your answer]

4. What is important for Raymond's decision?

   what is best for himself | what is best for his mother | what is best for his father | what is best for the family [circle your answer]

5. How important is it to tell the truth?

   very important | important | not important [circle your answer]

New Homework Assignments

(a) Answer the questions at Andrew's problem situation[8]

---

[7] This problem situation is an adaptation of Reggie's problem situation as it has been published in Gibbs et al. (1995) and in Goldstein et al. (1998).

[8] This problem situation is an adaptation of Antonio's problem situation as it has been published in Gibbs et al. (1995) and in Goldstein et al. (1998).

Andrew is busy with writing an exam. Suddenly says the teacher: “I’m gone for a few minutes.” After the teacher has left, Ed, Andrew’s friend, whispers to him: “Let me see your answers, Andrew.”

What could Andrew say or do?

1. Should Andrew let Ed copy his answers?

   yes | no | no opinion [circle your answer]

2. What if Ed whispers that cheating is not bad and that he knows a lot of people who always do it? Must Andrew then let Ed copy his answers?

   yes | no | no opinion [circle your answer]

3. What if Andrew knows that Ed will fail because he is not studying? Should Andrew then let Ed copy his answers?

   yes | no | no opinion [circle your answer]

4. What if you were the teacher? Would you want Andrew to let Ed copy?

   yes | no | no opinion [circle your answer]

5. Is it possible to have a good friendship with someone who often copies?

   yes | no | no opinion [circle your answer]

6. Let’s change the situation a bit. What if Andrew hardly knows Ed? Should Andrew then let Ed copy?

   yes | no | no opinion [circle your answer]

7. How important is it not to deceive?

   very important | important | not important [circle your answer]

8. Is it correct that teachers punish cheaters?
   yes | no | no opinion [circle your answer]

(b) Describe how you have solved a moral problem that you had to face:

- What did the problem situation look like [where, when, with whom]? ………………………………………………………………………………
- Between which two options did you have to choose?

   1. ………………………………………………………………………………
   2. ………………………………………………………………………………

- Which option did you choose and why? ……………………………………………
- How did you finally solve the problem? ……………………………………………
- Were you satisfied with your solution and why? ………………………………………

(c) Describe the next week a situation where you have applied skill 1, 2, 3, 4, or 5.

- Who was it? ……………………………………………………………………………
- Where were you? ………………………………………………………………………
- What day was it? ………………………………………………………………………
- What did they say or do? ………………………………………………………………
- What did you do well? …………………………………………………………………
- What else could you improve? …………………………………………………………

Plan of Session 15

Goals

- Discussing homework assignments
- Practicing Vincent's problem situation
- Explaining new homework assignments

Agenda

0:00	Opening
0:05	Discussing homework assignments
0:35	Practicing Vincent's problem situation
1:15	Explaining new homework assignments
1:20	Evaluation of the session
1:30	Closing

Course

Opening

- Brief discussion of the session plan.

Homework Assignments

- The trainer asks two participants to report on the homework assignments:

> In Andrew's problem situation, it concerns loyalty to a friend versus honesty [1, 2, 3, and 6] and the punishment that comes when Andrew is caught [4]. It also raises the question whether you can be friends with someone who commits fraud during an exam [7, 8].

- The trainer asks all participants what they have learned from the homework assignments.
- The trainer records the reports.

Vincent's Problem Situation

- The trainer asks all participants to read the text about Vincent's problem situation. Then the questions about this will be discussed and one situation is exercised in role-play. The trainer emphasizes that this exercise is not about good or bad reactions.

In Vincent's problem situation it is about unreliable behavior and loyalty to a partner. To what extent is a white lie allowed to save a relationship, especially if there are children? If someone promises to do better and yet is unfaithful again, then is a lie allowed for a good reason such as saving a relationship? In this problem situation, we also discuss the extent to which Dawn has to accept Vincent's unfaithful behavior.

New Homework Assignments

(a) Describe how you have solved a moral problem that you had to face.
(b) Describe the next week another situation where you have applied skill 1, 2, 3, 4, or 5.

Evaluation

- The trainer asks each participant what he has learned from the session.

For the Participants

Exercise

Vincent's Problem Situation

Vincent lives with Dawn. Before he started living together, Vincent was a real womanizer and partygoer. He had a lot of girlfriends before Dawn. Recently, Vincent encountered an attractive colleague at a company party, who was also charmed by him. Both spent the night in a hotel room. At home, Dawn asks if it had been a fun party.

1. What should Vincent have to say when he knows that Dawn will forgive him for cheating?

   ....

2. Should Vincent say something if he knows that Dawn will become very angry and possibly leave him?

   yes | no | no opinion [circle your answer]

3. Should Vincent say something when Dawn and he now have two children?

   yes | no | no opinion [circle your answer]

4. Dawn has Vincent forgiven his cheating but warned him that it should not happen again. However, Vincent does cheat for the second time. Should Vincent say something to Dawn?

   yes | no | no opinion [circle your answer]

5. What does Vincent have to say when Dawn finds out that Vincent was cheating for the second time?
6. When is a white lie allowed?
7. If someone is cheating, is a white lie allowed if a break up threatens in the relationship?

   yes | no | no opinion [circle your answer]

8. Do you think that cheating is always known by the partner?

   yes | no | no opinion [circle your answer]

New Homework Assignments

(a) Describe how you have solved a moral problem that you had to face:

- What did the problem situation look like [where, when, with whom]? ....
  ....
- Between which two options did you have to choose?

  1. ....
  2. ....

- Which option did you choose and why? ....
- How did you finally solve the problem? ....
- Were you satisfied with your solution and why? ....

(b) Describe the next week a situation where you have applied skill 1, 2, 3, 4, or 5.

- Who was it? ....
- Where were you? ....
- What day was it? ....
- What did the other person say or do? ....
- What did you do well? ....
- What else could you improve? ....

10.5 Extended Program: Prosocial Thinking

Plan of First Prosocial Thinking Session: Not Putting Yourself in Somebody Else's Shoes

Goals

- Discussing homework assignments
- Announcing the Prosocial module Thinking
- Announcing the theme for the session: Not putting yourself in somebody else's shoes
- Practicing William's problem situation
- Explaining new homework assignments

Agenda

0:00	Opening
0:05	Discussing homework assignments
0:15	Explaining the goal of the module Prosocial Thinking
0:20	Theme: Not putting yourself in somebody else's shoes
0:25	William's problem situation
0:45	Role-play
1:20	Explaining new homework assignments
1:25	Evaluation of the session
1:30	Closing

Course

Opening

- Brief discussion of the session plan

Homework Assignments

- The trainer asks two participants to report on the homework assignments.
- The trainer asks all participants what they have learned from the homework assignments.
- The trainer records the reports.

Explanation of the Goal of the Module Prosocial Thinking

- The trainer explains the goal of the Prosocial Thinking module, namely learning thoughts that may lead to antisocial behavior to convert into thoughts that may lead to prosocial behavior.
- The following cognitions will be discussed: Not putting yourself in somebody else's shoes, Egocentricity, Denial, Suspicious, and Blaming others.

Theme: Not Putting Yourself in Somebody Else's Shoes

- The trainer asks all participants to read William's problem situation. Then the questions will be discussed, where the participants must convert antisocial thoughts in prosocial ones. Preferably the situation is acted out in role-play.
- Finally, the trainer defines putting yourself in somebody else's shoes. That is the willingness to imagine how it is for someone when something serious happens to him or her.

Role-Play

- The trainer asks participants to describe a situation in which they were unable to control their aggression.
- In a role-play, a participant shows how he behaves himself or herself in the problem situation. The other participants and trainers provide feedback.
- The other participants show how they would behave in the problem situation.
- Finally, the participant who brought the problem situation forward, excercises again.

New Homework Assignments

(a) Exercise a situation with the management of your aggression.
(b) Describe a situation in which you did not put yourself in somebody else's shoes and indicate which thoughts you had or which thoughts you have changed.

Evaluation

- The trainer asks each participant what he has learned from the session.

For the Participants

Exercise

Answer the Questions at William's Problem Situation

James brings his grandparents home after a birthday party. As soon as he opens their front door, he immediately sees that there has been a break-in. The place is in a huge mess. Personal things are thrown everywhere on the floor, a glass dish is in pieces and pictures are torn up. All the cabinets have been broken open. Some jewelry appears to have been stolen.

1. What should William do first and why?
2. How do you think his grandparents feel? Has anyone ever stolen something from you and if so, how did you feel then?
3. Can William leave his grandparents alone in their house that night, and why do you think so? Do you think his grandparents may feel unsafe or upset? Have you ever felt that way and if so, what did you think?
4. Do you think that William's grandparents will have their jewelry recovered? Or do you think the insurance will pay up? Does that matter? Explain why you think so.
5. Who are the victims in this situation? What will be the effect on the victims physically, mentally, and financially and in daily life?
6. Who are the offenders in this situation? Do you think those offenders have thought that William's grandparents suffer from such a theft? Explain why you think so.
7. Have you ever been the victim of a crime and if so, from whom? Do you know others who have been victims? What was the effect on them physically, mentally, and financially and in daily life?
8. What did you think when you committed a crime yourself and why? How do you think about it now and why?

New Homework Assignments

(a) Describe a situation where you could manage your annoyance, irritation, anger, or aggression or a situation where you did not succeed.

- The situation was? ....
- Who was it? ....
- Where were you? ....
- What did the other person say or do? ....
- What did you think or feel? ....
- What did you say or do? ....
- How the other person reacted? ....
- Were you satisfied with how you managed this situation? ....

(b) Describe a situation in your unit, your work, your school or at home where something bad happened to others.

- The situation was? ....
- Who was it? ....
- Where were you? ....
- What happened to others? ....
- How did those others experience that? ....
- What did you think? ....
- What did you say to those others? ....
- How did they respond to this? ....
- Were you satisfied with what you said and if not, what would you rather have said?...
- When I put myself in somebody's shoes, then the advantages for me and the other people are: .... and the disadvantages for me and the other people are: ....
- When I do not put myself in somebody's shoes, then the advantages for me and the other people are: .... and the disadvantages for me and the other people are: ....

Prosocial Thinking Session: Egocentrism

For the Participants

Exercise

Susan's Problem Situation

Susan walks with her daughter in a quiet street. With her right hand she pushes the stroller with her little daughter, and in her left hand, she carries her handbag. Peter and his friend Patrick want to buy a new mobile phone, but they have too little money. That is why they decide to rob someone. They drive on their scooter in search of a suitable victim. Then they see Susan carrying a handbag. Peter accelerates and Patrick is ready to grasp the bag. He is lucky. Susan remains confused and upset.

1. Why did Peter and Patrick rob Susan?
2. What are their thoughts when they decided to rob someone? Were they only thinking of themselves or also of others? Explain why you think so.
3. Do you think that Susan can be blamed for not holding her handbag more firmly?
4. Do you find that it makes a difference whether you rob a young mother with child (such as Susan), an old woman, or a strong young guy? And why do you think so?
5. What do you think was the effect of the robbery on Susan physically, mentally, and financially?
6. In case Peter and Patrick were aware of the impact of the robbery on Susan, would that have led to the abandonment of their plan? Explain why you think that.
7. If people are careless with their stuff it is no wonder that they are robbed? Were you ever robbed or do you know a friend or family member who was robbed? What was the motive of the offender? How was it for you, your friend or your family member to be robbed?
8. What are the benefits of the theft for Peter and Patrick? And what are the drawbacks?
9. What are the consequences for Peter and Patrick as Susan can give a detailed description of them to the police?
10. What are the chances that Peter and Patrick will be arrested by the police? What are your estimates?

New Homework Assignments

(a) Describe a situation where you could manage your annoyance, irritation, anger, or aggression or a situation where you did not succeed.

- The situation was? ....
- Who was it? ....

- Where were you? ....
- What said or did the other person? ....
- What did you think or feel? ....
- What did you say or do? ....
- How did the other person react? ....
- Were you satisfied with how you managed this situation? ....

(b) Describe a situation in your unit, your work, your school or at home where you initially thought: "I can do what I want, I do not have to take anybody into account."

- The situation was? ....
- Who was it? ....
- Where were you? ....
- What goal did you want to achieve? ....
- What did you think and why? ....
- What did you do and/or say? ....
- How did the other person respond? ....
- Did you reach your goal? ....
- What was the effect of what you did or said on the other person? ....
- Were you satisfied with what you did or said and, if not, what would you rather have done or say? ....
- If you would rather have handled the situation differently, what would you have been able to think better in the first instance? ....
- If I only think about myself, then the advantages for me and the other are: .... and the disadvantages for me and the other are: ....
- If I also think of others, then the advantages for me and the other are: .... and the disadvantages for me and the other are: ....

Prosocial Thinking Session: Denial

For the Participants

Exercise

Achmed's Problem Situation

Achmed is addicted to hard drugs. He has no work and no more money left from his welfare check. Therefore, he decides to commit a robbery. Late at night, he went to a Chinese restaurant that is located on a quiet street. He has a balaclava over his face, grabs his imitation pistol and runs while screaming inside. Achmed commands the owner, the waitress, and the cook to lie down flat on the ground and tells them not to move. Then he takes all the money from the cash register and runs away. But the police are faster on the scene than Achmed had expected, and he is caught. At the police station, he claims that the robbery means nothing because his gun was not real. Also, he did not lay a finger on the restaurant staff.

1. What was the reason that Achmed started the robbery?
2. What kind of preparations were undertaken? Explain why these precautions were taken.
3. Is the owner of the restaurant to be blamed for opening the restaurant so late at night and not having undertaken any security measures?
4. Do you think that Achmed would not have executed his plan to rob the restaurant if he had thought about the negative impact of his action on the staff? Explain why you think so.
5. What was the effect of the attack on the owner, the waitress and the cook of the restaurant? Include their current feelings and thoughts.
6. Do you find that people who pay too little attention to their safety actually provoke a robbery?
7. What do you think about Achmed's statement that such a robbery with a plastic gun and without physical injury means nothing?
8. What are the benefits of the robbery for Achmed? And what are the drawbacks?
9. What are the advantages and disadvantages for Achmed if the police had not been able to arrest him?
10. If you were a judge what punishment would you apply and why? Specify your charges. Why is your punishment not higher or not lower?

New Homework Assignments

(a) Describe a situation where you could manage your annoyance, irritation, anger, or aggression or a situation where you did not succeed.

- The situation was? ....
- Who was it? ....

- Where were you? ....
- What did the other person say or do? ....
- What did you think or feel? ....
- What did you say or do? ....
- How the other person reacted? ....
- Were you satisfied with how you managed this situation? ....

(b) Describe a situation in your unit, your work, your school or at home where you initially thought: "What I say or do is not harmful to the other, because it does not mean anything."

- The situation was? ....
- Who was it? ....
- Where were you? ....
- What goal did you want to achieve? ....
- What did you think and why? ....
- What did you do and/or say? ....
- How did the other person respond? ....
- Did you reach your goal? ....
- What was the effect of what you did or said on the other person? ....
  ....
- Were you satisfied with what you did or said and, if not, what would you rather have done or said? ....
- If you would rather have handled the situation differently, what would you have been able to think better in the first instance? ....
- When I minimize the consequences of my actions for others (making the consequences for others unimportant), then the advantages for me and the other person are: .... and the disadvantages for me and the other person are: ....
- When I face the consequences of my actions for others (making the consequences important), then the advantages for me and the other person are: ....and the disadvantages for me and the other person are: ....

Prosocial Thinking Session: Suspicious

For the Participants

Exercise

Stevens's Problem Situation

Steven goes with his girlfriend and some friends to a nightclub. There he notices that a boy at the bar is flirting with his girlfriend. It looks very much that this guy wants to befriend his girlfriend. Steven approaches the guy and says that he should leave her alone. And he pushes him lightly as a warning. But the guy's friends cannot leave that alone. After a while, Steven's friends also start interfering and quarreling. Now a noisy quarrel is imminent, and both parties are removed by the security staff from the disco. Outside the nightclub the groups beat each other. Suddenly everyone runs away. Steven lies unconscious on the street. The security staff call the police and an ambulance. When the police arrive none of the fighters are to be seen.

1. Why did Steven strike the guy at the bar?
2. What were his thoughts when he decided to strike the guy at the bar? Explain why you think so.
3. Do you think that Steven had good reasons to strike that guy? Or do you think that there are other ways to solve that situation?
4. Was Stephen right when he believed that the guy at the bar wanted to approach his girlfriend? Or did that guy signal that he only liked the girl without further intentions?
5. Would Stephen have abandoned his actions if he knew that it ended in a fight? Say why you think so.
6. What was the impact of the fight on all participants, and on particular Steven physically, mentally, and financially?
7. Do you think that guys/men have the right to approach other people's girlfriend? Or do you think right that people are too suspicious with other people's sexual intentions?
8. What are the benefits of the fight for Steven? And what are the drawbacks?
9. What are the advantages and disadvantages for Steven's friends? What kind of punishment do you find that the fighters should get and why?

New Homework Assignments

(a) Describe a situation where you could manage your annoyance, irritation, anger, or aggression or a situation where you did not succeed.

- The situation was? ....
- Who was it? ....
- Where were you? ....

- What did the other person say or do? ....
- What did you think or feel? ....
- What did you say or do? ....
- How did the other person react? ....
- Were you satisfied with how you managed this situation? ....

(b) Describe a situation in your unit, your work, your school or at home where you initially thought: "What I say or do is the other person's fault, because he provoked it himself by what he said or did."

- The situation was? ....
- Who was it? ....
- Where were you? ....
- What goal did you want to achieve? ....
- What did you think and why? ....
- What did you do and/or say? ....
- How did the other person respond? ....
- Did you reach your goal? ....
- What was the effect of what you did or said for the other person? ....
- Were you satisfied with what you did or said and if not, what would you rather have done or said? ....
- If you would rather have handled the situation differently, what would you have been able to think better in the first instance? ....
....
- When I always distrust others, then the advantages for me and the other person are: ....
- and the disadvantages for me and the other person: ....
- When I first check what others mean and do not immediately assume the worst, the advantages are for me and the other: .... and the disadvantages for me and the other: ....

Prosocial Thinking Session: Blaming Others

For the Participants

Exercise

Wesley's Problem Situation

Wesley has a new girlfriend recently, Latifa. They have had sex already a few times. Wesley's friends know that, and they think that Latifa is a slut. One day Wesley and his friends hang around at the flat where he lives. His friends ask him if they also can have sex with Latifa. Wesley and Latifa have no firm courtship, so what does it matter? Wesley is not enthusiastic but dares not refuse. He thinks "You need to help your friends if possible" and he is not sure about how his relationship with Latifa will develop. When Latifa appears, his friends ask if they can have sex with her. Wesley has no objections. Latifa declines and is upset. Nevertheless, his friends push her into a bike shelter and force her to oral sex. Wesley does nothing at all. Later on, Latifa does not report this event to the police. Wesley's friends are acquaintances or distant relatives of hers. Wesley wants not to offend his friends and keeps silent.

1. Why did Wesley not protest when his friends mentioned wanting to have sex with Latifa?
2. Why did Wesley's friends ask Wesley if they could have sex with Latifa, while they knew that Latifa and Wesley were together? What is in your opinion the reason?
3. Do you find that Latifa provoked the rape herself because she went to bed with Wesley shortly after she had met him? Is that the reason that one might call her a slut?
4. What might be the effect of the rape on Latifa physically and mentally?
5. Do you think it was right that Wesley had sex with Latifa shortly after they had met? And if you do not approve of that, who is to blame? Wesley, Latifa, or both?
6. Do you like that men are entitled to sex even when a girl or woman refuses?
7. On television one sees that women sometimes like to have sex, even though they declined sex earlier. Do you believe that women who say "no" actually mean "yes," or is that a fairy tale?
8. Do you think that a girl/woman with a history of several relationships or who quickly go to bed with someone is a slut? When do you think a woman is a slut?
9. What are the consequences of the rape for Wesley?
10. What are the consequences for Wesley if Latifa reports the rape to the police?
11. What are the consequences for Latifa if she reports the rape?
12. What punishment do you think that Wesley's friends should get and why?
13. What punishment do you think that Wesley should get and why?
14. Do you think that Latifa with Wesley can continue their relationship? Give your reasons.

New Homework Assignments

(a) Describe a situation where you could manage your annoyance, irritation, anger, or aggression or a situation where you did not succeed.

- The situation was? ....
- Who was it? ....
- Where were you? ....
- What did the person say or do? ....
- What did you think or feel? ....
- What did you say or do? ....
- How did the person react? ....
- Were you satisfied with how you managed this situation? ....

(b) Describe a situation in your unit, your work, your school or at home where you initially thought: "What I say or do is the fault of others, because they let that happen."

- The situation was? ....
- Who was it? ....
- Where were you? ....
- What goal did you want to achieve? ....
- What did you think and why? ....
- What did you do and/or say? ....
- How did the other person respond? ....
- Did you reach your goal? ....
- What was the effect of what you did or said on the other person? ....
- Were you satisfied with what you did or said and, if not, what would you rather have done or said? ....
  ....
- If you would rather have handled the situation differently, what would you have been able to think better in the first instance? ....
  ....
- When I always blame others for what happens, then the advantages are for me and the other person are: ....
- and the disadvantages for me and the other person are: ....
- When I do not blame others, then the advantages for me and the other person are: .... and the disadvantages for me and the other person: ....

10.6 Extended Program: Consequences of Behavior

Plan of First Consequences of Behavior Session: Responsibility

Goals

- Discussing homework assignments
- Announcing the module Consequences of Behavior
- Announcing the theme for the session: Responsibility
- Practicing Dick's problem situation
- Explaining new homework assignments

Agenda

0:00	Opening
0:05	Discussing homework assignments
0:15	Explaining the goal of the module Consequences of Behavior
0:20	Theme: Responsibility
0:25	Dick's problem situation
0:45	Role-play
1:20	Explaining new homework assignments
1:25	Evaluation of the session
1:30	Closing

Course

Opening

- Brief discussion of the session plan.

Homework Assignments

- The trainer asks two participants to report on the homework assignments.
- The trainer asks all participants what they have learned from the homework assignments.
- The trainer records the reports.

Explanation of the Goal of the Module Consequences of Behavior

- The trainer explains the goal of the Consequences of Behavior module, namely learning to focus on the short-term and long-term consequences of prosocial and antisocial behavior.

- Five themes are discussed and exercised, namely Responsibility, Subservience, Respect, Cooperation, and Honesty.

Theme: Responsibility

- The trainer asks all participants to read Dick's problem situation. Then the questions are discussed, where the participants must convert antisocial thoughts in prosocial ones. Preferably the situation is acted out in role-play.
- Finally, the trainer defines responsibility as the willingness to be accountable for your behavior without blaming others.

Role-Play

- The trainer asks participants to describe a situation in which they were unable to control their aggression.
- In a role-play, a participant shows how he behaved himself in the problem situation. The other participants and trainers provide feedback.
- The other participants show how they would behave in the problem situation.
- Finally, the participant who brought the problem situation forward, excercises again.

Homework Assignments

(a) Exercise a situation with the management of your aggression.
(b) Describe a situation in which you have taken responsibility or have avoided taking responsibility and indicate the consequences for yourself and others.

Evaluation

- The trainer asks each participant what he has learned from the session.

For the Participants

Exercise

Answer the Questions at Dick's Problem Situation

When Dick comes home from school, his only interest is to snuggle on the couch, listen to music, or watch television. But the agreement with his parents was that he takes his little brother Ben from school, and prepares dinner for both of them. His parents work and come home around 8 o'clock. But Dick thinks that Ben is quite able to walk home by himself and to buy some snacks or French fries. If Ben does so, Dick can do what he likes and everything runs smoothly.

1. What are Dick's responsibilities?
2. If you are one of his parents, do you think that Dick will keep the agreement?
3. What happens when Dick fails to fulfill this agreement?
4. Who do you think is to blame when Dick's brother Ben comes late at home and is not able to do his homework?
5. Suppose that Dick does what he likes most and fails his agreement?
6. In that case, what is the impact of Dick's behavior on the other family members?
7. Does his failure to pick up Ben have an impact on his relationship with his parents and his little brother?

New Homework Assignments

(a) Describe a situation where you could manage your annoyance, irritation, anger, or aggression or a situation where you did not succeed.

- The situation was? ....
- Who was it? ....
- Where were you? ....
- What did the other person say or do? ....
- What did you think or feel? ....
- What did you say or do? ....
- How did the other person react? ....
- Were you satisfied with how you managed this situation? ....

(b) Describe a situation in your unit, your work, your school or at home where you are responsible for a certain task.

- I am responsible for: ....
- I take my responsibility when I: ....
- I avoid my responsibility when I: ....
- If I take my responsibility, then the advantages for others are: .... and the disadvantages for others: ....
- If I take my responsibility, then the advantages for me are: .... and the disadvantages for me are: ....
- If I avoid my responsibility, then the advantages for others are: .... and the disadvantages for others are: ....
- If I shirk my responsibility, then the advantages for me are: ....and the disadvantages for me are: ....

Consequences of Behavior Session: Subservience

For the Participants

Exercise

Andy's Problem Situation

Andy works as a volunteer in a retirement home in his neighborhood. He does errands and talks in a friendly way with the residents who look forwards to him visiting weekly. Andy volunteers so well that the staff of the retirement home offers him a paid job. At the beginning of the New Year, Andy's friends ask him to go to a party and to have some fun in the city. But that is precisely on a night that he works in the retirement home. His friends insist because they find that Andy is a nice guy and Andy a member of their group to have fun with.

1. What is Andy obliged to answer and why?
2. Does it matter if Andy's grandmother is also resident in the retirement home? Why?
3. What should Andy do if he has only worked for a month in the retirement home? And what if he works there for 2 years? Would that make a difference and why?
4. What should Andy do when a resident he has befriended is dying and has only some weeks to live?
5. What should Andy do as his friends put pressure on him by saying they no longer want to deal with him if he does not come with them?
6. What are the benefits for Andy if he just goes to work in the retirement home and does not go to party with his friends?
7. Do you find it important to work as a volunteer and why?

New Homework Assignments

(a) Describe a situation where you could manage your annoyance, irritation, anger, or aggression or a situation where you did not succeed.

- The situation was? ....
- Who was it? ....
- Where were you? ....
- What did the other person say or do? ....
- What did you think or feel? ....
- What did you say or do? ....
- How did the other person react? ....
- Were you satisfied with how you managed this situation? ....

(b) Describe a situation in your unit, your work, your school or at home where you have offered someone help at a certain task.

- I have [fill in a name] ……… helped with: ……………………………………………
- I offered help because: …………………………………………………………….
- Before I felt: ……………………………………………………………………….
- Afterwards I felt: ……………………………………………………………………
- Was giving help important and if so for whom? ………………………………….
- How would that person have carried out the task if you had not helped? …………
  ………………………………………………………………………………………
- If I offer someone my help, then the advantages for the other person are:………………………… and the disadvantages for the other person are: .....
  ………………………………………………………………………………………
- If I offer someone my help, then the advantages for me are: …………………… and the disadvantages for me are: …………………………………………………
- If I do not offer help to someone while he or she needs it, then the advantages for the other person are: ……………………………………… and the disadvantages for the other person are: ………………………………………………………
- If I do not offer help to someone while he or she needs it, then the advantages for me are: ……………………………………………………… and the disadvantages for me are: ……………………………………………………………………

Consequences of Behavior Session: Respect

For the Participants

Exercise

David's Problem Situation

David works 4 days a week as a trainee painter at a company and is at school 1 day a week. The mentor at school has made an appointment for an interview with David. His performance at school is below what is expected. Also, his employer complained that David always comes too late. On the day of his appointment David reports 15 min late to the mentor. During the interview, he keeps his coat and his cap on.

1. Why did David have to come on this occasion right on time?
2. Is David obliged to say sorry and say why he is late, or should he just wait and see how the mentor responds?
3. What do you think of the fact that David keeps his jacket and cap on during the interview?
4. How might David react if the mentor starts the conversation with telling what in his opinion is at stake? Should he first listen carefully or start with defending himself?
5. How should David react to the comments by the mentor? Why?
6. In case the mentor gives David no opportunity to respond, how should David react?
7. What can David say if he disagrees with the mentor's arguments?
8. What can David say if the mentor says that he is likely to be removed from school and consequently has to quit his job as a trainee?
9. How can David react if the mentor says that he finds David a softy because he does not even get out of bed on time?
10. Suppose that David needs the money very much to support his grandparents financially and thus cannot stop working at the company. How will he respond in this case?

New Homework Assignments

(a) Describe a situation where you could manage your annoyance, irritation, anger, or aggression or a situation where you did not succeed.

- The situation was? ....
- Who was it? ....
- Where were you? ....
- What did the other person say or do? ....
- What did you think or feel? ....

- What did you say or do? ....
- How did the other person react? ....
- Were you satisfied with how you managed this situation? ....
- How would you manage the situation next time? ....

(b) Describe a conversation situation in your unit, your work, your school or home in which you have paid attention to behave respectfully.

- Who was it? ....
- Who took the initiative in the conversation and why? ....
- Why did you do your best to behave respectfully? ....
- What did you want to achieve? ....
- How did you feel beforehand? ....
- What did you say or did? ....
- How did the other respond? ....
- How did you feel afterwards? ....
- Did you reach your goal in the conversation and if not why? ....
- How would you deal with such a situation the next time? ....
- If I behave respectfully, then the advantages for the other person are: ....and the disadvantages for the other person are: ....
- If I behave respectfully, then the advantages for me are: ....and the disadvantages for me are: ....
- If I behave disrespectfully, then the advantages for the other person are: .... and the disadvantages for the other person are: ....
- If I behave disrespectfully, then the advantages for me are: ....and the advantages for me are: ....

Consequences of Behavior Session: Cooperation

For the Participants

Exercise

Marco's Problem Situation

Coach Marco has called up for the national team three young soccer players: Ary on the left side, John in the center, and Robin as a player on the right side. During a practice game against England, they lose and none of them could score. John complains that he did not get any balls by Ary and Robin. Ary believes that the attacks should take place preferably on the left side, while Robin says that on the right is better given the weakness in the English defense. After the game, the coach asks the three players with him because they blame each other for the defeat.

1. What might Marco say to the players to improve their cooperation? Explain your suggestion.
2. How do you think that the three players will react to your suggestion and why?
3. How do you think the three players have to respond for a chance of better cooperation in the future, and why?
4. Ary and John are from the countryside, and both have a moderate temperament. Robin grew up in a big city and is hot tempered. Will that make a difference in their reactions to Marco?
5. What should Marco do to get the players work together?
6. During the next game, Ary and John work much better together, but Robin still keeps all the balls for himself. What should Marco do?
7. What can Marco do as in the next match Robin still keeps all the balls for himself but scored two goals?
8. In the following match, Robin gets injured, and Marco calls Rudy as a replacement. Rudy, Ary, and John play very well together. What should Marco do?

New Homework Assignments

(a) Describe a situation where you could manage your annoyance, irritation, anger, or aggression or a situation where you did not succeed.

- The situation was? ....
- Who was it? ....
- Where were you? ....
- What did the other person say or do? ....
- What did you think or feel? ....
- What did you say or do? ....
- How did the other person react? ....
- Were you satisfied with how you managed this situation? ....

(b) Describe a situation in your unit, your work, at school or at home where you have cooperated with others.

- Who did you work with? ……………………………………………………..
- What was the task or assignment? ……………………………………………
- Why did you decide to participate? ……………………………………………
- What did you want to achieve together? ……………………………………..
- How did you feel beforehand? …………………………………………………
- What was your share in the cooperation? ……………………………………
- How did the others respond to this? …………………………………………..
- How did you feel afterwards? …………………………………………………
- Did you reach your goal and if not why? ……………………………………..
- How would you deal with such a situation the next time? ……………………
- If I work together, then the advantages for the other person are: …………………………… and the disadvantages for the other person are: ……………………………………………………………………………………
- If I work together, then the advantages for me are: …………………………… and the disadvantages for me are: ……………………………………………
- If I refuse to cooperate, then the advantages for the other person are: ……………………………………………… and the disadvantages for the other person are: ……………………………………………………………
- If I refuse to cooperate, then the advantages for me are: …………………… and the disadvantages for me are: ……………………………………………………

Consequences of Behavior Session: Honesty

For the Participants

Exercise

Thomas' Problem Situation

Thomas keeps a cash journal so that the institution can monitor the daily income and expenses. One day Thomas' cash journal is not in order: There is $20 more spent than received, but he cannot figure out to who he has paid that money. Thomas decides to reduce the spend money with $20 so that his cash book is in order again.

1. What should Thomas say as the controller discovers that his cash book is not correct?
2. How do you think the controller will respond and why?
3. Suppose that small differences do sometimes occur in a cash book. What can Thomas say then?
4. Assume that the controller asks Thomas to investigate how and why this difference of $20 did occur. What can Thomas say then?
5. Suppose that Thomas has lent the $20 to a friend who cannot pay him back because he is broke. What should Thomas say in that case to the controller?
6. And what would Thomas say about his friend?
7. How important is it, in this case, to be honest? Do you think it would be a good idea if Thomas fails to mention that he has lent the money?
8. Do you think that Thomas' friend himself should tell the controller that he had borrowed $20 from Thomas? Explain your response.

New Homework Assignments

(c) Describe a situation where you could manage your annoyance, irritation, anger, or aggression or a situation where you did not succeed.

- The situation was? ....
- Who was it? ....
- Where were you? ....
- What did the other person say or do? ....
- What did you think or feel? ....
- What did you say or do? ....
- How did the other person react?..
- Were you satisfied with how you managed this situation? ....

(d) Describe a situation in your unit, your work, your school or home where you have been honest, even though you found that unpleasant.

- Who have you been honest with? ....

- What was the reason to be honest? ....
- What did you want to achieve? ....
- How did you feel beforehand? ....
- What did you say and/or do? ....
- How did the other person respond? ....
- How did you feel afterwards? ....
- Did you reach your goal and if not why? ....
- How would you deal with such a situation the next time? ....
- If I am honest, then the advantages for the other person are: ....
  and the disadvantages for the other person are: ....
- If I am honest, then the advantages for me are: ....
  and the disadvantages for me: ....
- If I am not honest, then the advantages for the other person are: ....
  and the disadvantages for the other person are: ....
- If I am not honest, then the advantages for me are: ....
  and the disadvantages for me are: ....

10.7 Extended Program: Prosocial Network

Plan of First Prosocial Network Session: Making Acquaintance

Goals

- Discussing homework assignments
- Announcing the module Prosocial Network
- Announcing the theme for the session: Making acquaintance
- Explaining new homework assignments

Agenda

0:00	Opening
0:05	Discussing homework assignments
0:15	Explaining the goal of the module Prosocial Network
0:30	Exercise: Making acquaintance
1:20	Explaining homework assignments
1:25	Evaluation of the session
1:30	Closing

Course

Opening

- Brief discussion of the session plan

Homework Assignments

- The trainer asks two participants to report on the homework assignments.
- The trainer asks all participants what they have learned from the homework assignments.
- The trainer records the reports.

Explanation of the Goal of the Module Prosocial Network

- The trainer explains the goal of the Prosocial Network module, namely learning how to engage in prosocial contacts and how to hold off or end antisocial contacts.

- Five problem situations are exercised, namely Making acquaintance, Making an appointment, Deepening a contact, Informing others about your rehabilitation or treatment program, and Responding to a rejection.

Theme: Making Acquaintance

- The trainer discusses the goals and criteria with the participants for Making acquaintance (Appendix 4).

Exercise: Making Acquaintance

- The trainer mentions three exercise situations from easy to difficult. For example, making acquaintance with a fellow offender or patient, with a group leader, and with the person responsible for the rehabilitation or treatment program.
- Each participant exercises, so far as available time that allows, all situations in order of difficulty. The other participants and trainers provide feedback.

New Homework Assignments

(a) Exercise a situation with the management of your aggression.
(b) Describe a situation in which you have made acquaintance with someone.
(c) Answer the questions at Pascal's problem situation.

Evaluation

- The trainer asks each participant what he has learned from the session.

For the Participants

New Homework Assignments

(a) Describe a situation where you could manage your annoyance, irritation, anger, or aggression or a situation where you did not succeed.

- The situation was? ....
- Who was it? ....
- Where were you? ....
- What did the other person say? ....
- What did you think or feel? ....
- What did you say or do? ....

- How did the other person react?...
- Were you satisfied with how you managed this situation? ....
- How would you manage the situation next time? ....

(b) Describe a situation in which you have made acquaintance with someone.

- The situation was? ....
- Who was it? ....
- Where were you? ....
- What did the other person say or do? ....
- What did you think or feel? ....
- What did you say or do? ....
- How did the other person react? ....
- Were you satisfied with how you managed this situation? ....
- How would you manage the situation next time? ....

(c) Answer the questions at Pascal's problem situation.

Pascal's Problem Situation

Pascal works 4 days a week at a carpenter company. One day a week he goes to school for further training. On his first working day, four workmates are playing cards in the canteen. Pascal wants to introduce himself and therefore goes to their table. However, the four colleagues pay no attention on him and continue with their game. In the end, Pascal gives it up and goes to another place in the canteen to eat his lunch alone.

1. What could Pascal have done to get the attention of the four colleagues? What could he say? ....
2. What could Pascal say when he sees that the four colleagues quit playing card? ....
3. Suppose that the four colleagues invite Pascal at their table. How could Pascal respond in that case? ....
4. Assume that there is a fifth workmate sitting quite by himself in the cafeteria lunch. What could Pascal do? ....
5. The fifth colleague demonstrates by his attitude that he prefers to sit alone. What could Pascal do? ....
6. The fifth colleague invites Pascal to sit at the table with him. What could Pascal talk about when they have lunch together? ....
7. The fifth colleague tells that the four card players do not get on well with the other colleagues. How could Pascal respond? ....
8. The boss of the company enters the canteen directly after Pascale. What could Pascal do?...
9. What are Pascal's thoughts and conclusions when he notices that his colleagues are not very friendly to a newcomer? ....

Prosocial Network Session: Making an Appointment

For the Participants

New Homework Assignments

(a) Describe a situation where you could manage your annoyance, irritation, anger, or aggression or a situation where you did not succeed.

- The situation was? ....
- Who was it? ....
- Where were you? ....
- What did the other person say or do? ....
- What did you think or feel? ....
- What did you say or do? ....
- How did the other person react? ....
- Were you satisfied with how you managed this situation? ....
- How would you manage the situation next time? ....

(b) Describe a situation in which you have made an appointment with someone.

- The situation was? ....
- Who was it? ....
- Where were you? ....
- What did the other person say or do? ....
- What did you think or feel? ....
- What did you say or do? ....
- How did the other person react? ....
- Were you satisfied with how you managed this situation? ....
- How would you manage the situation next time? ....

(c) Answer the questions at Rachid's problem situation.

Rachid's Problem Situation

Rachid is a member of a soccer club. After a match, he used to go for a drink in the canteen. Several times he talks there with Andrew and his wife, Rita. Rita accompanies her husband at every game. During their talks, it appears that they all like the same kind of movies. Rachid suggests to go to a new film together. Andrew and Rita find that a good idea but they are rather busy at the moment. They will tell him when they have more time.

1. How could Rachid invite Andrew and Rita to go with him to a movie? What could he say? ....
2. Andrew and Rita say that they are very busy at this time. How could Rachid respond? ....

3. After several weeks Andrew and Rita have still not indicated that they have time to go to the movie. How could Rachid respond? ....
4. One day Andrew calls Rachid to make an appointment. Unfortunately, it is Rachid's sister's birthday. How could Rachid respond? ....
5. Another time after a match Andrew and Rita suggest going out to a restaurant. Rachid does not know if his wife has the interest to come with them. What could he do? How could he respond? ....
6. Rachid has made an appointment with Andrew and Rita. A day in advance Rachid has to accompany his very ill brother to the hospital. How could Rachid act? ....
7. Rita calls and says that they have to cancel the appointment because they are too busy with a lot of things. How could Rachid respond? ....
   ....

Prosocial Network Session: Deepening a Contact

For the Participants

New Homework Assignments

(a) Describe a situation where you could manage your annoyance, irritation, anger, or aggression or a situation where you did not succeed.

- The situation was? ....
- Who was it? ....
- Where were you? ....
- What did the other person say or do? ....
- What did you think or feel? ....
- What did you say or do? ....
- How did the other person react? ....
- Were you satisfied with how you managed this situation? ....
- How would you manage the situation next time? ....

(b) Describe a situation in which you have deepened a contact with someone.

- The situation was? ....
- Who was it? ....
- Where were you? ....
- What said or did the other person? ....
- What did you think or feel? ....
- What did you say or do? ....
- How the other person reacted? ....
- Were you satisfied with how you managed this situation? ....
- How would you manage the situation next time? ....

(c) Answer the questions at Bram's problem situation.

Bram's Problem Situation

Bram and Chris had already gone to the movies a few times. Afterwards, both of them go for a snack in the neighborhood. Chris has visited Bram several times, and they have similar interests. Bram would like to meet Chris more frequently, but he knows that Chris is a rather popular guy and has many friends already.

1. How can Bram show that he likes to go out more often with Chris? What could Bram say? ....
2. Chris says he appreciates the contact with Bram and likes to go to the movies with him now and then. How could Bram respond? ....
3. Bram and Chris have already met each other several times. Chris has indicated that he wants to talk with Bram about the problems of one of his friends. How could Bram respond? ....

4. Bram and Chris have talked a few times about the problems of one of Chris's friends. Bram says that he also wants to tell something personal. Namely, that some time ago he was in a forensic psychiatric hospital. In what way could Bram say that? ....
5. Bram and Chris know each other now some months. However, Bram has recently a new girlfriend. What could Bram tell Chris? ....
6. Bram notes that things are not going well with Chris. Chris loses his friends one by one, has more and more problems at work, and alienates himself from his parents. How could Bram intervene?...
7. After some time, Bram has the same problems that were the reason for his treatment in a forensic psychiatric hospital. His physician has referred him to a forensic psychiatric outpatient clinic. What could he tell Chris? ....

Prosocial Network Session: Informing Others About Your Rehabilitation or Treatment Program

For the Participants

New Homework Assignments

(a) Describe a situation where you could manage your annoyance, irritation, anger, or aggression or a situation where you did not succeed.

- The situation was? ....
- Who was it? ....
- Where were you? ....
- What did the other person say or do? ....
- What did you think or feel? ....
- What did you say or do? ....
- How did the other person react? ....
- Were you satisfied with how you managed this situation? ....
- How would you manage the situation next time? ....

(b) Describe a situation in which you have informed someone about your rehabilitation or treatment program.

- The situation was? ....
- Who was it? ....
- Where were you? ....
- What did the other person say or do? ....
- What did you think or feel? ....
- What did you say or do? ....
- How did the other person react? ....
- Were you satisfied with how you managed this situation? ....
- How would you manage the situation next time? ....

(c) Answer the questions at Dwayne's problem situation.

Dwayne's Problem Situation

Dwayne is socializing for some time with a married couple, Elliott and Aicha. Dwayne visits them regularly, and they know each other well. Dwayne did advise them when their relationship was deteriorating. Elliott and Aicha have said several times that they appreciated his efforts because it did improve their relationship very much. Dwayne believes that it is now time to tell them that he has been a patient at a forensic psychiatric hospital.

1. Tell what Dwayne could say. ....
2. When Dwayne tells them, they react very upset and do now know what to say. Givesomesuggestionshow Dwaynemightrespond....................................

3. Elliott and Aicha respond compassionate, but they have a lot of questions. Give some examples of the questions they might have. ....
4. In case Dwayne has committed a sexual offense. What and how could he tell them? Does it matter what kind of sexual offense? ....
5. Dwayne was admitted because he has committed several violent robberies. Elliott and Aicha have two small children. They worry about the negative impact of Dwayne's past behavior on them. How might Dwayne respond? ....
   ....
6. Elliott and Aicha often have visitors at home. It is possible that the conversation drifts to talk about the criminality in the neighborhood. What agreements could Dwayne make with the couple in case the topic of the conversation is criminality?
   ....
   Dwayne has told an uncle and aunt about his forensic psychiatric past. Both reacted compassionately, but Dwayne is afraid that in no time the whole family will be informed. What would he say? ....
7. Dwayne has noticed that the daughter of his brother started to avoid him. In the past, they got on well with each other. He suspects that she is informed by her parents that he was institutionalized. What would Dwayne do or say? ....
   ....

Prosocial Network Session: Responding to a Rejection

For the Participants

New Homework Assignments

(a) Describe a situation where you could manage your annoyance, irritation, anger, or aggression or a situation where you did not succeed.

- The situation was? ....
- Who was it? ....
- Where were you? ....
- What did the other person say or do? ....
- What did you think or feel? ....
- What did you say or do? ....
- How did the other person react? ....
- Were you satisfied with how you managed this situation? ....
- How would you manage the situation next time? ....

(b) Describe a situation in which you have responded on a rejection.

- The situation was? ....
- Who was it? ....
- Where were you? ....
- What did the other person say or do? ....
- What did you think or feel? ....
- What did you say or do? ....
- How did the other person react? ....
- Were you satisfied with how you managed this situation? ....
- How would you manage the situation next time? ....

(c) Answer the questions at Fabian's problem situation.

Fabian's Problem Situation

Fabian works 4 days a week at a large shopping company. Only his boss knows that he has a criminal history. The boss thinks it is the time to inform Fabian's three colleagues with whom he works together. The colleagues and Fabian are called to the boss's office and the boss informs them about Fabian's past criminal history. One of the colleagues, George, says he has had no problems so far with Fabian. Another colleague, Hassan, keeps his mouth shut, but the third colleague, Iwan, is dismissive and asks the boss for another workplace. He says he does not want to have anything to do with Fabian.

1. Could Fabian have contributed to the conversation with his boss and colleagues? Give some examples of what you could have said. ....
   ....

2. What kind of preparations could have been made by Fabian before this conversation? ....
3. After the conversation, George tells Fabian that he has no problems with Fabian's past. What can Fabian say? ....
4. At lunch break, a few days after this talk Fabian take a seat at the table near Hassan. What could Fabian say to Hassan? ....
5. On one day Fabian meets Iwan at work. What can Fabian say? What can Fabian do if Iwan does not respond and walks away? ....
6. After the talk, Fabian goes to his boss to tell what he thinks of the conversation with his colleagues. What could Fabian tell his boss? ....
7. People have talked about Fabian's criminal past, and several workers are now avoiding Fabian. What kind of actions might Fabian undertake? ....
....
8. There is a lot of gossip about Fabian at the shopping company. How should Fabian deal with it? What can he do about it? ....
9. At the start of his day, Fabian sees a paper on his locker with the text: "Convict fuck off." How could Fabian respond? ....
10. One day the chef comes to Fabian with the message that the situation is untenable. A lot of colleagues have asked the boss to dismiss Fabian. How could he respond to his chef? What kind of actions might Fabian undertake? ....
....

10.8 Extended Program: Contact with Women

Plan of the First Contact with Women Session: Showing Your Need for Intimacy

Goals

- Discussing homework assignments
- Announcing the module Contact with women
- Announcing the theme for the session: Showing your need for intimacy
- Explaining new homework assignments

Agenda

0:00	Opening
0:05	Discussing homework assignments
0:15	Explaining the goal of the module Contact with Women
0:30	Exercise: Showing your need for intimacy
1:20	Explaining homework assignments
1:25	Evaluation of the session
1:30	Closing

Course

Opening

- Brief discussion of the session plan.

Homework Assignments

- The trainer asks two participants to report on the homework assignments.
- The trainer asks all participants what they have learned from the homework assignments.
- The trainer records the reports.

Explanation of the Goal of the Module Contact with Women

- Trainer explains the goal of the Contact with Women module, namely learning how to behave respectfully towards women.
- Five problem situations are exercised, namely Showing your need for intimacy, Responding to a rejection, Responding to an approach, Talking about sex, and Deepening intimacy.

Theme: Showing Your Need for Intimacy

- The trainer discusses the goals and criteria with the participants for showing your need for intimacy (Appendix 5).

Exercise: Showing your Need for Intimacy

- The trainer mentions three exercise situations from easy to difficult. For example: Your need for intimacy at a superficial acquaintance, a good acquaintance, and a girlfriend.
- Each participant exercises, as far as the available time that allows all situations in order of difficulty. The other participants and trainers provide feedback.

New Homework Assignments

(a) Exercise a situation with the management of your aggression.
(b) Describe a situation in which you have showed your need for intimacy.
(c) Answer the questions at Jesse's problem situation.

Evaluation

- The trainer asks each participant what he has learned from the session.

For the Participants

New Homework Assignments

(a) Describe a situation where you could manage your annoyance, irritation, anger, or aggression or a situation where you did not succeed.

- The situation was? ....
- Who was it? ....
- Where were you? ....
- What did the other person say or do? ....
- What did you think or feel? ....
- What did you say or do? ....
- How did the other person react? ....
- Were you satisfied with how you managed this situation? ....
- How would you manage the situation next time? ....

(b) Describe a situation in which you have showed your need for intimacy.

- The situation was? ....
- Who was it? ....
- Where were you? ....
- What did the other person say or do? ....
- What did you think or feel? ....
- What did you say or do? ....
- How did the other person react? ....
- Were you satisfied with how you managed this situation? ....
- How would you manage the situation next time? ....

(c) Answer the questions at Jesse's problem situation.

Jesse's Problem Situation

Jesse and Kristi do like to walk to the beach, and they do so frequently. When they just knew each other, they took an espresso at a café located near the beach. The last weeks they go to Jesse's home for some refreshments. Jesse does like to have a more intimate relationship. He finds Kristi sexually attractive and fun. He would like to have sex with Kristi. He has reason to believe that she loves him too. At this moment they are having a drink at Jesse's home, and Jesse wants to express his feelings for Kristi.

1. To show that he likes her, what might Jesse say or do during their walks on the beach or when saying goodbye when she goes home? ....
2. How could Jesse observe (looks, behavior, talk) that Kristi finds him also attractive? ....
3. How could Jesse express his desire for more intimate contact with Kristi? ....
4. Jesse said to Kristi that he likes her very much. But Kristi is shy and does not seem to know how she should react. What might Jesse say? ....
5. Kristi says she also would like to have more contact with Jesse, but that their current friendship is enough for her. How can Jesse respond? ....
6. Kristi says that more frequent contact with Jesse is fine. However, she has a relationship with her friend now for several years. She is not sure how he would react. How can Jesse respond? ....

Contact with Women Session: Responding to a Rejection

For the Participants

New Homework Assignments

(a) Describe a situation where you could manage your annoyance, irritation, anger, or aggression or a situation where you did not succeed.

- The situation was? ....
- Who was it? ....
- Where were you? ....
- What did the other person say or do? ....
- What did you think or feel? ....
- What did you say or do? ....
- How did the other person react?..
- Were you satisfied with how you managed this situation? ....
- How would you manage the situation next time? ....

(b) Describe a situation in which you have responded to a rejection.

- The situation was? ....
- Who was it? ....
- Where were you? ....
- What did the other person say or do? ....
- What did you think or feel? ....
- What did you say or do? ....
- How did the other person react? ....
- Were you satisfied with how you managed this situation? ....
- How would you manage the situation next time? ....

(c) Answer the questions at Julian's problem situation.

Julian's Problem Situation

Julian and Jean are dating for almost a year. They see each other regularly and go partying together. On occasion, Jean sleeps with Julian. Initially, their sexual contact was excellent, but the last time Jean had less interest in sex. Jean even went to her own home after a less pleasant evening.

1. How might Julian respond to the current situation? ....
2. Jean says that for her a pleasant evening does not necessarily have to result in sex. How would Julian respond? ....
3. Jean has made remarks that Julian does not shave and showers himself frequently enough. But her comments did not make a difference. She says that therefore she is reluctant to have physical contact with Julian. How might Julian respond? ....

4. Julian finds it no longer necessary to use condoms because they know each other long enough. Moreover, he says Jean must start using the pill. Jean disagrees strongly. In her view, it is too early in their relationship for that kind of methods. How can Julian respond? ....
5. One evening Jean says that they have to talk. She tells him that she has met another guy. So far, they had no sexual contact. But she makes clear that she likes this guy very much and even more so than Julian. She would like to stay friends with Julian but not having sex with him. How can Julian respond? ....

   ....
6. Julian tells Jean that he has met another girl. From the first moment, they did like each other very much with the result that they did sleep with each other the same evening. Jean is very upset and angry. She says that this is the end of their friendship. How can Julian respond? ....

Contact with Women Session: Responding to an Approach

For the Participants

New Homework Assignments

(a) Describe a situation where you could manage your annoyance, irritation, anger, or aggression or a situation where you did not succeed.

- The situation was? ....
- Who was it? ....
- Where were you? ....
- What did the other person say or do? ....
- What did you think or feel? ....
- What did you say or do? ....
- How did the other person react? ....
- Were you satisfied with how you managed this situation? ....
- How would you manage the situation next time? ....

(b) Describe a situation in which you have responded to an approach.

- The situation was? ....
- Who was it? ....
- Where were you? ....
- What did the other person say or do? ....
- What did you think or feel? ....
- What did you say or do? ....
- How did the other person react? ....
- Were you satisfied with how you managed this situation? ....
- How would you manage the situation next time? ....

(c) Answer the questions at Coen's problem situation.

Coen's Problem Situation

Coen has a new girlfriend named Mariska. They met at the Athletic Association. Koen was detained for 1 year and is now free for about 9 months. Koen and Mariska see each other regularly, and sometimes they end up embracing and kissing. Mariska says one evening that she wants to have sex with Coen. Coen is excited but also has his concerns. He wonders whether Mariska also has sex with other men. If so, it is not for him.

1. How can Coen respond? ....
2. Mariska admits she has also sex with other men, but they are always using a condom. She says Coen that she likes him very much but do not want a permanent relationship. How might Coen respond? ....
   ....

3. One evening Mariska says that she does not only want to kiss and cuddle with Coen but she also wants to have sex with him. But only if they have a permanent relationship from then on. How can Coen respond? ....
   ....
4. Since he has come out of jail Coen has several one-night stands. For several months he is friends with Mariska, but he has also regularly had sex with other women. If on one evening Mariska says that she wants to have sex with him, Coen says that he likes it very much, but that she must not conclude that they have a permanent relationship. Mariska says that she has not that expectation because she prefers to have sex with other men regularly. What should Coen say?
   ....
5. Coen and Mariska are madly in love and know each other for almost a year. The relationship goes without any major problems, and the sex is fine for both of them. Mariska live in a rather small apartment, while Coen has a spacious four-room flat. Mariska says that it is time to move in and live together. How might Coen react? Explain why he does so. ....
   ....

Contact with Women Session: Talking About Sex

For the Participants

New Homework Assignments

(a) Describe a situation where you could manage your annoyance, irritation, anger, or aggression or a situation where you did not succeed.

- The situation was? ....
- Who was it? ....
- Where were you? ....
- What did the other person say or do? ....
- What did you think or feel? ....
- What did you say or do? ....
- How did the other person react? ....
- Were you satisfied with how you managed this situation? ....
- How would you manage the situation next time? ....

(b) Describe a situation in which you have talked with a woman about sex.

- The situation was? ....
- Who was it? ....
- Where were you? ....
- What did the other person say or do? ....
- What did you think or feel? ....
- What did you say or do? ....
- How did the other person react? ....
- Were you satisfied with how you managed this situation? ....
  ....
- How would you manage the situation next time? ....

(c) Answer the questions at Mikel's problem situation.

Mikel's Problem Situation

Mikel and Natasha are friends for already more than half year. They kiss and snuggle, but have not yet been to bed with each other. One evening they are so excited by each other that it is now or never. Mikel says that he would like to have sex with her. Natasha says that she likes it very much, but first, she wants to talk about what she likes and do not like.

1. How might Mikel respond? ....
2. Natasha says she wishes that they take first a shower and that she wants to start with only oral sex. How might Mikel respond? ....
3. Sometime later Mikel and Natasha want to have intercourse. But Natasha does not wish to become pregnant and asks Mikel to use a condom and spermicide.

Mikel has no condoms and has never used one. How might Mikel respond? ....

4. Natasha is distraught by Mikel's obscene cries during intercourse. She has asked him several times to stop. Mikel says that that excites him and it is the only way for him to ejaculate. Natasha doubts if there are no other ways for Mikel to do so. How would Mikel respond? ....
5. Before they have intercourse, Mikel prefers to look at a pornographic movie with Natashsa, because that excites him very much. Natasha finds these films annoying because the sex is much too harsh and the women are sluts. She asks Mikel what she could do so he is more excited by her. How might Mikel respond? ....
6. Natasha told Mikel that she wants to have intercourse but that the vaginal penetration is always painful for her. How would Mikel respond? ....
7. Mikel regularly has no erection. Natasha asks him to satisfy her orally. Mikel does that, but he thinks himself a failure when that is the case. Natasha says that she does not mind. How might Mikel respond? ....

Contact with Women Session: Deepening Intimacy

For the Participants

New Homework Assignments

(a) Describe a situation where you could manage your annoyance, irritation, anger, or aggression or a situation where you did not succeed.

- The situation was? ....
- Who was it? ....
- Where were you? ....
- What did the other person say or do? ....
- What did you think or feel? ....
- What did you say or do? ....
- How did the other person react? ....
- Were you satisfied with how you managed this situation? ....
- How would you manage the situation next time? ....

(b) Describe a situation in which you have deepened your intimacy with a woman.

- The situation was? ....
- Who was it? ....
- Where were you? ....
- What did the other person say or do? ....
- What did you think or feel? ....
- What did you say or do? ....
- How did the other person react? ....
- Were you satisfied with how you managed this situation? ....
- How would you manage the situation next time? ....

(c) Answer the questions at Omar's problem situation.

Omar's Problem Situation

Omar and Dana moved in together recently. Omar works as a salesman at an Electronics Shop and spends many evenings with his friends. Dana works in a nursing home and has irregular shifts. Omar has the feeling that their relationship is not going well. The main obstacle is that they see each other too little.

1. How might Omar discuss this problem with Dana? What can he say? ....
   ....
2. It turns out that Dana agrees with Omar. She finds it also annoying that he is often not at home when she returns from her evening shift. Omar dislikes that he has to cook his meal most days. But Dana says she does not want to give up her work for their relationship. How might Omar respond? ....
   ....

3. If Dana returns from her work, she is very talkative and has whole stories about what she has experienced that day. Omar finds his job boring and is annoyed about his experiences with difficult customers. Dana asks if there was something nice at work and if he had sometimes fun with his colleagues. How might Omar respond? ....

....
4. If Dana's girlfriend Silvana is visiting. Both women are enthusiastic talkers. While Omar Silvana's husband, Philip, do not know what to say to each other. When they are gone, Omar says to Dana that he did not like their visit. But Dana says that he has to demonstrate more interest in Philip and Silvana. How might Omar respond? ....

....
5. Dana says one evening that she wants to do more things together in their free time. She has arranged that she only has to work during the day and has no more night shifts. She asks that Omar should stop with meeting his friends every night or in the weekend. How might Omar respond? ....

....
6. Dana is pregnant, and Omar wants to look for a more substantial house. He has found an attractive house in an advertisement. Their joint income is just enough for a mortgage. Dana says that Omar bills are too high. She would prefer to rent a house for the time being, also because eventually they may have a second child. In that case, they would have to move again. How might Omar respond? ....

....
7. Dana notes that Omar comes home often bad-tempered from his work. Right after dinner, he leaves for his friends, most of the time without saying anything. Dana has already said several times that they should talk more about his tedious work. She also would like it very much if he helps out more in the household. How might Omar respond? ....

....
8. When Dana comes home from work late, Omar is reading his computer magazines and his dirty clothes are laying around. Dana has often requested him to help her with the household. According to Omar that is no job for men. From that moment Dana stops cleaning up Omar's mess. How might Omar respond to solve this problem? ....

....

10.9 Extended Program: Work and Leisure

Plan of First Work and Leisure Session: Responding to a Compliment and Maintaining Contact

Goals

- Discussing homework assignments
- Announcing the module Work and Leisure
- Announcing the theme for the session: Responding to a compliment and maintaining contact
- Explaining new homework assignments

Agenda

0:00	Opening
0:05	Discussing homework assignments
0:15	Explaining the goal of the module Work and Leisure
0:30	Exercise: Responding to a compliment and Maintaining contact
1:20	Explaining new homework assignments
1:25	Evaluation of the session
1:30	Closing

Course

Opening

- Brief discussion of the session plan.

Homework Assignments

- The trainer asks two participants to report on the homework assignments.
- The trainer asks all participants what they have learned from the homework assignments.
- The trainer records the reports.

Explanation of the Goal of the Module Work and Leisure

- The trainer explains the goal of the Work and Leisure module, namely learning skills for performing paid work or unpaid voluntary work, and learning skills for practicing recreation in the form of sports, hobby, or the like.

Theme: Responding to a Compliment and Maintaining Contact

- The trainer discusses the goals and criteria for Responding to a compliment and Maintaining contact (Appendix 3).

Exercise: Responding to a Compliment and Maintaining Contact

- Trainer mentions three exercise situations from easy to difficult. For example: responding to a compliment from a colleague and maintaining contact, responding to a compliment from your boss and maintaining contact, and responding to a compliment from your employer and maintaining contact.
- Each participant exercises, so far as the available time allows, all situations in order of difficulty. The other participants and trainers provide feedback.

New Homework Assignments

(a) Describe a situation in which you respond to a compliment from a colleague and, if possible, maintain contact.
(b) Describe a situation where you respond to a compliment from your boss and, if possible, maintain contact.

Evaluation

- The trainer asks each participant what he has learned from the session.

For the Participants

New Homework Assignments

(a) Describe a situation in which you respond to a compliment from a colleague and, if possible, maintain contact:

- The situation was? ....
- Who was it? ....

- Where were you? ....
- What did the other person say or do? ....
- What did you think or feel? ....
- What did you say or do? ....
- How did the other person react?..
- Were you satisfied with how you managed this situation? ....
- How would you manage the situation next time? ....

(b) Describe a situation where you respond to a compliment from your boss and maintain contact:

- The situation was? ....
- Who was it? ....
- Where were you? ....
- What did the other person say or do? ....
- What did you think or feel? ....
- What did you say or do? ....
- How did the other person react? ....
- Were you satisfied with how you managed this situation? ....
- How would you manage the situation next time? ....

Work and Leisure Session: Standing Up for Yourself and Responding on a Refusal

Exercises

- The trainer mentions three exercise situations from easy to difficult. For example: You remind a colleague of an appointment and he refuses to comply, you remember your boss to an appointment and he refuses to comply, and you remember your employer to an appointment and he refuses to comply.
- Each participant exercises, so far as the available time allows, all situations in order of difficulty. The other participants and trainers provide feedback.

For the Participants

New Homework Assignments

(a) Describe a situation in which you remind a colleague to an appointment and he refuses to comply.

- The situation was? ....
- Who was it? ....
- Where were you? ....
- What did the other person say or do? ....
- What did you think or feel? ....
- What did you say or do? ....
- How did the other person react? ....
- Were you satisfied with how you managed this situation? ....
- How would you manage the situation next time? ....

(b) Describe a situation where you remind your boss of an appointment and he refuses to comply.

- The situation was? ....
- Who was it? ....
- Where were you? ....
- What did the other person say or do? ....
- What did you think or feel? ....
- What did you say or do? ....
- How did the other person react? ....
- Were you satisfied with how you managed this situation? ....
- How would you manage the situation next time? ....

Work and Leisure Session: Refusing and Giving Your Opinion

Exercises

- The trainer mentions three exercise situations from easy to difficult. For example, you refuse to help a colleague with a job and give your opinion about his commitment, you refuse your boss to help a colleague with a job and give your opinion about his commitment, and you refuse a group of colleagues to help with a job to help and give your opinion about their commitment.
- Each participant exercises, so far as the available time allows, all situations in order of difficulty. The other participants and trainers provide feedback.

For the Participants

New Homework Assignments

(a) Describe a situation where you refuse a colleague to help with a job and give your opinion on his commitment.

- The situation was? ....
- Who was it? ....
- Where were you? ....
- What did the other person say or do? ....
- What did you think or feel? ....
- What did you say or do? ....
- How did the other person react? ....
- Were you satisfied with how you managed this situation? ....
- How would you manage the situation next time? ....

(b) Describe a situation where you refuse a request of your boss to help a colleague with a job and give your opinion about the colleague's commitment.

- The situation was? ....
- Who was it? ....
- Where were you? ....
- What did the other person say or do? ....
- What did you think or feel? ....
- What did you say or do? ....
- How did the other person react? ....
- Were you satisfied with how you managed this situation? ....
- How would you manage the situation next time? ....

Work and Leisure Session: Responding to Criticism and Asking for Help

Exercises

- The trainer mentions three exercise situations from easy to difficult. For example: You respond to criticism from a colleague and asks him to help you, you respond to criticism from your boss and ask which colleague you could help, and you respond to criticism from your employer and ask which colleagues could help you.
- Each participant exercises, so far as the available time allows, all situations in order of difficulty. The other participants and trainers provide feedback.

For the Participants

New Homework Assignments

(a) Describe a situation where you respond to criticism from a colleague and ask him for help.

- The situation was? ....
- Who was it? ....
- Where were you? ....
- What did the other person say or do? ....
- What did you think or feel? ....
- What did you say or do? ....
- How did the other person react? ....
- Were you satisfied with how you managed this situation? ....
- How would you manage the situation next time? ....

(b) Describe a situation where you respond to criticism from your boss and ask him which colleague could help you.

- The situation was? ....
- Who was it? ....
- Where were you? ....
- What did the other person say or do? ....
- What did you think or feel? ....
- What did you say or do? ....
- How did the other person react? ....
- Were you satisfied with how you managed this situation? ....
- How would you manage the situation next time? ....

Work and Leisure Session: Criticizing and Complimenting Someone

Exercises

- The trainer mentions three exercise situations from easy to difficult. For example: You criticize a colleague at a certain job and then compliment him because he does it better, you criticize your boss because a colleague fails at a certain job and then compliment him when he has done something about it, and you criticize your employer for bad working conditions and compliment him if he improved them.
- Each participant exercises, so far as the available time allows, all situations in order of difficulty. The other participants and trainers provide feedback.

For the Participants

New Homework Assignments

(a) Describe a situation where you criticize a colleague at a certain job and then compliment him because he does better.

- The situation was? ....
- Who was it? ....
- Where were you? ....
- What did the other person say or do? ....
- What did you think or feel? ....
- What did you say or do? ....
- How did the other person react? ....
- Were you satisfied with how you managed this situation? ....
- How would you manage the situation next time? ....

(b) Describe a situation where you criticize your boss because a colleague fails at a certain job and compliment him when he has done something about it.

- The situation was? ....
- Who was it? ....
- Where were you? ....
- What did the other person say or do? ....
- What did you think or feel? ....
- What did you say or do? ....
- How did the other person react? ....
- Were you satisfied with how you managed this situation? ....
- How would you manage the situation next time? ....

10.10 Evaluation

Plan of First Evaluation Session

Goals

- Discussing homework assignments
- Evaluation of the program

Agenda

0:00	Opening
0:05	Discussing homework assignments
0:25	Evaluation of the program
1:30	Closing

Course

Opening

- Brief discussion of the session plan.

Homework Assignments

- The trainer asks two participants to report on the homework assignments.
- The trainer asks all participants what they have learned from the homework assignments.
- The trainer records the reports.

Evaluation of the Program

- The trainer evaluates the program by ratings on the evaluation scale. For that purpose, the scores of all participants are inventoried per item, after which they can explain their scores. The trainer ensures that the participants give each other positive feedback as much as possible.

For the Participants

Evaluation Scale

1 = not applicable at all 5 = strongly applicable

1	I actively participated in the program.	1	2	3	4	5
2	I learned a lot by practicing myself.	1	2	3	4	5
3	I learned to pay more attention to what others say and do.	1	2	3	4	5
4	I have learned to behave calmer and in a more satisfactory way with others.	1	2	3	4	5
5	Now I have a better understanding of the effect of my behavior in the short and long term.	1	2	3	4	5
6	I have learned to achieve my goals without harming others.	1	2	3	4	5
7	Now I understand better that it is sometimes disadvantageous for yourself to put your self-interest first.	1	2	3	4	5
8	I learned that you cannot judge everyone equally hard.	1	2	3	4	5
9	I better notice what damage you can do to others with aggressive behavior.	1	2	3	4	5
10	Now I know that when you're dealing with others you cannot always get it your way.	1	2	3	4	5
11	I feel that I can continue to work on what I learned during the program.	1	2	3	4	5
12	I find the information that I have received clearly	1	2	3	4	5
13	I have had enough information at the beginning about what would happen in the program.	1	2	3	4	5
14	I think that the subjects which were practiced during the program fit well with the problems that I have (and had) in dealing with others.	1	2	3	4	5
15	I think we had enough time during the sessions.	1	2	3	4	5
16	I think that there could be practiced sufficiently.	1	2	3	4	5

Plan of Second Evaluation Session

Goals

- Evaluation of individual participants.

Agenda

0:00	Opening
0:05	Evaluation of individual participants
1:25	Presenting certificate of participation
1:30	Closing

Course

Opening

- Brief discussion of the session plan.

Evaluation of Individual Participants

- Trainers distribute the reports to the referrer. All participants get to read each other's report and become invited to give each other and the trainers feedback. Finally, agreements are made about adjustments of the text. When the opinion of a participant is different from the opinion of the trainers, both opinions are included in the report.
- Distribution of certificates.
- Finally, all participants receive a certificate as proof of participation.

Appendix 1: Observing

This program is aimed at improving the way you interact with others. If you want to change how you deal with others, you need to be first of all aware of your behavior. In other words, you need to observe what you do and say. By looking and listening to yourself, it is easier to assess what you want to change and improve in your behavior. Also, in interacting with others, it is also important to observe what others are doing. This brochure is about the behavior of observing.

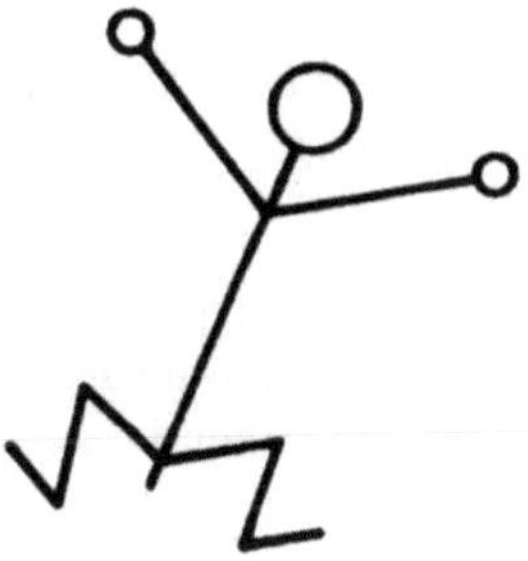

What Is Observing?

Observation is a description of what you hear and see. For example, someone who looks at the above drawing might say that the person of this figure is happy. What he or she really sees or observes is a hodgepodge of lines and circles, which is similar to a person with legs apart and diagonally up straight arms. Someone who says: "This is a happy person" is interpreting. This means that he does not describe what he sees when he looks at the drawing, but what he infers or thinks to see. Interpreting is to describe situations, persons, and events as to how one thinks that they are; that is to say one concludes what one actually sees and hears.

A few examples of observations and interpretations

- Joe has his mouth pinched together and said not a word to his supervisor/Joe is angry at his supervisor.
- Maria frequently moves from the left to the right in her chair/Maria is nervous.
- Fred got an A for his exam/Fred is doing everything well.
- Frank goes whistling through the apartment/Frank is cheerful.
- Ellen shouts at her child/Ellen is a lousy parent.
- Rita started crying when the dentist entered the waiting room/Rita is neurotic.

Some of the examples described here will probably raise questions with you. For example, "Joe is angry at his supervisor;" you can see this clearly on his face! The answer to this is that you actually do not know if Joe is angry at his supervisor. Perhaps he is afraid of him. What you can probably see, is that he pinches his mouth together and is silent. Thus, you cannot see that Joe is angry. If you say that he is angry, you interpret or conclude what you see. Of course, you may think that Joe is angry at his supervisor. But this does not clarify Joe's feelings (angry or afraid?), and you might be wrong in your reactions. A rather concrete description of what someone is doing makes it is also evident to other persons what he or she was doing (observations). Also, the disadvantage of an interpretation is that various meanings and the following actions are possible. Acting upon the one that is not relevant leads to misunderstandings.

Observation in Situations in Which You Are Emotionally Involved

We have discussed so far only examples, where the actions of other people were observed. If you participate in a situation and feel insecure, anxious, angry, or disappointed, then it is even more challenging to observe. Let us consider what Carl said about attending a birthday party: "Listen. I was at a birthday party, and nobody noticed me. I was quite upset." It is clear that by saying "nobody noticed me" Carl does not describe what he saw and heard. It is unlikely that no one has noticed him. In this case, Carl interpreted. Let us go further and question what happened? "Well, I can tell you, I felt terrible. I came in and congratulated the guy who gave the birthday party. I looked around and saw about 30 people in a room decorated with garlands. These people stood together in small groups and talked. I stood there quite alone and looked at the ground. I went after 5 min without saying something to anybody." The latter is a report of Carl's observations. You may perhaps have noticed now that his report contains statements such as "I have felt terrible" (observation of his emotion). This shows how Carl has felt at the moment. Your own feelings are observations too. Therefore, observations are descriptions of what one sees, hears, and feels itself.

Some examples of observations that relate to what you feel:

- "I was very insecure during the examination."
- "I am sick."
- "Last night I was furious at my father."
- "I'm very irritated by the child's yelling."

In examples above, the feeling is named (such as insecure, sick, and angry), and it is indicated clearly that it is me ("I") and when (during the examination, last night). In the next example, Thomas describes what he experienced while shopping. Thomas' statements are both observations and interpretations. Only the observations are printed in italics: "It was a disaster in the supermarket. *The woman behind me has hit me with her shopping cart.* I can't stand just that. *I felt irritated. I touched the man who stood in front of me. He turned around and said: 'You are in a hurry?'* I blacked out *and left quickly. Other supermarkets had already been closed.* Such things happen to me again and again. "That is what upsets me."

Exercises

We give some examples of someone's reported experiences. Try to identify the observations and underline them.

1. I can say it again and again: That secretary will never learn it. Always the same errors in her letters. I went to her, and she did not even look up from her computer. I said "hello." Even then she did not look up. I repeated my hello, and after some time she asked: "What's the matter?" I was furious. I showed her the letter and the misspellings and asked her what that was about. She said, "If you are not satisfied, I can write another one." The whole affair makes me pissed.
2. Yesterday I met the girl next door in front of our house. She always behaves as if I do not exist. I thought: "Give it a try." And said: "Good evening." She looked up and quickly looked the other way. She finds me not attractive enough.
3. It is always the same. Before I realize it is a huge pile of work that has to be completed. He obviously wants to annoy me. He comes out to me and asks if I have time to type just a few letters. Of course, I will be fired, if I don't do it. He obviously thinks that I work too slowly. I can see it on his face.
4. Nobody likes me. Yesterday I got a letter from my mother. She writes nothing else than: Do you eat properly? Do you learn enough? Did you write to your aunt? Always being negative. As if there is nothing else in the world. The last 14 days I was every night quite alone, and do not think that anyone thinks to visit me. In any case, I've seen nobody for the last 14 days.

Appendix 2: Anger Management

Introduction

Below we explain how anger may lead to maladaptive (aggressive), but also to adapted (assertive) behavior. Anger is a feeling. For instance, you are furious at someone because what you wanted to happen did not happen. You feel that you have been wronged or think that the other person has offended you. Anger is a very strong emotion, less strong emotions are annoyance or irritation. If you can control your anger in such a way that you react appropriately, you will reach your goal more often and you will feel less agitated. To clarify the connection between anger and maladapted behavior, we use the following behavior chain: Behavior chain: *Antecedent → Thoughts → Tension → Emotion → Behavior → Consequences*

1. Behavior

Aggressive behavior is an example of inappropriate behavior because the direct result is often positive, but in the long run, you get into difficulties. You get annoyed by others or, in the worst case, you come into contact with the law. Therefore, we call aggressive behavior inappropriate behavior. It is better to stand up for yourself in an assertive way. Assertive behavior means that you act according to your interests without affecting other people's rights. Assertive behavior is an adaptive behavior. In our interaction with each other, we have to apply specific values and norms of our society. Standards and values are social rules that ensure that people are pleasant, polite, and respectful of each other. With assertive behavior, you take into account those values and norms, even if you stand up for yourself.

2. Antecedent

Emotions such as anger usually have to do with what someone else says or does. We speak of an antecedent event when the behavior of another person can give rise to irritation, anger, or rage. These emotions may lead you to behave aggressively, for instance by scolding, threatening, or beating. To be able to act appropriately, it is essential to realize what happens precisely: What does or says that other person exactly. In a situation, it is best to first carefully observe what you hear or what you see and what you feel yourself. We call those observations. Behavior chain: *Antecedent → Behavior.*

Example: Wesley has just made coffee, but the coffee can is still on the counter. However, Nancy wants to do the dishes. Nancy says to Wesley in an angry voice: "Can't you store that coffee in the closet right away? Then at least I can do the dishes."

Behavior chain: Coffee can at the kitchen counter → Nancy scolds Wesley. Alternative behavior chain: Coffee can at the kitchen counter → Nancy asks Wesley to store the coffee.

3. Thoughts

Observations are followed by thoughts (interpretations). It is important to make a distinction between what you observe (antecedent) and the interpretations you make (thoughts). Interpretations are thoughts that you have about the antecedent. A thought can be: "She has the pick on me" or "He is forgetful again." Behavior chain: *Antecedent → Thoughts → Behavior.*

Example: Daphne is not home yet at 7 o'clock in the evening, while she always stops working at half past five. Dennis looks at the clock and thinks: "She's cheating." As soon as Daphne comes home, Dennis scolds her. Behavior chain: Daphne is not home yet at 7 o'clock → Dennis thinks: "She has an affair." → Dennis scolds Daphne when she returns home. Alternative behavior chain: Daphne is not home yet at 7 o'clock. → Dennis thinks: "She can take care of herself." → Dennis asks Daphne when she comes home why she is late and if she wants to call from now on when she has to work overtime.

4. Physical Tension

When people perceive someone's behavior as a threat, they usually do not get angry right away. It takes a while before they know exactly what is happening. They do notice that their physical tension immediately increases. This tension can occur in different ways: faster heartbeat, perspiration, stretching muscles, shaking, blushing, and the like. An increase in physical tension is entirely reasonable in social situations in which, in our opinion, something unpleasant happens. Behavior chain: *Antecedent → Thoughts → Tension → Behavior.*

Example: Patrick walks into the hall with a bag full of groceries. Marian is running ahead of him. Marian does not keep the door open for Patrick. Patrick thinks: "What a bitch" and gets completely riled up. The next time Patrick does not keep the door open for Marian. Behavior chain: Marian does not keep the door open for Patrick → Patrick thinks: "What a bitch" → Patrick gets worked up → Next time, Patrick bangs the door shut in front of Marian's nose. Alternative behavior chain: Marian does not keep the door open for Patrick → Patrick thinks: "She is with her thoughts elsewhere." → Patrick relaxes → Patrick says something about the fact that Marian did not keep the door open for him and asked her to show some consideration with him the next time.

5. Emotions

Behavior is partly determined by the feelings that precede it. Negative feelings may lead to maladaptive behavior: Feeling down to depression, anger to aggression, suspicion to social isolation. Negative feelings are not always wrong. Death comes with grief, and deception comes with bitterness. These feelings are temporary. Behavior chain: *Antecedent → Thoughts → Tension → Emotions → Behavior.*

Example: Gerald is waiting in the bakery for his turn. Then arrives a woman who immediately addresses the saleswoman and asks for her order. The saleswoman does not dare to refuse because she and the woman are good acquaintances. Gerald thinks: "What a rude person, acquaintances have certain privileges here." He gets it completely hot under the collar. Gerald feels completely ignored and walks angrily out of the shop. Behavior chain: Woman pushes forward in the bakery → Gerald thinks: "What a rude person, acquaintances are allowed to do this." → Gerald gets it hot under the collar → Gerald feels ignored and angry → Gerald runs out of the store. Alternative behavior chain: A woman pushes forward → Gerald thinks: "She does not notice me." → Gerald relaxes → Gerald feels fairly calm → Gerald says that it is his turn first.

6. Consequences

Behavior is mainly determined by the consequences it has. It is essential to make a distinction between (a) consequences immediately after the end and (b) consequences after some time. Some behaviors directly produce a positive result but have negative consequences in the longer term. For instance, good food can lead to getting too fat. In yet other cases, the result is negative in the short term but the effect is positive after months or years. Going to school means that you cannot spend all day with your friends but you obtained a diploma later on. Consideration is not always easy. This is partly because you can be more assured of a direct result than of a long-term consequence. Many people find it difficult to see beyond the end of their noses.

Aggressive behavior almost always has immediate positive consequences. You immediately get your way, the other one caves in. You have been able to take revenge, your prestige in the group becomes more prominent, etc. The consequences, in the long run, are hardly visible at the time. It is only after some time that the other person is likely to mobilize his friends and, in turn, he will pay you back. In the worst case, you come into contact with the law. Often it takes months before you are convicted and even longer if you have to serve a sentence. In the long run, aggressive behavior is always disadvantageous for all those involved. Aggression always leads to even stronger aggression, to social isolation, and to crime. Behavior chain: *Antecedent → Thoughts → Tension → Emotions → Behavior → Consequences.*

Example: Dwight is queuing at the supermarket. The woman for Dwight asks the cashier after the checkout how it goes with her children. Dwight thinks: "I'll be here until tomorrow" and is getting tense. He is annoyed and says to the cashier and the woman: "Can't you hurry up? I have something else to do than to listen to your chatting." The cashier gets scared and says: "I will help you immediately." Dwight is immediately helped but later feels uncomfortable because he was in no hurry. Behavior chain: A woman is talking with cashier → Dwight thinks: "I'll be here until tomorrow." → Dwight gets tense → Dwight gets annoyed → He makes an angry remark to the cashier → Dwight is helped immediately but later feels uncomfortable. Alternative behavior chain: A woman is talking with cashier → Dwight thinks: "I have some time, if it does not last too long." → Dwight relaxes → He stays calm → Dwight says to the women: "Aren't you chatting a bit too long?" → Dwight feels comfortable because the women look at him kindly and take him into account.

Appendix 3: Social Skills for Module Prosocial Skills and Module Work and Leisure: Goals and Criteria

1. Making and Maintaining a Contact

What do I want to achieve?

- Starting a conversation with the other person
- Telling something about myself
- Asking something from the other person
- Showing that I appreciate the contact with the other person
- Letting the other person know that I pay attention to what he or she says

What do I pay attention to?

- That I show why I want to make acquaintance.
- That I am direct by starting sentences with "I".
- That I say that I appreciate the contact.
- That I am clear about that I am talking about us together.
- That I am short and concise.
- That I align my nonverbal behavior with what I say.

2. Ending a Situation

What do I want to achieve?

- Stopping the conversation with the other person.
- Showing the other person that I will return to the discussion soon or in due time.
- Emphasizing that stopping does not mean that I find the discussed subject unimportant.
- Allowing myself the time to think about what has been discussed.
- Letting the other person know that I find the continuation of good contact important.
- Ensuring that the other person knows that he or she can also return to the discussion.

What do I pay attention to?

- That it is clear what I want to convey, namely that I want to think about what we discussed and that I consider the continuation of good contact important.
- That I am clear by starting sentences with "I."
- That I am clear about what and who I am talking about, namely what we just discussed.
- That I am short and concise.
- That I align my nonverbal behavior with what I say.

3. Asking for Help (Making a Request)

What do I want to achieve?

- Asking the other person to help me with a certain activity.
- Showing the other person that I cannot do it alone, and that I think it is important that the activity takes place.
- Thanking the other person afterwards for his or her help.
- Ensuring that the other person knows that he or she can also appeal to me if necessary.

What do I pay attention to?

- That it is clear what I ask help for.
- That I am direct by starting sentences with "I".
- That I am clear about what and about which activity I am talking and how the other person can help me.
- That I am short and concise.
- That I align my nonverbal behavior with what I say.

4. Refusing

What do I want to achieve?

- Doing what I want to do.
- Preventing me from doing things that I do not want to do.
- Teaching the other person to look for a solution himself or herself.
- Preventing me from raising expectations with another person, as a result of which he may make me too many and unreasonable requests.
- Preventing me from doing something against my will.
- Preventing people from benefiting from me.
- Ensuring that the other person takes into account my interests.
- Making it clear to the other person that I will refuse and reject his request and not his person and future requests.

What do I pay attention to?

- That I refuse or say "no".
- That the refusal is direct, that is to say, that "I" does not want something.
- That the refusal is specific, which means that I indicate precisely what I refuse.
- That I make clear that I have decided to refuse and do not defend myself.
- That I align my nonverbal behavior to what I say.

5. Responding to a Refusal

What do I want to achieve?

- Showing that I understand that the other person refuses and why.
- Accepting that my request is rejected and not my person.
- Indicating that I assume that the refusal concerns only this request.
- Investigating whether I can achieve my goal differently.

What do I pay attention to?

- That I express my feelings of disappointment.
- That I remain calm and do not continue to urge the other person.
- That I ask if I can appeal to him or her in other situations.
- That I align my nonverbal behavior to what I say.

6. Criticizing

What do I want to achieve?

- To give the other person an insight into his or her behavior with the intention to stop an annoying habit.
- By criticizing somebody to make him or her something clear.
- To show the other the consequences of his or her behavior.
- Give the other alternatives for his or her behavior.
- Making it clear to others that my criticism is focused on his or her behavior and not on his or her person.
- Opening up my feeling about something, instead of holding it back.
- To let someone know to what extent he or she can count on me.
- Preventing people from trifling with me.
- Satisfying myself with an achieved goal.

What do I pay attention to?

- That I say that I am dissatisfied with someone's behavior or way of doing things.
- That my criticism is an assertion and not a question.
- That I directly say that "I" am bothered by it.
- That my criticism is directed at the other by saying "you".
- That I am concise and concise.
- That I am specific in what I am talking about and do not associate my criticism with other situations.
- That my criticism may be accompanied by request for change in a positive direction.
- That I align my nonverbal behavior to what I say.

7. Responding to Criticism

What do I want to achieve?

- Letting the other person know that I have listened.
- Giving the other person room for his criticism, even though I do not agree with it.
- Wondering seriously if I should change something in my behavior.
- Asking the other which alternatives he or she thinks of.
- Making it clear that I do not interpret the criticism as directed at my person but at my behavior or activity.

What do I pay attention to?

- That I show that I have understood to which behavior or activity the criticism relates (for example by summarizing what the other person has said).
- That I say briefly and concisely what I think of the criticism.
- That I express any feelings of disappointment.
- That I may thank the other person for his or her remarks.
- That I align my nonverbal behavior to what I say.

8. Giving Your Opinion

What do I want to achieve?

- Making clear what my position is.
- Showing that I have a point of view.
- Presenting my ideas, even though I may not know everything about it.
- Giving space to the other person's point of view.
- Trying to improve the relationship with the other person.
- Trying the other to convince of something.
- Provoking a discussion with the other person because I find that interesting.
- Ensuring that others take account of me or my opinion.
- Showing who I am.
- Learning something, becoming wiser.

What do I pay attention to?

- That I make it clear that it is my point of view, by saying "I like," "I agree with you because ……," "I do not agree with you, because …," "I think that …… ," "I believe that ……," and so on.
- That I say briefly and concisely what my opinion is.
- That I am clear in what I think.
- That I listen to what the other person says and possibly summarize this.
- That I let the other person finish.
- That I align my nonverbal behavior with what I say.

9. Standing Up for Yourself

What do I want to achieve?

- Getting what I think is due to me.
- Ensuring that another person keeps to his agreements.
- Giving myself the feeling that I have achieved something.
- Making it clear to the other person that I think I am entitled to something.
- Making it clear to the other person that from now on I want to return what is mine without asking for it.
- Making sure that the other person takes account of me.
- Making it clear to the other person that I find it annoying when wronging me.
- Achieving my own goals.
- Preventing me from being used or misused.

What do I pay attention to?

- That I state specifically when I want that something happens.
- That I am direct by saying that "I" wants something.
- That I say briefly and concisely what I want.
- That I do not do my request as an order or assignment, so for example: "I would like …" instead of: "Do this or do that."

10. Complimenting Someone

What do I want to achieve?

- Making the other person feel good; improving the relationship with another person.
- Promoting that the other also does something for me in return.
- Letting the other person know that I pay attention to what he or she says or does.
- Promoting that the other makes fewer demands on himself.
- Allowing myself the space to give a positive opinion, even if the other does not agree with it.

What do I pay attention to?

- That it is positive what I say.
- That I am direct by starting sentences with "I".
- That is clear about what and who I am talking about, namely about the other person.
- That I am short and concise.
- That I align my nonverbal behavior with what I say.

11. Complimenting Yourself (Making Positive Self-Statements)

What do I want to achieve?

- Making me feel good.
- Rewarding myself with the goal of performing the activity in the future more often.
- Communicating the pleasant feeling that I have to others.
- Giving the other person a compliment about myself.
- Letting someone else know that I am happy with myself.
- Letting someone else know that I have met the demands that I made to myself.

What do I pay attention to?

- That it is positive what I am saying about myself.
- That I am direct, namely that "I" finds something.
- That I am clear, so say exactly what I am talking about and who I am talking about, namely myself.
- That I am short and concise.
- That I align my nonverbal behavior with what I say.

12. Responding to a Compliment

What do I want to achieve?

- Showing my feelings about the compliment that the other person expresses.
- Showing that the valuation makes me feel well.
- Ensuring that another person gives his or her compliment more often.
- Making the other person feel good.
- Ensuring that I continue with what I did/do.
- Letting the other person know that I pay attention to what he or she says.
- Letting the other person know that I have listened.
- Making me feel good.
- If necessary, adapt my high requirements because of the others compliment.
- Allowing the other person to give his positive opinion, even though I do not agree with it.

What do I pay attention to?

- That it is positive what I say, about the fact that the other person gives the compliment whether or not I agree with what the other person says.
- That I am direct by starting sentences with "I".
- That I am clear about what and who I am talking about, namely about myself.
- That I am short and concise.
- That I align my nonverbal behavior with what I say.

Appendix 4: Social Skills for Module Prosocial Network: Goals and Criteria

1. Making Acquaintance

What do I want to achieve?

- Starting a conversation with the other person.
- Telling something about myself.
- Asking something to the other person.
- Showing that I appreciate the contact with the other person.
- Letting the other person know that I pay attention to what he or she says.

What do I pay attention to?

- That I have thought in advance of a topic for a short conversation.
- That I explain why I want to become acquainted.
- That I am direct by starting sentences with "I".
- That I say that I appreciate the contact.
- That I ask open questions.
- That I am short and concise.
- That I align my nonverbal behavior with what I say.

2. Making an Appointment

What do I want to achieve?

- Making an appointment to get to know the other person better.
- Letting the other person know what my interest is.
- Asking the other person what his or her interest is.
- Checking whether we have common interests.
- Showing that I appreciate the contact with the other person.
- Letting the other person know that I will appreciate a continuation of the contact.

What do I pay attention to?

- That I explain why I want to become acquainted.
- That I am direct by starting sentences with "I".
- That I say that I appreciate the contact.
- That I am clear about that I am talking about us together.
- That I take the time to tell something about my interests and to let the other person tell something about his or her interests.
- That I align my nonverbal behavior with what I say.

3. Deepening a Contact

What do I want to achieve?

- Getting a better contact with the other person.
- Telling the other about certain subjects that are confidential to me.
- Letting the other tell about confidential matters for him or her.
- Showing that I want to intensify contact with the other person.
- Letting the other person know that I am interested in him or her as a person.
- Letting the other person know that in the future I want to continue to see the other person regularly.

What do I pay attention to?

- That I show that I want a better contact with the other person.
- That I gradually bring up confidential topics.
- That I let it be appreciated as the other person enters confidential matters for him or her.
- That I am direct by starting sentences with "I".
- That I show to appreciate it that the other is interested in me.
- That I am clear about who I am talking about, namely about us together.
- That I take the time to quietly discuss confidential subjects.
- That I align my nonverbal behavior with what I say.

4. Informing Others About Your Rehabilitation or Treatment Program

What do I want to achieve?

- Informing the other about the fact that I undergo (have undergone) an obliged rehabilitation or treatment program.
- Showing that I appreciate it if the other person wants to listen to my story.
- Correcting any misconceptions about imprisonment or obligatory forensic psychiatric treatment.
- Enabling the other person to ask questions about my previous history.
- Showing that I would appreciate it if the contact is not broken.
- Showing that I understand the other person's difficulty with my pre-history.
- *What do I pay attention to?*
- That I announce in advance that a difficult subject will be mentioned.
- That I tell the other person in a direct way and without rancor that I undergo (have undergone) an imprisonment or obligatory forensic psychiatric treatment.
- That I show understanding for any difficulty the other person may have with my background.
- That I tell exactly what happened on questions about my prior history.

- That I say to appreciate it that the other person wanted to listen to my story.
- That I say I hope that the contact is not broken.
- That I ask the other person to use the information I have provided confidentially.
- That I align my nonverbal behavior with what I say.

5. Responding to a Rejection

What do I want to achieve?

- Showing that I understand that the other person does not accept my previous history.
- Accepting that only the other person rejects my person and not everyone.
- Making it clear that I assume that the other person wants to break the contact.

What do I pay attention to?

- That I express my feelings of disappointment.
- That I remain calm and do not insist on the other person.
- That I request nevertheless to keep confidential with the information provided by me.
- That I align my nonverbal behavior with what I say.

Appendix 5: Social Skills for Module Contact with Women: Goals and Criteria

1. Showing Your Need for Intimacy

What do I want to achieve?

- More intimate contact with my girlfriend/boyfriend.
- Telling something about my sexual preferences.
- Knowing the other person's sexual preferences.
- Touching, kissing, and making love.
- Showing that I will not impose anything.
- Showing the other person that you find her/him sexually attractive.

What do I pay attention to?

- That I state what I need, namely intimacy.
- That I am direct by starting sentences with "I would like …;"
- That I say how attractive she/he is.
- That I do not force anything if my girlfriend/boyfriend responds negatively.
- That during or after touching, kissing and lovemaking, I ask my girlfriend/boyfriend if she/he liked it.
- That I am clear about who I am talking about, namely us together.
- That I align my nonverbal behavior with what I say.

2. Responding to a Rejection

What do I want to achieve?

- Letting the other know that I understand that the other does not share my needs at that time.
- Accepting that I may proceed too energetically and that my initiative at that time is rejected, but not my person.
- Making it clear that I assume that my girlfriend/boyfriend indicates when she/he does need more intimacy.

What do I pay attention to?

- That I express my feelings of disappointment.
- That I remain calm and do not continue to urge my girlfriend/boyfriend.
- That I ask my girlfriend to indicate the moment she/he needs more intimacy.
- That I do not blame my girlfriend/boyfriend but respect her/his opinion.
- That I align my nonverbal behavior with what I say.

3. Responding to an Approach

What do I want to achieve?

- Letting the other know that I appreciate the approach.
- Saying to the other person that I find her attractive.
- Saying that I have strong feelings or are excited.
- Showing that I want to have sexual contact.
- Showing that I will take the other person into account as she/he thinks that I react too directly.

What do I pay attention to?

- That I say that the approach is pleasant.
- That I tell the other person to find her/him be (sexually) attractive.
- That I indicate the need for sexual contact.
- That I am direct by starting sentences with "I".
- That I respect the opinion of the other person who thinks that I am too fast.
- That I take ample time to go into the approach and to say what I think of it.
- That I align my nonverbal behavior with what I say.

4. Talking About Sex

What do I want to achieve?

- Exchanging experiences with pleasant and unpleasant sexual actions.
- Exchanging habits around sex.
- Discussing the use of contraceptives.
- Discussing any sexual problems like premature ejaculation, erection problems, or not able to achieve orgasm.
- Discussing any tools such as porn movies, challenging clothes, and the like.

What do I pay attention to?

- That I state my sexual preferences.
- That I make sure my girlfriend/boyfriend can say what her sexual preferences are.
- That I take ample time to discuss topics as the use of contraceptives.
- That I show understanding for the possible sexual problems from my girlfriend/boyfriend.
- That I do not want to force anything and that I ask my girlfriend/boyfriend to say it right away if I do something she/he does do not like.
- That I tell my girlfriend/boyfriend immediately about my possible sexual problems and expect her/him to show understanding.
- That I align my nonverbal behavior with what I say.

5. Deepening Intimacy

What do I want to achieve?

- Improving further the relationship with my girlfriend/boyfriend.
- Saying that I need more and more intimate contact.
- Discussing possibilities to continue with improving the relationship.
- Asking my girlfriend/boyfriend if she/he also needs more intimacy.
- Discussing the conditions for a better relationship.
- Letting the other person know that I care much about further improvement of the relationship.

What do I pay attention to?

- That I say that it is important to me that the relationship further improves.
- That I indicate being prepared to do a lot to achieve that.
- That I ask my girlfriend/boyfriend how she/he thinks about it.
- That I ask my girlfriend/boyfriend what possibilities she/he sees in a further improvement of the relationship.
- That I am direct by sentences with "I would like to start …."
- That I take plenty of time for the conversation.
- That I align my nonverbal behavior with what I say.

References

Gibbs, J. C., Potter, G. B., & Goldstein, A. P. (1995). *The EQUIP program: Teaching youth to think and act responsibly through a peer-helping approach.* Champaign, IL: Research Press.

Goldstein, A. P., Glick, B., & Gibbs, J. C. (1998). *Aggression Replacement Training: A comprehensive intervention for aggressive youth* (2nd ed.). Champaign, IL: Research Press.

Chapter 11
Treatment Modules for Sexually Violent Offenders

Ruud H. J. Hornsveld and Floris W. Kraaimaat

11.1 Introduction

The modules described in this chapter can be part of a treatment program according to the need of the participants. However, we recommend that the Basic program is performed as described in Chap. 10 for the violent offenders, except that the Anger Management module is replaced by the Emotion Management module for the child sexual abusers. The rapists follow the Basic program for the non-sexually violent offenders. Rapists and child sexual abusers together follow the Specific program with the Psychoeducation, Cognitive Distortions, and Management of Risk Situations modules. For the Psychoeducation module, a plan for the first session and session 2–10 has been described, while for the Cognitive Distortions and Management of Risk Situations modules, the plans of all sessions are provided. The Specific program continues with three modules of the Extended program for non-sexually violent offenders, namely Prosocial Network (Sect. 10.7), Contact with Women (Sect. 10.8), and Work and Leisure (Sect. 10.9). Almost all modules include exercises and homework assignments. Also, reference is sometimes made to information brochures (Appendix in this chapter or Appendices 10.1–10.5 from Chap. 10). It is advisable to compose a workbook for the participants in which these exercises, assignments, and brochures are included.

It should be noted that the information about the different aspects of sexuality in the Psychoeducation module is quite explicit and not included in this book but available via https://www.agressiehanteringstherapie.nl/nl/menu/boeken. Some trainers will find parts of this information less suitable for sexually violent offenders.

R. H. J. Hornsveld (✉)
Erasmus University Medical Center, Rotterdam, The Netherlands
e-mail: ruud.hornsveld@ziggo.nl

F. W. Kraaimaat
Radboud University Nijmegen, Nijmegen, The Netherlands

R. H. J. Hornsveld et al. (eds.), *Assessment and Obligatory Treatment of Violent and Sexually Violent Offenders*, Advances in Preventing and Treating Violence and Aggression, https://doi.org/10.1007/978-3-030-27840-3_11

Incidentally, it is not intended that trainers restrict themselves to the text offered, but use the module for a discussion in the group about the normative and moral aspects of sexuality such as the equality of sexes and the acceptance of individuals with a non-heterosexual orientation.

Trainers have to be prepared that the implementation of a program is often difficult. Sex offenders often find that their sexual desires and activities are justified. Child sexual abusers sometimes believe that sexual contact of a minor with an adult is good for the emotional development of the young person. In their opinion, pedosexuality must be seen as a sexual orientation that must be socially accepted as heterosexuality or homosexuality. Such opinions can sometimes lead to an unpleasant atmosphere in the group. Therefore, trainers must sometimes schedule their confrontations in such a way that the continuity of the group is not jeopardized. For some participants, participation in the group will hardly lead to further insight into their problems or behavior change but will only result in further insights for the trainers into the seriousness of their problems.

11.2 Basic Program: Emotion Management

Plan of Session 1

Goals

- Welcoming the participants.
- Announcing the module Emotion Management.
- Learning to distinguish between interpretations and observations.
- Explaining new homework assignments.

Agenda

0:00	Opening.
0:05	Making acquaintance.
0:35	Appointments and introduction of portfolio.
0:40	Announcing the module Emotion Management.
0:45	Observation exercise 1: Distinction between observations and interpretations.
1:00	Observation exercise 2: State only observations/facts.
1:15	Explaining new homework assignments.
1:20	Evaluation of the session.
1:30	Closing.

Course

Opening

- Welcoming the participants.
- Brief discussion of the session plan.

Making Acquaintance

- Each participant briefly tells something about himself, to begin with, some biographical data ("What is your profession? Do you have a family? What are your plans for the future?"). Then the trainer asks each participant why he has to follow the program ("What is the latest offense for which you have been convicted? What punishment have you received?"), which problems he has with managing emotions, and in what way these emotions are now verbally and nonverbally expressed.
- The trainer explains what is understood by rapists and child sexual abusers. The victims of *rapists* are female or male adults, who have not consented to commit

sexual acts. The victims of *child sexual abusers* are related or unrelated children, girls or boys, below a certain age (usually 16 years).

Appointments and Portfolio

- The trainer discusses the goal and method of the program, confidentiality during the sessions, consequences of absence, and reporting the referrer.
- The trainer gives a portfolio to each participant. The participants are asked to bring along this portfolio every session.

Announcing the Module Emotion Management

- The trainer explains the goal of the Emotion Management module.

Observation Exercise 1

- The trainer explains the purpose of the exercise: Learning to look and listen to the behavior of others (and yourself) and to describe this behavior concretely. Both goals are conditions for accomplishing behavior change. This will be exercised with a role-play.
- The trainer instructs the participants about the role-play "in the subway." The trainer intends that the participants watch what happens and then write it down. The trainer will indicate the start and end of the role-play. Trainer "makes a subway" by facing two chairs.
- Situation: The trainer sits down in one of the chairs and is reading a magazine. Seeks extensively in his pockets, cannot find it, and grumbles "Where have I left it, that's too crazy? I just had it," without saying what he is looking for. Finally, he mutters: "I do not understand anything" and continues reading.
- The trainer asks the participants to write down what has happened and gives them the time to do so. The trainer asks the participants their explanation of the situation and writes this using bullet points on a blackboard in two columns. Next, the trainer asks the participants what the difference is between both columns. If the participants do not notice it, the trainer helps. Then, the columns are labelled as observations (facts) and interpretations (impressions, conclusions).
- The trainer asks the participants what the purpose of the exercise might be: Making a distinction between what you see or hear and what you think it means.

Observation Exercise 2

- The trainer performs a second role-play with a similar instruction. After the end of the role-play, the participants have to record only observations (facts).
- Situation: The trainer is waiting on the street and shows nonverbally impatient behavior, walks back and forth, looks up his watch, looks into the distance and murmurs: "I am on time, am I in the wrong place?", without to say who or what he is waiting for. The trainer looks in his diary and decides finally to leave, muttering: "Well, that's it."
- The trainer gives participants the opportunity to write down observations, which are then discussed one by one and tested for observation versus interpretation.

Homework Assignments

- The trainer explains the homework assignments and the information in the portfolio. The homework assignments are:
  (a) Read the information in the brochure Observing (Chap. 10, Appendix 10.1) and do the exercises.
  (b) Observe someone in the next week and make a report of your observations and interpretations.
  (c) Do the same exercise again.

Evaluation

- The trainer asks each participant what he has learned from the session.

For the Participants

Exercise

- Observation exercise 1
  In the subway. What is happening? ……………………………………………..
- Observation exercise 2
  Walking on the street. What do you observe? ……………………………….…

Homework Assignments

(a) Read the information in the brochure Observing (Chap. 10, Appendix 10.1). Underline on the last page in the four situations the sentences that are observations or facts.
(b) Observe someone you know in the next week without that person noticing that you are observing him or her. You only have to be brief looking at him or her, for example, at most a half minute. When you have done that, you write down what you saw and what you heard, by asking the questions below.

- Who did you look at (first name)? ....
- Where was it that you looked at him or her? ....
- Which day was it? ....
- What did the other person do while you looked at him or her (facts/observations)?..
- What did the other person say? ....
- What conclusion did you draw while you looked at the other person (conclusions/interpretations)? ....

(c) Do the same exercise again. Write down what you saw and what you heard by answering the questions below.

- Who did you look at (first name)? ....
- Where was it that you looked at the other person? ....
- Which day was it? ....
- What did the other person do while you looked at him or her (facts/observations)? ....
- What did the other person say? ....
- What conclusion did you draw while you looked at the other person (conclusions/interpretations)? ....

Plan of Session 2

Goals

- Discussing homework assignments.
- Learning to consider alternative interpretations.
- Learning to recognize observations/interpretations in case of emotion-eliciting situations and thinking of alternative interpretations.
- Discussing the behavior chain.
- Explaining new homework assignments.

Agenda

0:00	Opening.
0:05	Discussing homework assignments.
0:35	Thoughts exercise 1: Considering alternative explanations.
0:55	Thoughts exercise 2: Considering alternative explanations in emotion-eliciting situations.
1:10	Discussing behavior chain: Antecedents.
1:15	Explaining new homework assignments.
1:20	Evaluation of the session.
1:30	Closing.

Course

Opening

- Brief discussion of the session plan.

Homework Assignments

- The trainer discusses the information in Observing as follows:
  * Invites participants to ask questions or to make comments.
  * Asks participants to summarize what matters briefly.
  * Discusses one of the exercise situations through short discussions per sentence: Observation or interpretation?
- The trainer asks one participant to read his report of the situation in which he briefly observed someone.
- The trainer asks all participants what they learned from the exercises.
- The trainer records the reports.

Thought Exercise 1

- The trainer reconsiders the distinction between observations and interpretations by emphasizing that interpretations are conclusions that you may draw from the situation and the behavior of the other person. This means that in the same situation often more than one interpretation is possible. The trainer explains this using a situation reported by a participant of a personal situation.
- The trainer asks the participants for each of the following situations to think of which different conclusions are possible.
  * Situation 1: You receive a gift voucher as a birthday present. You think: "Ugh, what a boring gift. He/she has no interest in me."
  * Situation 2: A family member makes you a compliment. You think: "What does he/she want from me?"
  * Situation 3: An acquaintance criticizes your clothes. You think: "He/she is teasing me."

Thought Exercise 2

- The trainer tells about an own situation in which he/she felt irritated and asks the participants to think about the possible interpretations by their questions about the observations.
- The trainer asks all participants to consider aloud a situation in which they felt annoyed and to write it down regarding observations and interpretations. A few situations are discussed for which different interpretations can be made.

Discussing the Behavior Chain

- The trainer asks the participants what may be the importance of the exercises and then discusses the behavior chain Antecedent → Thoughts → Behavior.
- Trainer gives an example of himself or herself.

New Homework Assignments

(a) Read the information in Emotion Management (Appendix) through Thoughts (paragraph 3).
(b) Describe next week a situation where you felt emotional with the aid of the previously mentioned behavioral chain and consider alternative interpretations/conclusions.
(c) Describe a second situation in the next week where you feel emotional.

Evaluation

- The trainer asks each participant what he has learned from the session.

For the Participants

Thought Exercise 1

- Situation 1: You receive a gift voucher as a birthday present. You think: "Ugh, what a boring gift. He/she has no interest in me."
- Situation 2: A family member makes you a compliment. You think: "What does he/she want from me?"
- Situation 3: An acquaintance criticizes your clothes. You think: "He/she is teasing me."

Thought Exercise 2

Antecedent

- Who was it? ....
- Where were you? ....
- What day was it? ....
- What did the other person say and do? ....

Thoughts

- What conclusion did you draw? ....
- What else could you have thought? ....
- What more could you have thought? ....

Behavior

- What did you say and do? ....

New Homework Assignments

(a) Read the information in Emotion Management (Appendix) through Thoughts (paragraph 3).
(b) Describe next week a situation where you felt irritated by answering the questions below:

For the Participants

Consequence Exercise 1

Problem Situation 1

Sean is 32 years old and works at a plastic factory. First, he has spent some time with a girlfriend but now he lives alone on a flat, and that is not easy. Recently, he learned from his boss at the factory that he has made a mistake. He finds this is unfair because his boss is responsible too. When he comes home, he finds a letter from the housing association that he must pay the overdue rent immediately otherwise, he will be expelled from the flat. Sean's reaction is:

(a) *Subassertive:* He has taken the letter from the housing association hard and puts him in a big pile. He does not say anything at work either. He becomes more and more depressed and starts drinking.
(b) *Assertive:* Sean calls the housing association and explains that he has forgotten the rent because he was very busy. At work, he will discuss the conflict with his boss.
(c) *Aggressive:* Sean becomes extremely angry, calls housing association and yells at the operator. When the next morning the boss asks him something, he says: "Do it yourself. You can go to hell."

Problem Situation 2

Miranda and Nancy, two sisters of 18 and 20 years old, go to a party where later in the evening cocaine is used. Miranda has not used it for some time and does not want to use it any more. When her sister, who still uses, offers her something, her response is:

(a) *Subassertive:* Miranda reminds her sister that she does not want to take it anymore. But after a lot of urging from her sister, she takes the coke anyway, because she wants to be part of the group.
(b) *Assertive:* Miranda refuses the coke. She explains that she is not using any more and that she does not want to start again. She stands up immediately and goes home.
(c) *Aggressive:* Miranda gets enraged that her sister brought her to a party with a group of users, and that she tries to persuade her to use. Miranda scolds her sister and says she will never go with her again to a party.

Problem Situation 3

Rob always has to get up early in the morning because he wants to be at work on time. In the evening when it is time to go to bed, the neighbor begins to play loud music and Rob cannot come to sleep. The music continues throughout the evening. Rob does the following:

(a) *Subassertive:* Rob goes to sleep on the couch in the living room so that he has less trouble with the music. He says nothing to the neighbor.
(b) *Assertive:* Rob goes to the neighbor's house and tells the neighbor he has to get up early. He asks if the music which can be softer. Together they find a solution.
(c) *Aggressive:* Furious, Rob calls the police. He demands that they make sure that his neighbor immediately plays the music softer. The neighbors blame for Rob that he did not warn them first.

Consequence Exercise 2

Antecedent

- Who was it? ....
- Where were you? ....
- What day was it? ....
- What did the other person do and say (observations)? ....

Thoughts

- What conclusion did you draw? ....

Tension

- How did you lower your physical tension? ....

Emotion

- How did you feel at that moment? ....

Behavior

- What did you say or do? ....

Consequences

- What were the consequences in the short term? ....
- What were the consequences in the long term? ....

New Homework Assignments

(a) Read the information in Emotion Management (Appendix) through paragraph Consequences (paragraph 6).
(b) Describe in the next week a situation where you felt very emotional by answering the questions below:

Antecedent

- Who was it? ....
- Where were you? ....
- What day was it? ....
- What did the other person say or do (observations)? ....

Thoughts

- What conclusion did you draw? ....

Tension

- How did you lower your physical tension? ....
- What was the result? ....

Emotion

- How did you feel at that moment? ....

Behavior

- What did you say or do afterwards? ....

Consequences

- What were the consequences in the short term? ....
- What were the consequences in the long term? ....

(c) Describe a second situation where you felt very emotional.

Antecedent

- Who was it? ....
- Where were you? ....
- What day was it? ....
- What did the other person say or do (observations)? ....

Thoughts

- What conclusion did you draw? ....

Tension

- How did you lower your physical tension? ....
- What was the result? ....

Emotion

- How did you feel at that moment? ....

Behavior

- What did you say or do afterwards? ……………………………………………..

Consequences

- What were the consequences in the short term? ……………………………………..
- What were the consequences in the long term? ………………………………………

Plan of Psychoeducation Sessions 2–10

Goals

- Discussing homework assignment.
- Theme(s): See next page.
- Explaining new homework assignment.

Agenda

0:00	Opening.
0:05	Discussing homework assignment.
0:15	Providing participants with information about aspects of sexuality.
1:20	Explaining new homework assignment.
1:25	Evaluation of the session.
1:30	Closing.

Course

Opening

- Brief discussion of the session plan.

Theme(s): See Next Page

- The trainer informs the participants about several aspects of sexuality. Participants are prompted to ask questions and to discuss the information with each other and with the trainers.

New Homework Assignment

- Read the text in your portfolio about the aspects of sexuality which have been discussed during the session.

Evaluation

- The trainer asks each participant what he has learned from the session.

Topics for the Psychoeducation Sessions 2–9

Session 2

- Information on sexuality, Chap. 1, The art of making love:
- 1.1 Making love without having intercourse
- 1.2 Having intercourse
- 1.3 Masturbation

Session 3

- Information on sexuality, Chap. 1, The art of making love:
- 1.4 Anal sex
- 1.5 Use of condoms
- Information on sexuality, Chap. 2, Difficulties in making love:

  2.1 No desire to make love
  2.2 Pain during sex

Session 4

- Information on sexuality, Chap. 2, Difficulties in making love:
- 2.3 Premature ejaculation
- 2.4 The squeeze technique
- 2.5 Not being able to have an orgasm (anorgasmia)
- 2.6 Erection problems

Session 5

- Information on sexuality, Chap. 2, Difficulties in making love:
- 2.7 Vaginismus
- Information on sexuality, Chap. 3, Sexual diversity:

  3.1 Heterosexuality
  3.2 Homosexuality
  3.3 Bisexuality
  3.4 Pedosexuality
  3.5 Exhibitionism
  3.6 Frotteurism
  3.7 Transvestism and transsexuality
  3.8 Voyeurism

Session 6

- Information on sexuality, Chap. 4, Sexually transmitted diseases (STDs):
- 4.1 Cheating and STD
- 4.2 Chlamydia
- 4.3 Genital warts

- 4.4 Gonorrhea
- 4.5 Herpes

Session 7

- Information on sexuality, Chap. 5, Contraception:
- 5.1 Condoms
- 5.2 Female condoms
- 5.3 The pill
- 5.4 Withdrawal
- 5.5 Periodic abstention
- 5.6 Morning-after pill (emergency pill)

Session 8

- Information on sexuality, Chap. 6, Pornography:
- 6.1 Definition
- 6.2 Problematic aspects
- 6.3 Sexual phantasies and masturbation

Session 9

- Information on sexuality, Chap. 7, Internet addiction to pornography:
- 7.1 Pornography and rape
- 7.2 Signs, symptoms, and treatment

Plan of Session 10

Goal

- Theme: Evaluation of the module Psychoeducation

Agenda

0:00	Opening.
0:05	Theme: Evaluation of the module by the participants.
1:30	Closing.

Course

Opening

- Brief discussion of the session plan.

Theme: Evaluation of the Module by the Participants

- Participants complete the evaluation scale. When everybody is ready, each participant's reactions are written on a blackboard. Then, notable outcomes are discussed.

Closing

- After the trainers have formulated their conclusions based on the evaluation of the participants, the module is closed.

For the Participants

Evaluation Scale

1 = not applicable at all, 5 = strongly applicable

1	I actively participated in the module.	1	2	3	4	5
2	I found the information in the portfolio clearly.	1	2	3	4	5
3	I benefitted from the information that I received on the subject: The art of making love.	1	2	3	4	5
4	I benefitted from the information that I received on the subject: Problems with making love.	1	2	3	4	5
5	I benefitted from the information that I received on the subject: Sexual diversity.	1	2	3	4	5
6	I benefitted from the information that I received on the subject: Sexually transmitted diseases (STD).	1	2	3	4	5
7	I benefitted from the information that I received on the subject: Anticonception.	1	2	3	4	5
8	I benefitted from the information that I received on the subject: Pornography.	1	2	3	4	5
9	I benefitted from the information that I received on the subject: Internet addiction.	1	2	3	4	5
10	The trainers took account of my wishes and preferences.	1	2	3	4	5
12	I can ask the trainers for advice.	1	2	3	4	5
13	I think the length of the module is just right.	1	2	3	4	5

11.4 Specific Program: Cognitive Distortions

Plan of Session 1

Goals

- Announcing the module Cognitive Distortions.
- Theme: Women are sexual objects.
- Practicing with problem situation.
- Explaining homework assignment.

Agenda

0:00	Opening.
0:05	Announcing the module Cognitive Distortions.
0:15	Peter's problem situation.
1:20	Explaining new homework assignments.
1:25	Evaluation of the session.
1:30	Closing.

Course

Opening

- Brief discussion of the session plan.

Announcing the Module Cognitive Distortions

- The trainer explains the goal of the Cognitive Distortions module, namely learning to convert thoughts that lead to sexual aggressive behavior into thoughts that lead to prosocial sexual behavior. The following five themes for rapists are addressed: women are sexual objects, women are unknowable, male sexual drive is uncontrollable, dangerous world, and entitlement. The five themes for the child sexual abusers are: children as sexual objects, nature of harm, male sexual drive is uncontrollable, dangerous world, and entitlement.

Theme: Women Are Sexual Objects

- Trainer asks all participants to read Peter's problem situation. Then, the different questions are discussed during which participants have to convert sexually antisocial thoughts into sexually prosocial thoughts.

Homework Assignment (Only for Rapists)

- Describe a situation in which you thought: "That woman wants sex."

Evaluation

- Trainer asks each participant what he has learned from the session.

For the Participants

Exercise

Peter's Problem Situation

Peter is a man of 38 years. He was born in the Caribbean but he and his mother came to Europe when he was 15 years old. Within a year, Peter has a sexual relationship with the girl next door. That relationship lasts one year. One day Peter found his mother gruesome and brutally murdered in her home. From that moment he starts living alone, loses contact with his relatives, and starts consuming alcohol. Peter behaves tougher and has frequent one-time sexual connections. He is successful in deceiving women as well as men, and cheating gives him a satisfying sense of power. At the age of 30, Peter has a long-lasting relationship with Caroline. After some time, he becomes domestically violent and increasingly aggressive but Caroline keeps it quiet and does not report anything. During their relationship, Peter has regularly short-term sexual relations with other women, for example, with Joke. He has had a few times sexual contact with Joke when his relationship with Caroline ends. Joke and Peter sleep regularly at Peters' place. When their relationship progresses, Peter hits her more often or forces her to sexual contact. Usually, this happens when he feels irritated, for example, when Joke asks for money to buy drugs. Finally, Joke reports Peter to the police because of physical and sexual violence. Still, Peter says to love Joke very much.

1. What is in your opinion Peters' main problem?
2. What do you think about the fact that Peter has all sorts of loose contacts before his enduring relationship with Caroline?
3. If there are problems within a relationship, do you find it then surprising that a man starts having other sexual contacts?

4. How come when Peter gets irritated, he also wants to have sex?
5. Do you think that the use of alcohol increases Peters' sex drive?
6. What do you think of the way Peter engages in his relationships?
7. How do you think that "power and control" play a role in a relationship?
8. In what ways could Peter stay out of trouble?

New Homework Assignment (Only for Rapists)

(a) Describe a situation in which you thought: "That woman wants sex."

- The situation was? ....
- Who was it? ....
- Where were you? ....
- What did the other person say or do? ....
- What did you think or feel? ....
- What did you say or do? ....
- How did the other person react? ....
- How do you look back on your behavior afterwards? ....
- What else could you have said or done? ....

Plan of Session 2

Goals

- Discussing homework assignment.
- Theme: Children are sexual objects.
- Practicing with problem situation.
- Explaining new homework assignment.

Agenda

0:00	Opening.
0:05	Discussing homework assignment.
0:15	Lars problem situation.
1:20	Explaining new homework assignment.
1:25	Evaluation of the session.
1:30	Closing.

Course

Opening

- Brief discussion of the session plan.

Theme: Children Are Sexual Objects

- Trainer asks all participants to read Lars' problem situation. Then, the different questions are discussed during which participants have to convert sexually antisocial thoughts into sexually prosocial thoughts.

New Homework Assignment

- Describe a situation in which you thought: "That girl/boy wants sex."

Evaluation

- Trainer asks each participant what he has learned from the session.

For the Participants

Exercise

Lars' Problem Situation

Lars is a single man of 36 years. He is often depressed and insecure in social contacts. Lars has no friends and only has contact with some family members. He feels at ease just in the company of underage boys. Lars is working on a voluntary basis as a classroom assistant at a primary school and as such comes in contact with young boys. Lars is aware that he is sexually attracted to some boys and he thinks of them when he masturbates at home. On the school playground, Lars talks with the 10-year-old Raymond. It turns out that they have a common interest, namely playing computer games. Lars has just bought a brand-new game console, and he invites Raymond to come to his home. When Raymond is playing this game, Lars asks him to give him a hand job. Raymond likes to keep playing the game very much and agrees to do so. Lars gets used to have underage boys at his home and Lars keeps on asking the boys to masturbate him or he has anal sex in exchange for computer games.

(a) What do you see as the main problem for Lars?
(b) What do you think about the fact that Lars only feels comfortable in the company of young boys?
(c) How do you think the boys felt when Lars asked them to satisfy him sexually?
(d) Do you think it a coincidence that Lars works as a volunteer at an elementary school and precisely as a classroom assistant?
(e) Do you think the boys liked to have sex with Lars?
(f) If a boy shows to be interested in sex, is Lars then allowed to respond to this interest?
(g) Do you think that Lars is interested in the boys or that he only used them for sex?
(h) Do you think that before his position as a volunteer Lars should have informed the school about his sexual orientation?
(i) Does it make a difference if Lars only touched the boys or also had sexual intercourse with them?

New Homework Assignment (Only for Child Sexual Abusers)

(a) Describe again a situation in which you thought: "That girl/boy wants sex."

- The situation was? ....
- Who was it? ....
- Where were you? ....
- What did the other person think or say? ....
- What did you think or feel? ....

- What did you say or do? ……………………………………………..………………...
- How did the other person react? ………………………………………………………..
- When you look back on your behavior now, what do you think about it? ………
  ……………………………………………………………………………..………
- What else could you have said or done? ……………………………….……………

Plan of Session 3

Goals

- Theme: Women/children are sexual objects.
- Discussing homework assignment.
- Explaining new homework assignment.

Agenda

0:00	Opening.
0:05	Discussing homework assignment.
1:20	Explaining new homework assignment.
1:25	Evaluation of the session.
1:30	Closing.

Course

Opening

- Brief discussion of the session plan.

Theme: Women/Children Are Sexual Objects

- On the basis of their homework assignment, participants explain to what extent the theme "Women/children are sexual beings" has played a role in their offense and discuss their current views with the other participants.

New Homework Assignment

- Describe again a situation in which you thought: "That woman fancies sex" or "That girl/boy fancies sex."

Evaluation

- The trainer asks each participant what he has learned from the session.

For the Participants

New Homework Assignment

(a) Describe again a situation in which you thought: "That woman wants sex" or "That girl/boy wants sex."

- The situation was? ....

- Who was it? ....
- Where were you? ....
- What did the other person say or do? ....
- What did you think or feel? ....
- What did you say or do? ....
- How did the other person react? ....
- When you look back on your behavior now, what do you think about it? ....
  ....
- What else could you have said or done? ....

Plan of Session 4

Goals

- Discussing homework assignment.

- Theme: Victims are not hurt.
- Practicing with problem situation.
- Explaining new homework assignment.

Agenda

0:00	Opening.
0:05	Discussing homework assignment.
0:15	Sam's problem situation.
1:20	Explaining new homework assignment.
1:25	Evaluation of the session.
1:30	Closing.

Course

Opening

- Brief discussion of the session plan.

Theme: Nature of Harm

- The trainer asks all participants to read Sam's problem situation. Then, the different questions are discussed during which participants have to convert sexually antisocial thoughts into sexually prosocial thoughts.

New Homework Assignment (Only for Child Sexual Abusers)

- Describe again a situation in which you thought: "Victims are not hurt"

Evaluation

- The trainer asks each participant what he has learned from the session.

For the Participants

Exercise

Sam's Problem Situation

Sam is a white 30-year-old male. As a child he was attracted to much younger girls. At the age of 14, Sam plaid sexual-oriented games with girls of about 8 years of age when he stroked their vagina. At the age of 18, Sam was convicted of indecent acts with underage girls. One year after that Sam is out of prison. He starts, on the advice of his mother, a relationship with Tanja. Tanja is a mature woman, and she has 6-year-old daughter Yvonne. Sam is not in love with Tanja but he marries her anyway. A few months after the wedding Sam starts cuddling and sexually touching Yvonne. Tanja discovers this and reports Sam to the police with the result that he has to begin counseling. Sam promises to refrain from sexually touching Yvonne, and the couple stays together. Sam keeps his promise and does not approach Yvonne or other girls sexually. A few years later, Tanja dies from lung cancer. Sam falls back into his old habits. He connects with underage girls to get an opportunity to grope them. Eventually, Sam raped an 8-year-old girl and is arrested.

(a) What do you see as Sam's main problem?
(b) Sam starts a relationship with mature women. What do you think about that?
(c) Is it not remarkable that Tanja has a 6-year-old daughter?
(d) Why continues Tanja the relationship with Sam?
(e) How do you value the fact that Sam has no contact with young girls as long as Tanja lives?
(f) How do you explain the relapse of Sam after the death of Tanja?
(g) How might young girls react to groping and to rape? Is there a difference between the short-term and the long-term consequences?
(h) Is a relationship with an adult woman an effective way for a pedosexual to stay out of trouble?
(i) What would you advice Sam to stay out of trouble in future?

New Homework Assignment (Only for Child Sexual Abusers)

(a) Describe a situation in which you thought: "Victims are not hurt."

- The situation was? ……………………………………………………………
- Who was it? ……………………………………………………………………
- Where were you? ………………………………………………………………
- What did the other person say or go? ……………………………………………
- What did you think or feel? ………………………………………………………
- What did you say or do? …………………………………………………………
- How did the other person react? …………………………………………………
- When you look back on your behavior now, what do you think about it? ………
  ……………………………………………………………………………………
- What else could you have said or done? …………………………………………

Plan of Session 5

Goals

- Discussing homework assignment.
- Theme: Women are unknowable.
- Practicing with problem situation.
- Explaining new homework assignment.

Agenda

0:00	Opening.
0:05	Discussing homework assignment.
0:15	Roy's problem situation.
1:20	Explaining new homework assignment.
1:25	Evaluation of the session.
1:30	Closing.

Course

Opening

- Brief discussion of the session plan.

Theme: Women Are Unknowable

- Trainer asks all participants to read Roy's problem situation. Then, the different questions are discussed during which participants have to convert sexually antisocial thoughts into sexually prosocial thoughts.

New Homework Assignment (Only for Rapists)

- Describe a situation in which you thought: "I cannot understand that woman."

Evaluation

- The trainer asks each participant what he has learned from the session.

For the Participants

Exercise

Roy's Problem Situation

Roy is a Pakistani Hindu man of 23 years. Roy spoke hardly English and was as a child frequently bullied because of his poor English. This harassment was one of the reasons that he did not complete school. Roy has no work and earns his money by dealing drugs. Roy's parents separated. His father is an alcoholic. During drunken tantrums, his father used to attack Roy with his belt. Roy has a relationship with Yolanda. Roy has more need for sex than Yolanda. At times when Yolanda refuses to have sex with Roy, he forces her to have sexual intercourse. After several months Yolanda reports him of rape to the police and Roy ends up in prison. In prison, Roy is told that his father is deceased. When Roy is released from prison, he decides to celebrate his release by a lot of alcohol and drug use. After that Roy visits a prostitute. Even with being very aroused he does not succeed to ejaculate during sex with the prostitute. He ends up with feeling ashamed and angry. On his way home, Roy raped a woman who was walking past by chance.

(a) What do you see as the main problem of Roy?
(b) What are the consequences for Roy of the regular beatings by his father?
(c) What do you think about it that Roy forces his wife to have sex?
(d) How do you see the connection between the mistreatment of Roy by his father and his raping of Yolanda?
(e) What is your opinion of Yolanda's new relationship with a drug dealer?
(f) What do you think about Roy's visit of a prostitute after using drugs and alcohol?
(g) What are Roy's views on women?
(h) What do you recommend to Roy if he wants to get his life back in order?

New Homework Assignment (Only for Rapists)

(a) Describe a situation in which you thought: "I cannot understand that woman."

- The situation was? ....
- Who was it? ....
- Where were you? ....
- What did the other person say or do? ....
- What did you think or feel? ....
- What did you say or do? ....
- How did the other person react? ....
- When you look back on your behavior now, what do you think about it? ....
  ....
- What else could you have said or done? ....

Plan of Session 6

Goals

- Theme: Nature of harm and Women are unknowable.
- Discussing the homework assignment.
- Explaining new homework assignment.

Agenda

0:00	Opening.
0:05	Theme: Nature of harm and Women are unknowable.
0:15	Discussing the homework assignment.
1:20	Explaining new homework assignment.
1:25	Evaluation of the session.
1:30	Closing.

Course

Opening

- Brief discussion of the session plan.

Theme: Victims Are Not Hurt and Women Are Unknowable

- On the basis of homework assignment, participants explain to what extent the theme "Nature of harm" and "Women are unknowable" have played a role in their offense and discuss their current views with the other participants.

New Homework Assignment

- Describe again a situation in which you thought: "Victims are not hurt" or "I cannot understand that woman."

Evaluation

- The trainer asks each participant what he has learned from the session.

For the Participants

New Homework Assignment

(a) Describe again a situation in which you thought: "Victims are not hurt" or "I cannot understand that woman."

- The situation was? ……………………………………………………………………
- Who was it? ……………………………………………………………………………
- Where were you? ………………………………………………………………………
- What did the other person say or do? ………………………………………………
- What did you think or feel? …………………………………………………………
- What did you say or do? ………………………………………………………………
- How did the other person react? ……………………………………………………
- When you look back on your behavior now, what do you think about it? ………
  ……………………………………………………………………………………………
- What else could you have said or done? ……………………………………………

Plan of Session 7

Goals

- Discussing homework assignment.
- Theme: Male sexual drive is uncontrollable.
- Practicing with problem situation.
- Explaining new homework assignment.

Agenda

0:00	Opening.
0:05	Discussing homework assignment.
0:15	Eric's problem situation.
1:20	Explaining new homework assignment.
1:25	Evaluation of the session.
1:30	Closing.

Course

Opening

- Brief discussion of the session plan.

Theme: Male Sexual Drive Is Uncontrollable

- The trainer asks all participants to read Eric's problem situation. Then, the different questions are discussed during which participants have to convert sexually antisocial thoughts into sexually prosocial thoughts.

New Homework Assignment

- Describe a situation in which you thought: "I am so horny; I must have sex."

Evaluation

- The trainer asks each participant what he has learned from the session.

For the Participants

Exercise

Eric's Problem Situation

Eric is a 24-year-old male. In his childhood, he was neglected by both parents. As an adolescent Eric often had fantasies about raping women. These fantasies occurred, especially during masturbation. Eric has never had stable relationships because he has difficulties to talk with women. He does have some friends, and they visit bars and discos regularly. During one of their nightly outings, Eric is out of money and lends $100 of his friends. To repay this money as soon as possible Eric breaks into a house the next night. When Eric walks into the living room, he sees a woman asleep on the couch. The woman is wearing only underwear, and Eric becomes very aroused. He rapes the woman and runs away. From this point in time Eric started of committing more burglaries in the hope to encounter sleeping women. Eventually, Eric raped three women in this way.

(a) What do you see as the main problem of Eric?
(b) When Eric is masturbating, he fantasizes about raping women. What do you think about that?
(c) What are the reasons that Eric has problems to make contact with women?
(d) How does Eric think about women?
(e) What do you think about Eric's burglary to get money?
(f) Why was Eric excited by the view of a sleeping woman in underwear?
(g) Some men start talking with women before they rape them. Why?
(h) How would women feel if that is the case?
(i) Give Eric some suggestions what he can do to stay out of trouble?

New Homework Assignment

(a) Describe a situation in which you thought: "I am so horny; I must have sex."

- The situation was? ....
- Who was it? ....
- Where were you? ....
- What did the other person say or do? ....
- What did you think or feel? ....
- What did you say or do? ....
- How did the other person react? ....
- When you look back on your behavior now, what do you think about it? ....
....
- What else could you have said or done? ....

Plan of Session 8

Goals

- Discussing homework assignment.
- Theme: Male sexual drive is uncontrollable.
- Discussion with participants.
- Explaining new homework assignment.

Agenda

0:00	Opening.
0:05	Theme: Male sexual drive is uncontrollable.
0:15	Discussing homework assignment.
1:20	Explaining new homework assignment.
1:25	Evaluation of the session.
1:30	Closing.

Course

Opening

- Brief discussion of the session plan.

Theme: Male Sexual Drive Is Uncontrollable

- On the basis of homework assignment, participants explain to what extent the theme "Male sexual drive is uncontrollable" has played a role in their offense and discuss their current views with the other participants.

New Homework Assignment

- Describe again a situation in which you thought: "I am so horny; I must have sex."

Evaluation

- The trainer asks each participant what he has learned from the session.

For the Participants

New Homework Assignment

(a) Describe again a situation in which you thought: “I am so horny; I must have sex.”

- The situation was? ……………………………………………………………………
- Who was it? ……………………………………………………………………………
- Where were you? ………………………………………………………………………
- What did the other person say or do? …………………………………………………
- What did you think or feel? ……………………………………………………………
- What did you say or do? ………………………………………………………………
- How did the other person react? ………………………………………………………
- When you look back on your behavior now, what do you think about it? ………
  ……………………………………………………………………………………………
- What else could you have said or done? ………………………………………………

Plan of Session 9

Goals

- Discussing homework assignment.
- Theme: Dangerous world.
- Practicing with problem situation.
- Explaining new homework assignment.

Agenda

0:00	Opening.
0:05	Discussing homework assignment.
0:15	Bert's problem situation.
1:20	Explaining new homework assignment.
1:25	Evaluation of the session.
1:30	Closing.

Course

Opening

- Brief discussion of the session plan.

Theme: Dangerous World

- The trainer asks all participants to read Bert's problem situation. Then, the different questions are discussed during which participants have to convert sexually antisocial thoughts into sexually prosocial thoughts.

New Homework Assignment

- Describe a situation in which you thought: "Everyone is against me; I take what I can take."

Evaluation

- The trainer asks each participant what he has learned from the session.

For the Participants

Exercise

Bert's Problem Situation

Bert is a white 26-year-old male. He comes from a broken family and has two younger sisters. After the separation of his parents, Bert discovers that his father is not his biological father. As a child he was an ill-disciplined boy and he spent time with a lot of older guys. At the age of 7 he commits his first theft, and from his 14th year on he used alcohol daily. Bert earns his money as a drug dealer. This job gives him a lot of money and a sense of power. He is an addicted gambler and a regular visitor to the pubs. Here he meets his friend Natasha who is 10 years older. She is a former prostitute and addicted to alcohol. To fund his gambling addiction Bert commits house break-ins. Bert plans these burglaries carefully and the victims are always young, single women. One evening he meets Jessica in one of the pubs. They have a drink, and later in the evening, Bert tries to kiss Jessica. Jessica refuses his advances and leaves home. Bert follows Jessica unseen to her house. When Jessica opens her front door, he goes inside. Bert pulls of Jessica's clothes and rapes her. After the rape Bert leaves with Jessica's handbag.

(a) What do you see as the main problem of Bert?
(b) How do you explain that Bert in his youth especially dealt with older guys?
(c) What do you think about Bert's alcohol abuse when he was only 14 years old?
(d) Bert started a relationship with an addicted 10 years older woman. What is your opinion?
(e) What about the way that Bert earns his money by dealing drugs and committing burglaries?
(f) Why does Bert burgle only young, single women?
(g) Why would Jessica not want to be kissed by Bert?
(h) Some men have a strong need for power. How does this influence their views of women?

New Homework Assignment

(a) Describe a situation in which you thought: "Everyone is against me; I take what I can want."

- The situation was? ....
- Who was it? ....
- Where were you? ....
- What did the other person say or do? ....
- What did you think or feel? ....
- What did you say or do? ....
- How did the other person react? ....
- When you look back on your behavior now, what do you think about it? ....
  ....
- What else could you have said or done? ....

Plan of Session 10

Goals

- Theme: Dangerous world.
- Discussion with participants.
- Explaining new homework assignment.

Agenda

0:00	Opening.
0:05	Discussing the homework assignment.
1:20	Explaining new homework assignment.
1:25	Evaluation of the session.
1:30	Closing.

Course

Opening

- Brief discussion of the session plan.

Theme: Dangerous World

- On the basis of homework assignment, participants explain to what extent the theme "Dangerous world" has played a role in their offense and discuss their current views with the other participants.

New Homework Assignment

- Describe again a situation in which you thought: "Everyone is against me; I take what I want."

Evaluation

- Trainer asks each participant what he has learned from the session.

For the Participants

New Homework Assignment

(a) Describe again a situation in which you thought: "Everyone is against me; I take what I want."

- The situation was? ……………………………………………………………………
- Who was it? ....
- Where were you? ……………………………………………………………………
- What did the other person say or do? ………………………………………………
- What did you think or feel? …………………………………………………………
- What did you say or do? ……………………………………………………………
- How did the other person react? ……………………………………………………
- How do you look back on your behavior afterwards? ………………………………
- What else could you have said or done? ……………………………………………

Plan of Session 11

Goals

- Discussing homework assignment.
- Theme: Entitlement.
- Practicing with problem situation.
- Explaining new homework assignment.

Agenda

0:00	Opening.
0:05	Discussing homework assignment.
0:15	John's problem situation.
1:20	Explaining new homework assignment.
1:25	Evaluation of the session.
1:30	Closing.

Course

Opening

- Brief discussion of the session plan.

Theme: Entitlement

- The trainer asks all participants to read John's problem situation. Then, the different questions are discussed during which participants have to convert sexually antisocial thoughts into sexually prosocial thoughts.

New Homework Assignment

- Describe a situation in which you thought: "They can do me something; I just grab her/him."

Evaluation

- The trainer asks each participant what he has learned from the session.

For the Participants

Exercise

John's Problem Situation

John is a white 54-year-old male. As a child, he clashed with his parents frequently. John emigrated to Spain at the age of 16. John got a Spanish girlfriend but he shared the bed almost every weekend with other women. After 7 years his girlfriend discovered John's infidelity, and they broke up. After the break, John met an 11-year-old neglected girl and takes her to his home. However, without the knowledge of her parents she stays with him a few days. The girl is reported missing, and John becomes sentenced to 6 years in prison for kidnapping. When John has served his sentence, he returns to his home country. John discovers that he is attracted to children. Nevertheless, he starts a photo studio and specializes in photographing children. Through this photo studio, John comes in contact with various child sexual offenders. John fantasizes about sex with children and starts exchanging child pornography with other child sexual abusers. To satisfy his need for sex with children he tries to win the confidence of the children during the photo sessions. With some children, he is successful and forces them to satisfy him sexually using a hand job or blow job. He threatens the children with physical violence if they talk about it. In the long run, John had sex with nine girls and two boys.

1. What do you see as the main problem for John?
2. Next, to his steady relationship with his Spanish girlfriend, he goes to bed with other women. What do you think about that?
3. It was only after 7 years that Johns girlfriend discovered that he was cheating. Why might that have been the case?
4. Why did John take an 11-year-old girl to his home?
5. It is realistic to start a photo studio if you are sexually attracted to children?
6. How would it come that the children initially approved of Johns' advances?
7. What do you think about it that John threatens the children?
8. Is John excited by his threats to the children? Does this add to his sexual arousal?

New Homework Assignment

(a) Describe a situation in which you thought: "They can do me something; I just grab her/him."

- The situation was? ....
- Who was it? ....
- Where were you? ....
- What did the other person say or do? ....
- What did you think or feel? ....
- What did you say or do? ....
- How did the other person react? ....
- When you look back on your behavior now, what do you think about it? ....
  ....
- What else could you have said or done? ....

Plan of Session 12

Goals

- Theme: Entitlement.
- Discussing homework assignment.
- Explaining new homework assignment.

Agenda

0:00	Opening.
0:05	Theme: Entitlement.
0:15	Discussing homework assignment.
1:20	Explaining new homework assignment.
1:25	Evaluation of the session.
1:30	Closing.

Course

Opening

- Brief discussion of the session plan.

Theme: Entitlement

- On the basis of homework assignment, participants explain to what extent the theme "Entitlement" has played a role in their offense and discuss their current views with the other participants.

New Homework Assignment

- Describe again a situation in which you thought: "They can do me something; I just grab her/him."

Evaluation

- The trainer asks each participant what he has learned from the session.

For the Participants

New Homework Assignment

(a) Describe again a situation in which you thought: “They can do me something; I just grab her/him.”

- The situation was? ....
- Who was it? ....
- Where were you? ....
- What did the other person say or do? ....
- What did you think or feel? ....
- What did you say or do? ....
- How did the other person react? ....
- When you look back on your behavior now, what do you think about it? ....
  ....
- What else could you have said or done? ....

Plan of Session 13

Goals

- Discussing homework assignment.
- Practicing with problem situation.
- Explaining new homework assignment.

Agenda

0:00	Opening.
0:05	Discussing homework assignment.
0:15	Dave's problem situation.
1:00	The ten cognitive distortions.
1:10	Explaining new homework assignment.
1:25	Evaluation of the session.
1:30	Closing.

Course

Opening

- Brief discussion of the session plan.

Dave's Problem Situation

- Trainer asks all participants to read Dave's problem situation. Then, the different questions are discussed during which participants have to convert sexually antisocial thoughts into sexually prosocial thoughts.

Cognitive Distortions

- Trainer writes on a blackboard the five cognitive distortions of rapists and the five cognitive distortions of child sexual abusers. For rapists these are: women are sexual objects, women are unknowable, male sexual drive is uncontrollable, dangerous world, and entitlement. For child sexual abusers these are: children are sexual objects, nature of harm, male sexual drive is uncontrollable, dangerous world, and entitlement.

New Homework Assignment

(a) Describe your latest offense and mention the cognitive distortions you probably had before, during, and after that moment.

Evaluation

- The trainer asks each participant what he has learned from the session.

For the Participants

Exercise

Dave's Problem Situation

Dave is 48 years old. As a child, he had a good relationship with his parents and many friends in school. In his first year of high school, Dave was two times sexually abused by several men. As far as Dave is concerned, there are no nasty memories of sexual abuse. At the age of 14, Dave had a relationship for the first time. Dave is not sexually attracted to his girlfriend but notes that he gets excited by his male peers. To satisfy his sexual needs, Dave plays all kind of sexual games with his male peers. At an older age, Dave is only sexually attracted to underage boys. Dave persuades boys to take part in sexual activities by offering them money or presents. However, as the boys want to stop or have no further interest, Dave becomes violent. Dave rapes the boys and forces them to oral sex. He records his sexual contact with young boys on a video camera. At last six boys goes to the police and report the rape. The other boys refuse to admit the abuse because they had sex with Dave voluntary.

1. What do you see as Dave's main problem?
2. What were the real consequences for Dave of the sexual abuse by different men?
3. Is it not odd that Dave starts a relationship with a girl while he is attracted to boys?
4. Should Dave have told his girlfriend of his attraction to boys?
5. The boys initially approved of Dave's advances. What do you think about that?
6. How was it for the boys when they were forced to oral sex?
7. What about Dave's recording of the sexual activities?
8. Why do you think that some boys did not report to the police?

New Homework Assignment

- Describe your latest offense and mention the cognitive distortions you probably had before, during, or after that moment.
- The situation was? ....
- Who was it? ....

- Where were you? ………………………………………………………………………
- What did the other person say or do? …………………………………………………
- What did you think or feel:
  - Women/children are sexual objects ………………………………………………
  - Women are unknowable/Nature of harm ……………………………………………
  - Male sexual drive is uncontrollable ………………………………………………
  - Dangerous world …………………………………………………………………
  - Entitlement ………………………………………………………………………
- What did you say or do? ………………………………………………………………
- How did the other person react? ………………………………………………………
- When you look back on your behavior now, what do you think about it? ………
………………………………………………………………………………………………
- How could you have corrected your cognitive distortions?
  - Women/children are sexual objects ………………………………………………
  - Women are unknowable/Nature of harm ……………………………………………
  - Male sexual drive is uncontrollable ………………………………………………
  - Dangerous world …………………………………………………………………
  - Entitlement ………………………………………………………………………
- What else could you have said or done? ………………………………………………

Plan of Session 14

Goals

- Discussing homework assignment.
- Theme: Presentation of offenses with distorted cognitions.
- Presentation of offenses.

Agenda

0:00	Opening.
0:05	Theme: Presentation of offenses with distorted cognitions.
1:25	Evaluation of the session.
1:30	Closing.

Course

Opening

- Brief discussion of the session plan.

Theme: Presentation of Offenses with Distorted Cognitions

- All participants present a summary of their latest offense and mention the cognitive distortions they had before, during, or after that moment.

Evaluation

- The trainer asks each participant what he has learned from the session.

Plan of Session 15

Goal

- Theme: Evaluation of the module Cognitive Distortions.

Agenda

0:00	Opening.
0:05	Theme: Evaluation of the module by the participants.
1:30	Closing.

Course

Opening

- Brief discussion of the session plan.

Theme: Evaluation of the Module by the Participants

- Participants complete the evaluation scale. When everybody is ready, the reactions of each participant are written on a blackboard. Then, striking outcomes are discussed.

Closing

- After the trainers have formulated their conclusions based on the evaluation of the participants, the module is closed.

For the Participants

Evaluation Scale

1 = not applicable at all, 5 = strongly applicable

1	I actively participated in the module.	1	2	3	4	5
2	I found the information in the portfolio clearly.	1	2	3	4	5
3	I have gained a better insight into my behavior by practicing it myself.	1	2	3	4	5
4	I received good advice from the trainers about my behavior.	1	2	3	4	5
5	Now I have a better understanding of the effect of my behavior in the short and long term.	1	2	3	4	5
6	I have been informed in advance about what happens in the module.	1	2	3	4	5
7	I think that the topics that are addressed in the module are useful.	1	2	3	4	5
8	The trainers have taken into account my wishes and preferences.	1	2	3	4	5
9	The trainers can be asked for advice.	1	2	3	4	5
10	I think the length of the module is just right.	1	2	3	4	5

11.5 Specific Program: Management of Risk Situations

Session 1

Goals

- Discussing homework assignment.
- Announcing the module Management of Risk Situations.
- Discussing the risk situations per participant.
- Explaining new homework assignment.

Agenda

0:00	Opening.
0:05	Discussing homework assignment.
0:15	Explaining the goal of the module Management of Risk Situations.
1:20	Explaining new homework assignments.
1:25	Evaluation of the session.
1:30	Closing.

Course

Opening

- Brief discussion of the session plan.

Homework Assignment

- The trainer asks two participants to report on the homework assignments.
- The trainer asks all participants what they have learned from the homework assignments.
- The trainer records the reports.

Explanation the Goal of the Module Management of Risk Situations

- The trainer explains the goal of the Management of Risk Situations module, namely applying learned skills in risk situations in order to reduce the recidivism risk.

Discussing the Risk Situations

- Five risk situations are set for each participant.

New Homework Assignment

(a) Apply an order from small to very large in five risk situations.
(b) Describe how you would react in a situation with a small risk of recidivism.

Evaluation

- The trainer asks each participant what he has learned from the session.

For the Participants

New Homework Assignments

(a) Apply an order from small to very large in five risk situations.
    1. The situation with a small risk of recidivism is: ....
    ....
    2. The situation with a little risk of recidivism is: ....
    ....
    3. The situation with a medium risk of recidivism is: ....
    ....
    4. The situation with a high risk of recidivism is: ....
    ....
    5. The situation with a very high risk of recidivism is: ....
    ....

(b) Describe how you would react in a situation with a small risk of recidivism.

- A situation with a small risk of recidivism is: ....
  ....
- What would you think in that situation? ....
  ....
- How would you feel in that situation? ....
  ....
- How would you react in that situation? ....
  ....
- What would you think afterwards? ....
  ....
- How would you feel afterwards? ....
  ....
- How else could you react in such a situation? ....
  ....
- What precautions could you take? ....
  ....

Session 2

Goals

- Discussing homework assignments.
- Discussing the risk situations per participant.
- Explaining new homework assignment.

Agenda

0:00	Opening.
0:05	Discussing homework assignments.
0:25	Practicing situations with a small risk of recidivism.
1:20	Explaining new homework assignment.
1:25	Evaluation of the session.
1:30	Closing.

Course

Opening

- Brief discussion of the session plan.

Homework Assignment

- The trainer asks two participants to report on the homework assignments.
- The trainer asks all participants what they have learned from the homework assignments.
- The trainer records the reports.

Practicing Situations with a Small Risk of Recidivism

- All participants exercise situations with a small risk of recidivism.

New Homework Assignment

(a) Describe how you would react in a situation with a little risk of recidivism.

Evaluation

- The trainer asks each participant what he has learned from the session.

For the Participants

New Homework Assignment

(a) Describe how you would react in a situation with a little risk of recidivism.

- A situation with a little risk of recidivism is: ....
....
- What would you think in that situation? ....
....
- How would you feel in that situation? ....
....
- How would you react in that situation? ....
....
- What would you think afterwards? ....
....
- How would you feel afterwards? ....
....
- How else could you react in such a situation? ....
....
- What precautions could you take? ....
....

Session 3

Goals

- Discussing homework assignment.
- Discussing the risk situations per participant.
- Explaining new homework assignment.

Agenda

0:00	Opening.
0:05	Discussing homework assignment.
0:25	Practicing situations with a little risk of recidivism.
1:20	Explaining new homework assignment.
1:25	Evaluation of the session.
1:30	Closing.

Course

Opening

- Brief discussion of the session plan.

Homework Assignment

- The trainer asks two participants to report on the homework assignments.
- The trainer asks all participants what they have learned from the homework assignments.
- The trainer records the reports.

Practicing Situations with a Little Risk of Recidivism

- All participants exercise situations with a little risk of recidivism.

New Homework Assignment

(a) Describe how you would react in a situation with a medium risk of recidivism.

Evaluation

- The trainer asks each participant what he has learned from the session.

For the Participants

New Homework Assignment

(a) Describe how you would react in a situation with a medium risk of recidivism.

- A situation with a medium risk of recidivism is: ....
....
- What would you think in that situation? ....
....
- How would you feel in that situation? ....
....
- How would you react in that situation? ....
....
- What would you think afterwards? ....
....
- How would you feel afterwards? ....
....
- How else could you react in such a situation? ....
....
- What precautions could you take? ....
....

Session 4

Goals

- Discussing homework assignment.
- Discussing the risk situations per participant.
- Explaining new homework assignment.

Agenda

0:00	Opening.
0:05	Discussing homework assignment.
0:25	Practicing situations with a medium risk of recidivism.
1:20	Explaining new homework assignment.
1:25	Evaluation of the session.
1:30	Closing.

Course

Opening

- Brief discussion of the session plan.

Homework Assignment

- The trainer asks two participants to report on the homework assignments.
- The trainer asks all participants what they have learned from the homework assignments.
- The trainer records the reports.

Practicing Situations with a Medium Risk of Recidivism

- All participants exercise situations with a medium risk of recidivism.

New Homework Assignment

(a) Describe how you would react in a situation with a great risk of recidivism.

Evaluation

- The trainer asks each participant what he has learned from the session.

For the Participants

New Homework Assignment

(a) Describe how you would react in a situation with a great risk of recidivism.

- A situation with a great risk of recidivism is: ....
....
- What would you think in that situation? ....
....
- How would you feel in that situation? ....
....
- How would you react in that situation? ....
....
- What would you think afterwards? ....
....
- How would you feel afterwards? ....
....
- How else could you react in such a situation? ....
....
- What precautions could you take? ....
....

Session 5

Goals

- Discussing homework assignment.
- Discussing the risk situations per participant.
- Explaining new homework assignment.

Agenda

0:00	Opening.
0:05	Discussing homework assignment.
0:25	Practicing situations with a great risk of recidivism.
1:20	Explaining new homework assignment.
1:25	Evaluation of the session.
1:30	Closing.

Course

Opening

- Brief discussion of the session plan.

Homework Assignment

- The trainer asks two participants to report on the homework assignments.
- The trainer asks all participants what they have learned from the homework assignments.
- The trainer records the reports.

Practicing Situations with a Great Risk of Recidivism

- All participants exercise situations with a great risk of recidivism.

Homework Assignment

(a) Describe how you would react in a situation with a very great risk of recidivism.

Evaluation

- The trainer asks each participant what he has learned from the session.

For the Participants

New Homework Assignment

(a) Describe how you would react in a situation with a very great risk of recidivism.

- A situation with a very great risk of recidivism is: ....
....
- What would you think in that situation? ....
....
- How would you feel in that situation? ....
....
- How would you react in that situation? ....
....
- What would you think afterwards? ....
....
- How would you feel afterwards? ....
....
- How else could you react in such a situation? ....
....
- What precautions could you take? ....
....

Session 6

Goals

- Discussing homework assignment.
- Discussing the risk situations per participant.
- Explaining new homework assignment.

Agenda

0:00	Opening.
0:05	Discussing homework assignment.
0:25	Practicing situations with a very great risk of recidivism.
1:20	Explaining new homework assignment.
1:25	Evaluation of the session.
1:30	Closing.

Course

Opening

- Brief discussion of the session plan.

Homework Assignment

- The trainer asks two participants to report on the homework assignments.
- The trainer asks all participants what they have learned from the homework assignments.
- The trainer records the reports.

Practicing Situations with a Very Great Risk of Recidivism

- All participants exercise situations with a very great risk of recidivism.

Evaluation

- The trainer asks each participant what he has learned from the session.

11.6 Evaluation

Plan of First Evaluation Session

Goals

- Discussing homework assignments.
- Evaluation of the program.

Agenda

0:00	Opening.
0:05	Discussing homework assignments.
0:25	Evaluation of the program.
1:30	Closing.

Course

Opening

- Brief discussion of the session plan.

Homework Assignments

- The trainer asks two participants to report on the homework assignments.
- The trainer asks all participants what they have learned from the homework assignments.
- The trainer records the reports.

Evaluation of the Program

- The trainer evaluates the program by ratings on the evaluation scale. To this end, the scores of all participants are inventoried per item, after which they can explain their scores. The trainer ensures that the participants give each other positive feedback as much as possible

For the Participants

Evaluation Scale

1 = not applicable at all, 5 = strongly applicable

1	I actively participated in the program.	1	2	3	4	5
2	I learned a lot by practicing myself.	1	2	3	4	5
3	I learned to pay more attention to what others say and do.	1	2	3	4	5
4	I have learned to behave calmer and in a more satisfactory way with others.	1	2	3	4	5
5	Now I have a better understanding of the effect of my behavior in the short and long term.	1	2	3	4	5
6	I have learned to achieve my goals without harming others.	1	2	3	4	5
7	Now I understand better that it is sometimes disadvantageous for yourself to put your self-interest first.	1	2	3	4	5
8	I learned that you cannot judge everyone equally hard.	1	2	3	4	5
9	I better notice what damage you can do to others with aggressive behavior.	1	2	3	4	5
10	Now I know that when you're dealing with others you cannot always get your way.	1	2	3	4	5
11	I feel that I can continue to work on what I learned during the program.	1	2	3	4	5
12	I find the information that I have received clearly.	1	2	3	4	5
13	I have had enough information at the beginning of what would happen in the program.	1	2	3	4	5
14	I think that the subjects which were practiced during the program fit well with the problems that I have (and had) in the dealing with others.	1	2	3	4	5
15	I think we had enough time during the sessions.	1	2	3	4	5
16	I think that there could be practiced sufficiently.	1	2	3	4	5

Plan of Second Evaluation Session

Goals

- Evaluation of individual participants.

Agenda

0:00	Opening.
0:05	Evaluation of individual participants.
1:25	Presenting certificate of participation:
1:30	Closing.

Course

Opening

- Brief discussion of the session plan.

Evaluation of Individual Participants

- Trainers distribute the reports to the referrer. All participants get to read each other's report and become invited to give each other and the trainers feedback. Finally, agreements are made about adjustments of the text. When the opinion of a participant is different from the opinion of the trainers, both opinions are included in the report.

Distribution of Certificates

- Finally, all participants receive a certificate as proof of participation.

Appendix: Emotion Management

Introduction

Below we explain how emotions may lead to maladaptive but also to adaptive behavior. Emotion is a feeling. For instance, you are furious at someone because what you wanted to happen did not happen. You feel that you have been wronged or think that the other person has offended you. If you can control your emotion in such a way that you react appropriately, you will reach your goal more often and you will feel calmer. To clarify the connection between emotion and maladapted behavior, we use the following behavior chain: Behavior chain: *Antecedent → Thoughts → Tension → Emotion → Behavior → Consequences.*

1. Behavior

Aggressive behavior is an example of inappropriate behavior because the direct result is often positive, but in the long run, you get into difficulties. It is better to stand up for yourself in an assertive way. Assertive behavior means that you act according to your interests without affecting other people's rights. Assertive behavior is an adaptive behavior. In our interaction with each other, we have to apply specific values and norms of our society. Standards and values are social rules that ensure that people are pleasant, polite, and respectful of each other. With assertive behavior, you take into account those values and norms, even if you stand up for yourself.

2. Antecedent

Emotions usually have to do with what someone else says or does. We speak of an antecedent event when the behavior of another person can give rise to an emotion. These emotions may lead you to behave emotionally, for instance by scolding, threatening, or beating. To be able to act appropriately, it is essential to realize what happens precisely: What does or says that other person exactly. In a situation, it is best to first carefully observe what you hear or what you see and what you feel yourself. We call those observations. Behavior chain: *Antecedent → Behavior.*

Example: Wesley has just made coffee but the coffee can is still on the counter. However, Nancy wants to do the dishes. Nancy says to Wesley in an angry voice: "Can't you store that coffee in the closet right away? Then at least I can do the dishes."

Behavior chain: Coffee can at the kitchen counter → Nancy scolds Wesley. Alternative behavior chain: Coffee can is at the kitchen counter → Nancy asks Wesley to store the coffee.

3. Thoughts

Observations are followed by thoughts (interpretations). It is important to make a distinction between what you observe (antecedent) and the interpretations you make (thoughts). Interpretations are thoughts that you have about the antecedent. A thought can be: "She has the pick on me" or "He is forgetful again." Behavior chain: *Antecedent → Thoughts → Behavior.*

Example: Daphne is not home yet at 7 o'clock in the evening, while she always stops working at half past five. Dennis looks at the clock and thinks: "She's cheating." As soon as Daphne comes home, Dennis scolds her. Behavior chain: Daphne is not home yet at 7 o'clock → Dennis thinks: "She has an affair." → Dennis scolds Daphne when she returns home. Alternative behavior chain: Daphne is not home yet at 7 o'clock. → Dennis thinks: "She can take care of herself." → Dennis asks Daphne when she comes home why she is late and if she wants to call from now on when she has to work overtime.

4. Physical Tension

When people perceive someone's behavior as unpleasant, they usually do not get emotional right away. It takes a while before they know exactly what is happening. They do notice that their physical tension immediately increases. This tension can occur in different ways: faster heartbeat, perspiration, stretching muscles, shaking, blushing, and the like. An increase in physical tension is entirely reasonable in social situations in which, in our opinion, something unpleasant happens. Behavior chain: *Antecedent → Thoughts → Tension → Behavior.*

Example: Patrick walks into the hall with a bag full of groceries. Marian is running ahead of him. Marian does not keep the door open for Patrick. Patrick thinks: "What a bitch" and gets completely riled up. The next time Patrick does not keep the door open for Marian. Behavior chain: Marian does not keep the door open for Patrick → Patrick thinks: "What a bitch" → Patrick gets worked up → Next time, Patrick bangs the door shut in front of Marian's nose. Alternative behavior chain: Marian does not keep the door open for Patrick → Patrick thinks: "She is with her thoughts elsewhere." → Patrick relaxes → Patrick says something about the fact that Marian did not keep the door open for him and asked her to show some consideration with him the next time.

5. Emotions

Behavior is partly determined by the feelings that precede it. Negative feelings may lead to maladaptive behavior: feeling down to depression, anger to aggression, suspicion to social isolation. Negative feelings are not always wrong. Death comes with grief, and deception comes with bitterness. These feelings are temporary. Behavior chain: *Antecedent → Thoughts → Tension → Emotions → Behavior.*

Example: Gerald is waiting in the bakery for his turn. Then arrives a woman who immediately addresses the saleswoman and asks for her order. The saleswoman does not dare to refuse because she and the woman are good acquaintances. Gerald thinks: "What a rude person, acquaintances have certain privileges here." He gets it completely hot under the collar. Gerald feels completely ignored and walks angrily out of the shop. Behavior chain: Woman pushes forward in the bakery → Gerald thinks: "What a rude person, acquaintances are allowed to do this." → Gerald gets it hot under the collar → Gerald feels ignored and angry → Gerald runs out of the store. Alternative behavior chain: A woman pushes forward → Gerald thinks: "She does not notice me." → Gerald relaxes → Gerald feels fairly calm → Gerald says that it is his turn first.

6. Consequences

Behavior is mainly determined by the consequences it has. It is essential to make a distinction between (a) consequences immediately after the end and (b) consequences after some time. Some behaviors directly produce a positive result but have negative consequences in the longer term. For instance, good food can lead to getting too fat. In yet other cases, the result is negative in the short term but the effect is positive after months or years. Going to school means that you cannot spend all day with your friends but you obtain a diploma later on. Consideration is not always easy. This is partly because you can be more assured of a direct result than of a long-term consequence. Many people find it difficult to see beyond the end of their noses. Behavior chain: *Antecedent* → *Thoughts* → *Tension* → *Emotions* → *Behavior* → *Consequences.*

Example: Dwight is queuing at the supermarket. The woman for Dwight asks the cashier after the checkout how it goes with her children. Dwight thinks: "I'll be here until tomorrow" and is getting tense. He is annoyed and says to the cashier and the woman: "Can't you hurry up? I have something else to do than to listen to your chatting." The cashier gets scared and says: "I will help you immediately." Dwight is immediately helped but later feels uncomfortable because he was in no hurry. Behavior chain: A woman is talking with cashier → Dwight thinks: "I'll be here until tomorrow" → Dwight gets tense → Dwight gets annoyed → He makes an angry remark to the cashier → Dwight is helped immediately but later feels uncomfortable. Alternative behavior chain: A woman is talking with cashier → Dwight thinks: "I have some time if it does not last too long." → Dwight relaxes → He stays calm → Dwight says to the women: "Aren't you chatting a bit too long?" → Dwight feels comfortable because the women look at him kindly and take him into account.

Correction to: Assessment and Obligatory Treatment of Violent and Sexually Violent Offenders

Ruud H. J. Hornsveld, Floris W. Kraaimaat, Luk A. C. L. Gijs, and Emma J. Palmer

Correction to: R. H. J. Hornsveld et al. (eds.), *Assessment and Obligatory Treatment of Violent and Sexually Violent Offenders*, Advances in Preventing and Treating Violence and Aggression, https://doi.org/10.1007/978-3-030-27840-3

The book was inadvertently published with an incorrect affiliation for one of the volume editors, Luk A. C. L. Gijs, as "Moet zijn KU Leuven, Leuven, Belgium". It has been updated as "KU Leuven, Leuven, Belgium" in the front matter and in Chapters 1 and 5.

The updated online version of these chapters can be found at
https://doi.org/10.1007/978-3-030-27840-3_1
https://doi.org/10.1007/978-3-030-27840-3_5
https://doi.org/10.1007/978-3-030-27840-3

R. H. J. Hornsveld et al. (eds.), *Assessment and Obligatory Treatment of Violent and Sexually Violent Offenders*, Advances in Preventing and Treating Violence and Aggression, https://doi.org/10.1007/978-3-030-27840-3_12

Glossary

Adherence Degree to which patients follow the instruction of practitioners or therapists. Sometimes called compliance.

Aggression Behavior intended to cause harm to another person.

Agreeableness One of the Big Five personality domains characterized by a tendency to be kind, generous, sympathetic, and unselfish.

Aggression Replacement Training Multimodal intervention to improve prosocial behavior in children and adolescents who perform aggressive and violent behavior.

Anger Emotion elicited by an actual or alleged provocation that is expressed in behaviors such as persistent, intense looking, loud talking, and standing nearby. Feelings that vary from mild irritation to intense fury and rage.

Antisocial behavior Any behavior that violates the social norms of appropriate behavior.

Antisocial personality Personality disorder involving a long-term, persistent pattern of impulsive, selfish, unscrupulous, even criminal behavior.

Arousal General level of activation that is reflected in several physiological systems and can be measured by electrical activity in the brain, heart action, muscle tension, and the state of many other organ systems.

Assertiveness Behavior that allows one to stand up for personal rights and express one's thoughts and feelings respectfully to others.

Big Five The five traits found in many factor-analytic studies of personality that have been proposed as the basic components of human personality: neuroticism, extraversion, openness to experience, agreeableness, and conscientiousness.

Case formulation Idiographic theory of the person and his or her life situation, which includes problems as well as triggering and maintaining variables, including cognitions (thoughts and beliefs), that have relevance for treatment planning.

Case study Detailed examination and description of an individual's current feelings, thoughts, and behaviors. It is especially useful for studying complex or relatively rare phenomena.

R. H. J. Hornsveld et al. (eds.), *Assessment and Obligatory Treatment of Violent and Sexually Violent Offenders*, Advances in Preventing and Treating Violence and Aggression, https://doi.org/10.1007/978-3-030-27840-3

MIX
Papier aus verantwortungsvollen Quellen
Paper from responsible sources
FSC® C105338

If you have any concerns about our products,
you can contact us on
ProductSafety@springernature.com

In case Publisher is established outside the EU,
the EU authorized representative is:
Springer Nature Customer Service Center GmbH
Europaplatz 3, 69115 Heidelberg, Germany

Printed by Libri Plureos GmbH
in Hamburg, Germany